Continued on inside back cover

MEDICAL-SURGICAL NURSING

Concepts for
Clinical Judgment
and Collaborative Care

CLINICAL COMPANION

MEDICAL-SURGICAL NURSING

Concepts for Clinical Judgment and Collaborative Care

11th EDITION

IGNATAVICIUS
REBAR
HEIMGARTNER

NICOLE M. HEIMGARTNER,
DNP, RN, CNE, CNEcl, COI, FAADN

Subject Matter Expert and Nursing
  Education Consultant
Louisville, Kentucky;
Associate Professor
Galen College of Nursing
Louisville, Kentucky

ELSEVIER

Elsevier
3251 Riverport Lane
St. Louis, Missouri 63043

Notice

Practitioners and researchers must always rely on their own experience and
knowledge in evaluating and using any information, methods, compounds or
experiments described herein. Because of rapid advances in the medical
sciences, in particular, independent verification of diagnoses and drug dosages
should be made. To the fullest extent of the law, no responsibility is assumed by
Elsevier, authors, editors or contributors for any injury and/or damage to
persons or property as a matter of products liability, negligence or otherwise, or
from any use or operation of any methods, products, instructions, or ideas
contained in the material herein.

Previous editions copyrighted 2021, 2018, 2016, 2013, 2010, 2006, and 2002.
International Standard Book Number: 978-0-323-87699-5

Executive Content Strategist: Lee Henderson
Senior Content Development Specialist: Rebecca Leenhouts
Publishing Services Manager: Julie Eddy
Senior Project Manager: Jodi Willard
Design Direction: Amy Buxton

Printed in India

Last digit is the print number: 9 8 7 6 5 4 3 2 1

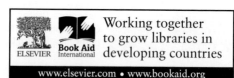

Welcome! The new edition of *Clinical Companion for Medical-Surgical Nursing: Concepts for Clinical Judgment and Collaborative Care* has been updated and streamlined to match content changes in the most current Ignatavicius, Rebar, and Heimgartner textbook. These revisions reflect an increased emphasis on patient-centered care, demonstrating evidence and principles of best practice within the nursing profession. Features new to this edition include a full-color design and color images, in addition to an enhanced layout for ease of use in the clinical setting.

The Clinical Companion uses an alphabetical, conceptual approach to organize content. Health care conditions are listed alphabetically, making them easy to locate within the resource. A conceptual presentation fosters the organization and delivery of safe patient care. In addition, the nursing process and the NCSBN Clinical Judgment Measurement Model are used throughout to foster best practice in the clinical setting.

Part I of this Clinical Companion provides a concise overview of professional nursing and health concepts that reflects the structure developed in the Ignatavicius, Rebar, and Heimgartner textbook.

Part II of this Clinical Companion provides, in alphabetical order, a concise, clinically oriented summary of conditions that are commonly seen in adults. Each condition contains an overview as well as an Interprofessional Collaborative Care section that includes Recognize Cues: Assessment and Take Actions: Interventions. Conditions that are concept exemplars follow an expanded format and are indicated throughout with an exemplar icon ✳. Be sure to organize care with these concepts in mind while still personalizing care based on each patient's individual needs. Remember, this Clinical Companion is designed for concise information. When additional detail is required, you will be referred to the main text—Ignatavicius, Rebar, and Heimgartner's *Medical-Surgical Nursing: Concepts for Clinical Judgment and Collaborative Care,* 11th edition. Be sure to look for the 🖼 icon for references to the main text when information beyond the scope of the Clinical Companion is needed.

Throughout Parts I and II, important aspects of care are highlighted within Patient-Centered Care boxes, such as Veteran Health, Genetics/Genomics, Heath Equity, Older Adult Health, Gender Health, and Cultural/Spiritual Health. These featured boxes help nurses and nursing students offer focused and individualized assessment and intervention. Nursing Safety Priority boxes are also included to highlight important information that can be used to foster best practice and avoid patient harm. These boxes are categorized as Drug

Alert, Action Alert, or Critical Rescue. In addition, boxes that high-light the Key Features of common disorders are included.

Medical-surgical nursing is a demanding specialty and is often considered the foundation of all nursing. Most adults will receive care from a medical-surgical nurse at some point during their lifetime. This resource is designed to provide concise information about both common and specialized conditions to support nurses and nursing students in providing quality care to a diverse adult population.

Nicole M. Heimgartner, DNP, RN, CNE, CNEcl, COI, FAADN

ACKNOWLEDGMENTS

Thank you, Donna and Cherie, for your mentorship, friendship, and continual support. I am so very thankful for both of you! Many thanks to Elsevier for transforming this manuscript into publication.

I am grateful for the support and love of my husband and beautiful twin girls. Alayna and Addi, it is a joy to be your mom! You all inspire me each day.

Students, I am so thankful for you and excited for the journey that lies ahead for you in the profession of nursing!

Nicole M. Heimgartner, DNP, RN, CNE, CNEcl, COI, FAADN

CONTENTS

APPENDIX

References, See http://evolve.elsevier.com/Iggy/

Professional Nursing and Health Concepts for Medical-Surgical Nursing

INTRODUCTION

Medical-surgical nursing, sometimes called *adult health nursing,* is a practice area that requires specialized knowledge and skills to manage patients from late adolescence throughout the adult life span (Academy of Medical-Surgical Nurses [AMSN], 2018). Medical-surgical nursing occurs within and across four "spheres" of health care delivery, which include (American Association of Colleges of Nursing [AACN], 2021) (Fig. 1.1):

- **Disease prevention/promotion of health and well-being**, which includes the promotion of physical and mental health for all patients and management of intermittent care needs of healthy patients.
- **Chronic disease care**, which includes chronic disease management and prevention of patient complications.
- **Regenerative or restorative care**, which includes critical/trauma care, complex acute care, acute exacerbations of chronic conditions, and treatment of physiologically unstable patients that generally requires care in a tertiary care center.
- **Hospice/palliative/supportive care**, which includes end-of-life and palliative care for patients requiring long-term care; those with complex, chronic disease states; and/or those requiring rehabilitative care.

The roles of the nurse in these spheres of care include care coordinator and transition manager, caregiver, patient educator, leader, and patient and family advocate. To function in these various roles, nurses need to have the knowledge, skills, attitudes, and abilities (KSAs) to keep patients and their families safe.

Health Promotion/Disease Prevention	Chronic Disease Care
Regenerative or Restorative Care	Hospice/Palliative/ Supportive Care

Fig. 1.1 Four "spheres" of health care delivery.

QUALITY AND SAFETY EDUCATION FOR NURSES (QSEN) COMPETENCIES

The Institute of Medicine (IOM, now the National Academy of Medicine [NAM]), a highly respected U.S. organization that monitors health care and recommends health policy, has published many reports over the past 30 years suggesting ways to improve patient safety and quality care. One of its classic reports, *Health Professions Education: A Bridge to Quality,* identified five broad core competencies for health care professionals to ensure patient safety and quality care (Institute of Medicine [IOM], 2003). All of these competencies are interrelated and include:

- Provide patient-centered care.
- *Collaborate* with the interprofessional health care team.
- Implement evidence-based practice.
- Use *quality improvement* in patient care.
- Use *informatics* in patient care.

Several years later, the QSEN initiative, more recently called the *QSEN Institute,* validated the IOM (NAM) competencies for nursing practice and added *safety* as a sixth competency to emphasize its importance.

In addition to the concepts identified by the IOM and QSEN, the authors have selected four professional nursing concepts to integrate throughout this clinical companion.

- Clinical Judgment
- Systems Thinking
- Health Equity
- Ethics

Each of these concepts plays an integral role in safe, effective management of care within the clinical setting. Table 1.1 provides a brief overview of each competency along with tangible clinical application examples. These competencies will be addressed throughout this resource, allowing focus on the knowledge, skills, and attitudes that are needed for safe nursing care. Keep in mind that these competencies do not exist in isolation. Rather, they are interdependent to form the foundation for safe nursing care. For more discussion of the competencies, review Chapter 1 in Ignatavicius, Rebar, and Heimgartner's *Medical Surgical Nursing: Clinical Judgment for Collaborative Care,* 11th edition.

TABLE 1.1 Professional Nursing Concepts

Competency	Overview	Clinical Application Examples
Patient-Centered Care (QSEN)	The patient is "the source of control and full partner in providing compassionate and coordinated care based on respect for the patient's preferences, values, and needs" (QSEN, 2022).	• Integrative Therapies: Massage therapy, guided imagery, music therapy, acupuncture • Care Coordination • Case Management • Transition Management
Safety (QSEN)	Safety is the ability to keep the patient and staff free from harm and to minimize errors in care.	• National Patient Safety Goals • The Joint Commission: Culture of Safety • Best Safety Practices: Assess unit protocols, memory checklists, and medication administration systems, such as the barcode administration systems
Evidence-Based Practice (QSEN)	Evidence-based practice (EBP) is the integration of the best current evidence and practices to make decisions about patient care. It considers the patient's preferences and values and one's own clinical expertise for the delivery of optimal health care (Melnyk & Fineout-Overholt, 2019; QSEN, 2022).	The best source of evidence is research! • Health care organizations receiving Medicare and/or Medicaid funding are obligated to follow the evidence-based interprofessional Core Measures to ensure that best practices are followed for selected health problems.

Continued

TABLE 1.1 **Professional Nursing Concepts—cont'd**

Competency	Overview	Clinical Application Examples
Teamwork and Interprofessional Collaboration (QSEN)	To provide patient and family-centered care, the nurse "functions effectively within nursing and interprofessional teams, fostering open communication, mutual respect, and shared decision-making to achieve quality patient care" (QSEN, 2022).	To improve communication between staff members and health care agencies, procedures for hand-off communication were established: • An effective procedure used in many agencies today is called *SBAR* or similar method. *SBAR* is a formal method of communication between two or more members of the health care team. The SBAR process includes: **S**ituation, **B**ackground, **A**ssessment, and **R**ecommendation/**R**equest. • TeamSTEPPS® is also a systematic communication approach for interprofessional teams that was designed to improve safety. STEPPS stands for **S**trategies and **T**ools to **E**nhance **P**erformance and **P**atient **S**afety.
Quality Improvement	Quality improvement (QI) is a process in which nurses and the interprofessional health care team use indicators (data) to monitor care outcomes and develop solutions to change and improve care.	When a patient care or system issue is identified as needing improvement, specific systematic QI models such as the **Plan-Do-Study-Act (PDSA)** may be used. The steps of the PDSA model include: 1. Identify and analyze the problem (Plan). 2. Develop and test an evidence-based solution (Do). 3. Analyze the effectiveness of the test solution, including possible further improvement (Study). 4. Implement the improved solution to positively impact care (Act).

TABLE 1.1 Professional Nursing Concepts—cont'd

Competency	Overview	Clinical Application Examples
Informatics (QSEN) and Technology	Informatics is defined as the access and use of information and electronic technology to communicate, manage knowledge, prevent error, and support decision making (QSEN, 2022).	Safety and quality of health care are the major purposes of informatics and technology. • Be mindful of patient and family privacy in the clinical setting.
Clinical Judgment	Clinical Judgment is an iterative process that uses nursing knowledge to observe and access presenting situations, identify a prioritized patient concern, and generate the best possible evidence-based solutions in order to deliver safe patient care (NCSBN, 2022).	In this clinical companion, elements of the clinical judgment measurement model (CJMM) developed by the National Council of State Boards of Nursing (NCSBN) are paired with steps of the nursing process, which are: • Recognize Cues: Assessment • Analyze Cues and Prioritize Hypotheses: Analysis • Generate Solutions and Take Actions: Planning and Implementation • Evaluate Outcomes: Evaluate
Systems Thinking	Systems Thinking is the ability to recognize, understand, and synthesize the interactions and interdependencies in a set of components designed for a specific purpose. In health care, the nurse must know how the components of a complex health care system influence the care of each patient.	• The nurse may identify a hospitalized older adult who is at an increased risk for falls. The nurse implements evidence-based interventions to prevent falls for that specific individual patient using Clinical Judgment. By expanding to Systems Thinking, the nurse may review the fall rate on the nursing unit where the patient is hospitalized and collaboratively plan interventions for all patients at risk for falls using a QI model. • For more examples, refer to Chapter 2 in Ignatavicius, Rebar, and Heimgartner's *Medical Surgical Nursing: Concepts for Clinical Judgment and Collaborative Care*, 11th edition.

Continued

TABLE 1.1 Professional Nursing Concepts—cont'd

Competency	Overview	Clinical Application Examples
Health Equity	Health equity is the ability to recognize differences in the resources and/or knowledge needed for individuals to fully participate in health care and achieve optimal outcomes (AACN, 2021).	• Health equity is achieved when all individuals have the opportunity to attain their full health potential. • Numerous factors can affect health equity, including social determinants of health.
Ethics	According to the American Nurses Association (ANA), ethics is "a theoretical and reflective domain of human knowledge that addresses issues and questions about morality in human choices, actions, character, and ends" (ANA, 2015, p. xii).	There are six essential *ethical principles* that nurses and other health care professionals should use as a guide for clinical decision making: • **Respect:** Implies that patients are treated as autonomous individuals capable of making informed decision about their care. This patient autonomy is referred to as *self-determination* or *self-management*. • **Beneficence:** Encourages the nurse to do good for the patient • **Nonmaleficence:** Emphasizes the importance of preventing harm and ensuring the patient's well-being • **Fidelity:** The agreement that nurses will keep their obligations or promises to the patient • **Veracity:** The obligation of nurses to tell the truth to the best their knowledge • **Social justice:** Refers to equality and fairness, that all patients should be treated equally and fairly

OVERVIEW OF HEALTH CONCEPTS FOR MEDICAL-SURGICAL NURSING

Introduction

Nurses care for adults in a variety of settings to help them meet a multitude of biopsychosocial needs. When these needs are not met, the nurse plans and implements care in collaboration with the interprofessional health team. This clinical companion alphabetically presents diseases and disorders that are commonly seen in adults. Selected diseases and disorders have been identified as exemplars, with expanded assessment and interventions presented with a conceptual focus.

Remember, conceptual thinking can be applied to many patient conditions. This section of this clinical companion provides a brief overview of the main concepts that will be emphasized throughout both this clinical companion and the main textbook, Ignatavicius, Rebar, and Heimgartner's *Medical Surgical Nursing: Concepts for Clinical Judgment and Collaborative Care, 11th edition*.

Key concepts will appear in ***bold italics*** throughout this clinical companion.

Throughout this clinical companion, this icon, 🖙, is used to refer the reader back to the main text for more details.

The health concepts included are:
- Acid-Base Balance
- Cellular Regulation
- Clotting
- Cognition
- Comfort
- Elimination
- Fluid and Electrolyte Balance
- Gas Exchange
- Glucose Regulation
- Immunity
- Infection
- Inflammation
- Mobility
- Nutrition
- Pain
- Perfusion
- Sensory Perception
- Sexuality
- Tissue Integrity

ACID-BASE BALANCE

Acid-base balance is the maintenance of arterial blood pH between 7.35 and 7.45 through control of hydrogen ion production and elimination. Blood pH represents a delicate balance between hydrogen ions (acid) and bicarbonate (base) and is largely controlled by the lungs and kidneys.

Recognize Cues: Assessment

Assess patient health history. Ask about recent signs and symptoms, such as excessive vomiting or diarrhea, that could predispose the patient to acidosis or alkalosis.

Take Actions: Interventions

Managing a patient with an acid-base imbalance depends on which type of imbalance is present. When possible, the health care team aims to diagnose and treat the underlying cause(s) of the imbalance.

*See Chapter 14 in the main text for more information on **acid-base balance.***

CELLULAR REGULATION

Cellular regulation is the process to control cellular growth, replication, and differentiation to maintain homeostasis. Cellular *growth* refers to division and continued growth of the original cell. Cell *replication* refers to making a copy of a specific cell. Cell *differentiation* refers to the process of the cell becoming specialized to accomplish a specific task.

Recognize Cues: Assessment

Assess for common risk factors of impaired cellular regulation. Perform a thorough patient history, extensive family history, and psychosocial history. Diagnostic tests such as radiographic examination, computed tomography (CT), or magnetic resonance imaging (MRI) may identify the location of any mass.

RISK FACTORS FOR IMPAIRED CELLULAR REGULATION

- Older age (55 years and older, with significant potential for abnormal cell development at ages >70)
- Smoking
- Poor nutrition
- Physical inactivity
- Environmental pollutants (such as air, water, soil)
- Radiation
- Selected medications (such as chemotherapy)
- Genetic predisposition or risk

Take Actions: Interventions

Interventions include primary and secondary prevention techniques. *Primary prevention* includes minimizing the risk of developing impaired cellular regulation. *Secondary prevention* includes proper and regular screening to identify early any risks or hazards that could be present. Screening also enables the primary health care provider to diagnose cancer early, which often increases the patient's chance for a cure or long-term survival. Collaborative care can include surgery, radiation, chemotherapy, targeted therapy, biologic therapy, hormonal therapy, and bone marrow or hemopoietic stem cell transplants.

See Chapter 18 in the main text for more information on **cellular regulation.**

CLOTTING

Clotting is a complex, multistep process by which blood forms a protein-based structure (clot) in an appropriate area of tissue injury to prevent excessive bleeding while maintaining whole body blood flow (perfusion). An inability to form adequate clots can result in bleeding and threaten a person's life.

Recognize Cues: Assessment

Assess for common risk factors for inadequate *clotting,* such as immobility and smoking. Observe patients for signs and symptoms of *decreased* clotting, especially purpuric lesions such as ecchymosis (bruising) and petechiae (pinpoint purpura). Notice whether bleeding is prolonged as a result of injury or trauma. Check urine and stool for the presence of occult or frank blood. Observe for frank bleeding from the gums or nose.

Take Actions: Interventions

Teach patients with *decreased* **clotting** ability to report unusual bleeding or bruising immediately. For many adults at increased risk for clotting, *anticoagulants* or *antiplatelet drugs* (also called *blood thinners* by many patients) are prescribed either in community or inpatient settings. Examples of medications that require frequent laboratory testing are sodium heparin and warfarin.

See Chapter 30 in the main text for more information on **clotting**.

NURSING SAFETY PRIORITY

Critical Rescue

An *arterial* thrombosis is not locally observable and is typically manifested by decreased blood flow (**perfusion**) to a distal extremity or internal organ. For example, a femoral arterial clot causes an occlusion (blockage) of blood to the leg. In this case, the distal leg becomes pale/ash gray and cool; distal pulses may be weak or absent; *this is an emergent problem requiring immediate intervention. Do not elevate the affected leg! If these symptoms are present, notify the primary health care provider or Rapid Response Team immediately.* If this condition continues, the leg may become gangrenous and require amputation. A mesenteric artery thrombosis can cause small bowel ileus and gangrene if not treated in a timely manner. A renal artery thrombosis can cause acute kidney injury.

COGNITION

Cognition is the complex integration of mental processes and intellectual function for the purposes of reasoning, learning, memory, and personality. *Reasoning* is a high-level thinking process that allows an individual to make decisions and judgments. *Memory* is the ability of an individual to retain and recall information for learning or recall of past experiences. *Personality* refers to the way an individual feels and behaves, often based on how that individual thinks.

Recognize Cues: Assessment

Assess for common risk factors for inadequate cognition, such as loss of short- and/or long-term memory; disorientation to person, place, and/or time; impaired language or reasoning; inappropriate or uncontrollable emotions; and delusions and/or hallucinations. Conduct a mental status assessment using one of several available mental health/behavioral health screening tools, such as the Confusion Assessment Method (CAM).

Differences in the Characteristics of Delirium and Dementia		
Variable	**Dementia**	**Delirium**
Description	A chronic, progressive cognitive decline	An acute, fluctuating confusional state
Onset	Slow	Fast
Duration	Months to years	Hours to less than 1 month
Cause	Unknown, possibly familial, chemical	Multiple, such as surgery, infection, drugs

Differences in the Characteristics of Delirium and Dementia—cont'd		
Variable	**Dementia**	**Delirium**
Reversibility	None	May be possible
Management	Treat signs and symptoms	Remove or treat the cause
Nursing interventions	Reorientation not effective in the late stages; use validation therapy (acknowledge the patient's feelings, and do not argue); provide a safe environment; observe for associated behaviors, such as delusions and hallucinations	Reorient the patient to reality; provide a safe environment

Take Actions: Interventions

Nursing interventions focus on *safety* to prevent injury and foster communication. For adults with delirium or mild dementia, provide orientation to person, time, and place. Collaborate with the interprofessional team to determine the underlying cause of delirium (e.g., psychoactive drugs, hypoxia). Patients with moderate or severe dementia cannot be oriented to reality because they have chronic confusion.

 See Chapter 4 in the main text for more information on **cognition**.

COMFORT

Comfort is a state of physical well-being, pleasure, and absence of pain or stress. This definition implies that comfort has physical and emotional dimensions. A primary role of the nurse is to promote basic care and comfort.

Recognize Cues: Assessment

Assess for common risk factors for decreased *comfort*, such as physical and/or emotional discomfort. Ask patients whether they are comfortable. If pain is the source of discomfort, assess the level of pain and plan interventions to manage it.

Take Actions: Interventions

Assess patients at risk for discomfort and plan interventions to alleviate it, depending on its source and cause. Collaborate care with members of the interprofessional health care team as needed.

 See Chapter 6 in the main text for more information on pain assessment to foster **comfort.**

ELIMINATION

Elimination is the excretion of waste from the body by the gastro-intestinal (GI) tract (as feces) and by the urinary system (as urine). *Bowel* elimination occurs as a result of food and fluid intake and ends with passage of feces (stool) or solid waste products from food into the rectum of the colon. *Urinary* elimination occurs as a result of multiple kidney processes and ends with the passage of urine through the urinary tract.

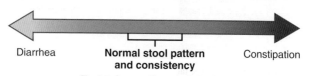

| Diarrhea | **Normal stool pattern and consistency** | Constipation |

Fig. 2.1 Scope of bowel elimination.

Recognize Cues: Assessment

Assess for common risk factors for changes in *elimination,* such as incontinence, diarrhea, and urinary retention. Monitor the frequency, amount, consistency, and characteristics of urine and stool. Listen to bowel sounds in all four quadrants for the presence of adequate bowel sounds. (See Fig. 2.1.)

Take Actions: Interventions

Maintaining normal *elimination* requires adequate nutrition and hydration. Teach adults to ensure a diet high in fiber, including eating fruits, vegetables, and whole grains, and drinking 8 to 12 glasses of water each day unless medically contraindicated. Adults with diarrhea or constipation need medical attention to determine the underlying cause. Adults who experience urinary incontinence need frequent toileting every 1 to 2 hours. Patients with urinary retention may require straight urinary catheterizations to empty the bladder until the usual voiding pattern returns.

📑 *See units in the main text related to the gastrointestinal system and the renal/urinary system for more on* ***elimination***.

FLUID AND ELECTROLYTE BALANCE

Fluid and electrolyte balance is the regulation of body fluid, fluid osmolality, and electrolytes by processes such as filtration, diffusion, and osmosis. To maintain balance or homeostasis in the body, fluid and electrolyte balance must be as close to normal as possible.

Common Fluid and Electrolyte Imbalances	
Common Fluid Imbalances	**Common Electrolyte Imbalances**
Fluid volume deficit (dehydration)	Hyponatremia (low serum sodium)
Fluid volume excess (overload)	Hypernatremia (high serum sodium)
	Hypokalemia (low serum potassium)
	Hyperkalemia (high serum potassium)
	Hypocalcemia (low serum calcium)
	Hypercalcemia (high serum calcium)
	Hypomagnesemia (low serum magnesium)
	Hypermagnesemia (high serum magnesium)

Recognize Cues: Assessment

Assess for common risk factors for fluid and electrolyte imbalance, such as acute illness (vomiting and diarrhea) or serious injury or trauma. Monitor vital signs, especially blood pressure, pulse rate and quality, fluid intake and output, and weight. *Changes in weight are the best indicator of fluid volume changes in the body.* Assess skin and mucous membranes for dryness and decreased skin turgor.

Take Actions: Interventions

Priority nursing interventions include maintenance of patient safety and *comfort* measures when managing fluid or electrolyte imbalances. For patients with a *fluid deficit,* the primary collaborative intervention is fluid replacement, either orally or parenterally. Depending on the cause of *fluid overload,* patients may require a fluid restriction (e.g., for those with chronic kidney disease). Diuretic therapy is often used for patients with fluid overload caused by chronic heart failure to prevent pulmonary edema, a potentially life-threatening complication.

*See Chapter 13 in the main text for more information on **fluid and electrolyte balance**.*

GAS EXCHANGE

Gas exchange is the process of oxygen transport to the cells and carbon dioxide transport away from the cells through ventilation and diffusion. Decreased *gas exchange* results in (1) inadequate transportation of oxygen to body cells and organs; and/or (2) retention of carbon dioxide. Inadequate oxygen results in cell dysfunction (ischemia) and possible cell death (necrosis or infarction). An excessive buildup of carbon dioxide combines with water to produce

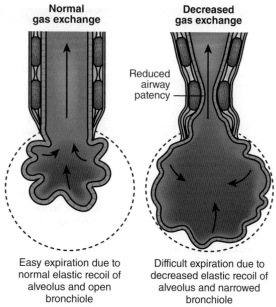

Fig. 2.2 Damaged inelastic alveoli common in patients with COPD cause decreases in oxygen and carbon dioxide diffusion.

carbonic acid. This increase in acid causes respiratory acidosis and lowers the pH of blood. (See Fig. 2.2.)

Recognize Cues: Assessment

Take a complete health history and perform a focused respiratory assessment. Ask the patient about current or history of lung disease or trauma. Assess the patient's breathing effort, oxygen saturation, capillary refill, thoracic expansion, and lung sounds anteriorly and posteriorly. Monitor for the presence of cough and/or sputum; reports of shortness of breath, dizziness, or chest *pain*; cyanosis; or adventitious lung sounds, such as wheezing, rhonchi, or crackles.

Take Actions: Interventions

Managing decreased *gas exchange* requires finding the underlying cause and treating it accordingly. Teach the patient about the need for deep breathing and coughing to further enhance lung expansion and decrease breathing effort. Teach patients how to correctly use incentive spirometry and inhalers if indicated. Administer oxygen therapy and monitor pulse oximetry to determine effectiveness.

Health Promotion Strategies to Maintain Gas Exchange and Prevent Decreased Gas Exchange

Teach patients the importance of using *infection* control measures (primarily proper handwashing), smoking cessation to prevent COPD, and getting immunizations as recommended to prevent influenza, pneumonia, and COVID-19. Instruct them to be aware of exposure to individuals with any of these respiratory conditions and to get tested if symptoms occur.

*See Chapters 22 through 26 in the main text for more on **gas exchange**.*

GLUCOSE REGULATION

Glucose regulation is the process of maintaining optimal blood glucose levels. With impaired glucose regulation, many acute and chronic health problems occur as life-shortening complications. Diabetes mellitus (DM) is a common, chronic, complex disorder of impaired nutrient metabolism, especially glucose; it is a disorder that can affect the function of every bodily system.

Recognize Cues: Assessment

Assess for risk factors related to diabetes mellitus, such as a history of gestational diabetes mellitus or glucose intolerance during pregnancy. Signs and symptoms of DM include fatigue, polyuria, and polydipsia.

Take Actions: Interventions

Teach patients and families to understand glucose regulation and the importance of glucose control in DM. The desired outcome is to help patients maintain blood glucose levels in the normal range *(euglycemia)* without causing either **hyperglycemia** (higher than normal blood glucose level) or **hypoglycemia** (lower than normal blood glucose level). Though this concept is not a primary concept used throughout this clinical companion, it is discussed in connection to multiple interrelated concepts with the *glucose regulation* concept exemplar diabetes mellitus.

*See Chapter 56 in the main text for more information on **glucose regulation**.*

IMMUNITY

Immunity is protection from illness or disease maintained by the body's physiologic defense mechanisms. *Natural active* immunity occurs when an antigen enters the body and the body creates antibodies to fight off the antigen. *Artificial active* immunity occurs via a vaccination or immunization. *Natural passive* immunity occurs when antibodies are passed from a mother to the fetus through the placenta or through colostrum or breast milk; *artificial passive* immunity occurs via a specific transfusion, such as immunoglobulins (Rogers, 2023).

Recognize Cues: Assessment

Assess for common risk factors for changes in *immunity*. A thorough history of the individual and the family is necessary to determine any of the previous risks associated with an immune problem.

COMMON RISK FACTORS FOR ALTERED IMMUNITY

Adult populations at risk for altered *immunity* include but are not limited to:
- Older adults (diminished immunity due to normal aging changes)
- Low socioeconomic groups (inability to obtain immunizations)
- Nonimmunized adults
- Adults with chronic illnesses that weaken the immune system
- Adults taking chronic drug therapy, such as corticosteroids and chemotherapeutic agents
- Adults experiencing substance use disorder
- Adults who do not practice a healthy lifestyle
- Adults who have a genetic risk for decreased or excessive immunity

Take Actions: Interventions

Handwashing, taking steps to avoid *infections*, and getting recommended immunizations are essential for promoting healthy immune function. Patients with a *decreased* immune system for any reason are very prone to infection. Remind them to wash their hands frequently and use hand sanitizer when water and soap are unavailable. Patients with an *excessive* immune function experience hypersensitivity reactions. Interprofessional collaborative management of these adults depends on the type and severity of the reaction.

 *See Chapter 16 in the main text for more on **immunity**.*

INFECTION

Infection is the invasion of pathogens (harmful microbes) into the body that multiply and cause disease or illness.

Recognize Cues: Assessment

When performing a nursing assessment, take a thorough history to determine the patient's risk for and exposure to *infection*. Observe for signs and symptoms of infection if visible, such as redness/hyperpigmentation, warmth, pain, and swelling. Ask about changes in elimination, including urinary burning and urgency, diarrhea, and nausea or vomiting. These changes may be indications of urinary or GI system infection.

Take Actions: Interventions

Health promotion related to *infection* may be categorized as primary and secondary prevention. *Primary* prevention includes measures to prevent infection, such as immunizations against common illnesses. *Secondary* prevention involves screening for existing infection. See the best practice box for strategies to prevent infection.

> ▶▶ **BEST PRACTICE FOR PATIENT SAFETY AND QUALITY CARE**
> *Primary Health Promotion Strategies to Prevent Infection*
>
> - Frequently wash hands or use an alcohol-based hand rub for at least 15 seconds (based on CDC recommendations).
> - Follow accepted recommended immunization guidelines for each adult age-group.
> - Provide self-care management, including a healthy lifestyle, to prevent or manage chronic disease.
> - Keep body mass index within the recommended range or lose weight, if needed, to help build immunity.
> - Keep open skin areas covered during the healing process.
> - Avoid direct contact with other people's wounds or other infections.
> - Do not share personal items such as razors or towels.
> - In health care, use Standard Precautions when caring for all patients
> - Employ appropriate Transmission-Based Precautions according to how the *infection* is transmitted (spread); for example, keep a social distance of at least 6 feet and wear a well-fitted mask when exposed to a patient with COVID-19 infection.

For some adults, infections resolve without medical or collaborative management. However, nursing and collaborative interventions may be needed to manage some types of *infection.* Collaborative interventions include:

- Antimicrobial drug therapy (type depends on type of pathogen)
- Increased fluids and electrolyte replacement
- Sufficient rest
- Adequate *nutrition*

 See Chapter 19 in the main text for more information on ***infection.***

INFLAMMATION

Inflammation is a syndrome of normal responses to cellular injury, allergy, or invasion by pathogens. This reaction may occur anywhere in the body and may not be observable. Inflammation may be categorized as either acute or chronic. *Acute* inflammation may be *localized* or *systemic*, and has a short duration (hours or days). *Chronic* inflammation continues for weeks, months, or possibly years. It is usually *systemic,* affecting a large portion of the body.

Recognize Cues: Assessment

Assess for signs and symptoms of inflammation, which can include redness/hyperpigmentation, warmth, swelling, and pain or discomfort. If the inflammation is not observable because it is confined to the inside of the body, monitor for signs and symptoms of organ dysfunction. For example, patients with chronic inflammatory bowel disease have frequent diarrhea.

Take Actions: Interventions

Manage the signs and symptoms of local inflammation in one or more extremities by applying RICE:

- **R**est
- **I**ce
- **C**ompression
- **E**levation

Drug therapy is often used for chronic systemic ***inflammation.***

 See Chapter 16 in the main text for more on ***inflammation.***

MOBILITY

Mobility is the ability of an individual to perform purposeful physical movement of the body. When individuals are able to move, they are usually able to perform activities of daily living (ADLs), such as eating, dressing, and walking. This ability depends primarily on the function of the central and peripheral nervous systems and the musculoskeletal system and is sometimes referred to as *functional ability.*

Recognize Cues: Assessment

Observe patients within the environment to determine their *mobility* level. The mobility level of patients is adequate if they can move purposely to walk with an erect posture and coordinated gait and perform ADLs without assistance. Assessment of patients who are most at risk for decreased mobility is critical.

Take Actions: Interventions

The nurse has a major role in promoting mobility and preventing immobility. For patients who are immobile or have decreased mobility, it is important to perform passive range of motion (ROM) exercises, turn and reposition every 1 to 2 hours, keep the patient's skin clean and dry, and encourage deep-breathing and coughing exercises. Interprofessional collaboration with a registered dietitian, physical therapist, and respiratory therapist should be anticipated.

 *See Chapter 7 in the main text for more on **mobility** assessment and rehabilitation.*

NUTRITION

Nutrition is the process of ingesting and using food and fluids to grow, repair, and maintain optimal body functions. Nutrients from food and fluids are used for optimal cellular metabolism and health promotion. Examples of nutrient groups are proteins, carbohydrates, fats, vitamins, and minerals.

Recognize Cues: Assessment

Conduct a complete patient and family history for risk factors that could cause impaired nutrition. Ask about current or recent GI symptoms such as nausea, vomiting, constipation, and diarrhea. Obtain the patient's height and weight, and calculate body mass index (BMI). Assess the patient's skin, hair, and nails. Malnutrition often causes very dry skin and brittle hair and nails. Serum laboratory testing depends on which nutrients are inadequate.

Take Actions: Interventions

Collaborative interventions to improve nutrition depend on the cause of decreased nutrition. For those with weight loss or low weight, common interventions include high-protein oral supplements, enteral supplements (either oral or by feeding tube), or parenteral nutrition. Collaborate with the registered dietitian for specific instructions regarding enteral feedings; consult with the pharmacist to administer parenteral therapy.

 See Chapter 45 in the main text for more information on nutritional screening.

PAIN

Pain is generally defined as an unpleasant sensory and emotional experience. Because pain is a subjective symptom, nurses and other health care professionals must respect the patient's description of pain.

Recognize Cues: Assessment

A comprehensive pain assessment includes these components (Jarvis & Eckhardt, 2024):

- Location of pain and whether it radiates or is referred to other areas of the body
- Intensity of pain, using one of several valid and reliable pain assessment tools
- Quality of pain (such as burning, stabbing, or sharp, in patient's own words)
- Onset and duration of pain
- Aggravating or precipitating factors that cause pain
- Effects of pain on quality of life and daily function
- Psychosocial effects of pain (such as anxiety, fear, and depression)

Take Actions: Interventions

Nursing and collaborative management of pain may be categorized by pharmacologic and nonpharmacologic interventions. Evidence-based pharmacologic interventions involve a variety of analgesics and are determined based on severity, type, and source of pain. Nonpharmacologic patient-centered interventions depend on the patient's preferences. Examples of these integrative therapies include imagery, acupressure, acupuncture, and aromatherapy.

*See Chapter 6 in the main text for more information on interventions for **pain**.*

PERFUSION

Perfusion is adequate arterial blood flow through the peripheral tissues (*peripheral* perfusion) and blood pumped by the heart to oxygenate major body organs (*central* perfusion). Perfusion is a normal physiologic process of the body; without adequate perfusion, cell death can occur (Fig. 2.3).

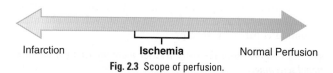

Infarction   **Ischemia**   Normal Perfusion

Fig. 2.3 Scope of perfusion.

Recognize Cues: Assessment

Conduct a complete patient and family history for risk factors and existing problems with perfusion. Assess for signs and symptoms of central perfusion, including dyspnea, dizziness or syncope, and chest pain. Signs and symptoms of decreased cardiac output include hypotension, tachycardia, diaphoresis, anxiety, decrease in cognitive function, and dysrhythmias.

Take Actions: Interventions

The nurse plays a vital role in promoting adequate perfusion and preventing impairment. Inadequate perfusion can cause serious and life-threatening consequences. For patients who have decreased perfusion, the primary health care provider may prescribe vasodilating drugs to promote blood flow. However, for many patients, a vascular intervention to open the occluded or narrowed artery may be performed.

 *See Chapters 29 and 30 in the main text for more on **perfusion**.*

SENSORY PERCEPTION

Sensory perception is the ability to perceive and interpret sensory input into one or more meaningful responses. Sensory input is usually received through the five major senses of vision, hearing, smell, taste, and touch.

Recognize Cues: Assessment

Conduct a thorough patient and family history to determine risk factors for vision or hearing loss. Ask the patient about the use of eyeglasses, contacts, or a magnifier to improve vision. Inquire whether the patient uses one or more hearing aids or amplifiers.

Take Actions: Intervention

Primary and secondary preventive interventions are used to promote vision and hearing and prevent sensory deficits. *Primary* measures focus on avoiding risk factors that cause vision and hearing loss or using protective devices to minimize risk. The purpose of *secondary* prevention is to perform screening and diagnostic tests for early detection of beginning sensory loss.

 *See Chapters 39 and 40 in the main text for more on alterations of **sensory perception**.*

SEXUALITY

Sexuality is a complex integration of physiologic, emotional, and social aspects of well-being related to intimacy, self-concept, and role relationships. It is not the same as *reproduction,* which is the process of conceiving and having a child. Sexuality involves sex, sexual acts, and sexual orientation; these terms are *not* the same as gender identity.

Recognize Cues: Assessment

Discussing sexuality, sexual health, and sexual intercourse is often difficult for both the patient and nurse. Ask patients about their perception of their sexuality, including both sexual activity and intimacy behaviors. Determine whether they have sex or intimacy with one or more partners. Ask about protection measures and any history of sexually transmitted infections (STIs) or problems during sexual intercourse.

Take Actions: Interventions

Interventions include STI screening and physical examinations to determine any physical cause of changes in sexuality. For patients with changes in sexuality, interventions depend on the cause of the sexual impairment.

See Chapter 65 in the main text for more on sexually transmitted infections (STIs).

TISSUE INTEGRITY

Tissue integrity is the intactness of the structure and function of the integument (skin and subcutaneous tissue) and mucous membranes. The skin is the largest organ of the body and has multiple functions, including protection from infection, fluid preservation, and temperature control.

Recognize Cues: Assessment

Take a thorough health history of previous and current chronic health problems and current medications (prescribed and over-the-counter [OTC]). Assess for change in skin color, moles or lesions, excessive skin dryness, bruising, and hair loss or brittle nails (indicating decreased tissue perfusion).

Take Actions: Interventions

The primary health promotion focus is on proper hygiene and nutrition to enhance tissue health. Teach patients at risk for impaired tissue integrity to inspect the skin every day. Keep the skin clean and dry; when needed, moisturize the skin to prevent excessive dryness. Interprofessional collaborative management of any *tissue integrity* alteration may include drug therapy (e.g., antibiotics, topical steroids, creams). Chemical or surgical wound debridement for necrotic tissue is essential to allow healing.

See Chapter 21 in the main text for more on wound care and skin assessment.

PART II

Diseases and Conditions

✳ ACIDOSIS: ACID-BASE BALANCE CONCEPT EXEMPLAR

Overview

- Acidosis is not a disease; it is a condition caused by a disorder or pathologic process. It can be caused by metabolic problems, respiratory problems, or both.
- In acidosis, the acid-base balance of the blood and other extracellular fluid (ECF) is upset by an excess of hydrogen ions (H^+). This is seen as an arterial blood pH below 7.35. The amount of acids present is greater than normal compared with the amount or strength of bases.

Metabolic Acidosis

- Four processes can result in metabolic acidosis: overproduction of hydrogen ions, underelimination of hydrogen ions, underproduction of bicarbonate ions, and overelimination of bicarbonate ions.

🕎 KEY FEATURES

Metabolic Acidosis: Expected Arterial Blood Gas Values

Test	Expected Value	Significance
pH	Below 7.35	Represents an increase in the free hydrogen ion concentration of arterial blood.
Pao_2	80–100 mm Hg	Represents the patient's normal value because oxygen intake is unimpaired
$Paco_2$	35–40 mm Hg	Retention of carbon dioxide is not a feature of metabolic acidosis because ventilation is not impaired. The value may be *low* because of respiratory compensation from a metabolic origin acidosis.
Bicarbonate	15–20 mEq/L (15–20 mmol/L) or lower	Loss of bicarbonate or inadequate production of bicarbonate is often the cause of metabolic acidosis, except for diabetic ketoacidosis.

$Paco_2$, partial pressure of arterial carbon dioxide; Pao_2, partial pressure of arterial oxygen

- Common causes of metabolic acidosis include:
  1. Diabetic ketoacidosis
  2. Starvation
  3. Hypoxia
  4. Seizure activity
  5. Aspirin or other salicylate intoxication

Respiratory Acidosis

- Respiratory acidosis results when respiratory function is impaired and the exchange of oxygen (O_2) and carbon dioxide (CO_2) is reduced. This problem causes CO_2 retention, which leads to the same increase in hydrogen ion levels and acidosis (Rogers, 2023). Respiratory acidosis results from only one cause— the retention of CO_2, causing increased production of free hydrogen ions.
- Common causes of respiratory acidosis include:
  1. Respiratory depression
  2. Reduced alveolar-capillary diffusion
     - Disorders include: pneumonia, pneumonitis, tuberculosis, emphysema, acute respiratory distress syndrome, chest trauma, pulmonary emboli, pulmonary edema, and drowning.
  3. Airway obstruction
  4. Inadequate chest expansion

Combined Metabolic and Respiratory Acidosis

- Metabolic and respiratory acidosis can occur at the same time (Emmett & Palmer, 2022; Rogers, 2023). For example, an adult who has diabetic ketoacidosis and chronic obstructive pulmonary disease has a combined metabolic and respiratory acidosis. Combined acidosis is more severe than either metabolic acidosis or respiratory acidosis alone.

 KEY FEATURES

Respiratory Acidosis: Expected Arterial Blood Gas Values

Test	Expected Value	Significance
pH	Below 7.35	Represents an increase in the free hydrogen ion concentration of arterial blood.
PaO_2	< 90 mm Hg	Represents greatly reduced gas exchange and inadequate oxygenation from the patient's underlying acute or chronic respiratory problems.

KEY FEATURES—cont'd

A

Respiratory Acidosis: Expected Arterial Blood Gas Values

Test	Expected Value	Significance
$Paco_2$	> 50 mm Hg and can even be above 100 mm Hg	Represents greatly reduced gas exchange and retention of CO_2 from the patient's underlying acute or chronic respiratory problems.
Bicarbonate	21–28 mEq/L (21–28 mmol/L) or higher	Bicarbonate is not lost in pure respiratory acidosis and the level is usually normal in acute respiratory acidosis. The level is elevated in chronic respiratory acidosis because of kidney compensation.

$Paco_2$, Partial pressure of arterial carbon dioxide; *Pao_2,* partial pressure of arterial oxygen.

Interprofessional Collaborative Care
Recognize Cues: Assessment
Signs and symptoms of acidosis are similar whether the cause is metabolic or respiratory (see Key Features: Acidosis). *Cognitive changes may be the first signs of acidosis.* Assess the patient's mental status for awareness of time, place, and person.

- *Respiratory changes* may cause the acidosis and can be caused by the acidosis. Assess the patient's rate, depth, and ease of breathing. Use pulse oximetry to determine how well oxygen is delivered to the peripheral tissues.
- If acidosis is metabolic in origin, the rate and depth of breathing increase as the hydrogen ion level rises. Breaths are deep and rapid and not under voluntary control (Kussmaul respiration).

 KEY FEATURES

Acidosis

Cardiovascular Signs and Symptoms
- Ranges from bradycardia to heart block
- Tall T waves
- Widened QRS complex
- Prolonged PR interval
- Hypotension
- Thready peripheral pulses

Central Nervous System Signs and Symptoms
- Depressed activity (lethargy, confusion, stupor, coma)

Continued

KEY FEATURES—cont'd

Acidosis

Neuromuscular Signs and Symptoms
- Hyporeflexia
- Skeletal muscle weakness
- Flaccid paralysis

Respiratory Signs and Symptoms
- Kussmaul respiration (in metabolic acidosis with respiratory compensation)
- Variable respirations (generally ineffective in respiratory acidosis)

Integumentary Signs and Symptoms
- Warm, flushed, dry skin in metabolic acidosis
- Pale/ash gray to cyanotic and dry skin in respiratory acidosis

Laboratory Assessment
- Arterial blood pH is the laboratory value used to confirm acidosis. Acidosis is present when arterial blood pH is less than 7.35. The serum potassium level is often high in acidosis as the body attempts to maintain electroneutrality during buffering.

NURSING SAFETY PRIORITY

Critical Rescue

Assess the cardiovascular system first in any patient at risk for acidosis because acidosis can lead to cardiac arrest from the accompanying hyperkalemia. If cardiac changes are present, respond by reporting these changes immediately to the primary health care provider.

Analyze Cues and Prioritize Hypotheses: Analysis
- Patients with acidosis have problems associated with decreased excitable tissues, including hypotension and decreased perfusion, impaired memory and cognition, and increased risk for falls. The priority patient problem for the patient experiencing respiratory acidosis is:
  1. Reduced gas exchange resulting from underlying pulmonary disease

Generate Solutions and Take Actions: Planning and Implementation
- Interventions for acidosis focus on correcting the underlying problem and monitoring for changes. Remember, acidosis is not a disease. It is a symptom of another health problem.

Metabolic Acidosis
- If the acidosis is caused by diabetic ketoacidosis, insulin is given to correct the hyperglycemia.
- Rehydration and antidiarrheal drugs are given if the acidosis is a result of prolonged diarrhea.
- Bicarbonate is given only if serum bicarbonate levels are low and the pH is less than 7.2.
- Continuously monitor:
  1. For signs of improvement or decline
  2. The cardiovascular and the skeletal systems (most sensitive to acidosis)
  3. Changes in ABG results

Respiratory Acidosis
- Interventions include drug therapy, oxygen therapy, pulmonary hygiene (positioning and breathing techniques), and ventilatory support. These interventions are the same as those used for a patient who has chronic obstructive pulmonary disease (COPD), which is the most common health problem associated with continuing risk for respiratory acidosis.
  1. Administer prescribed drug therapy to improve ventilation and *gas exchange* rather than alter pH.
     - Drug categories useful for respiratory acidosis include bronchodilators, corticosteroids, antiinflammatories, and mucolytics
  2. Administer oxygen as prescribed; carefully monitor oxygen saturation levels
  3. *Ventilation support* with mechanical ventilation may be needed for patients who cannot keep their oxygen saturation at 90% or who have respiratory muscle fatigue.
  4. *Prevent complications by* monitoring respiratory status hourly and intervening when changes occur.
     - Assess the following:
       - Respiratory rate and depth
       - Oxygen saturation (Spo_2) and ABG values to maintain a normal range of oxygenation (Spo_2 greater than 90% to 92% and Pao_2 greater than 90 mm Hg)
       - Effort of breathing, including use of accessory muscles
       - Nail beds and mucous membranes for cyanosis (late finding)

Care Coordination and Transition Management
- Because respiratory acidosis is a symptom or complication of another health problem, most often COPD, care during the acute phase occurs in a hospital setting.

Evaluate Outcomes: Evaluation

- Indications that the patient's underlying disease process is well managed and that the imbalance is reduced include the expected outcomes that the patient:
  1. Maintains adequate gas exchange
  2. Has an arterial pH above 7.2 and closer to 7.35
  3. Has a Pao_2 level above 90 mm Hg or at least 10 mm Hg higher than admission level
  4. Has a $Paco_2$ level below 45 mm Hg or at least 15 mm Hg below admission level

See Chapter 14 in the main text for more information on acid-base balance.

ACUTE CORONARY SYNDROMES: PERFUSION CONCEPT EXEMPLAR

Overview

- The term *acute coronary syndrome* (ACS) is used to describe patients who have either unstable angina or an acute myocardial infarction (MI or AMI).
  1. *Unstable angina* is chest pain or discomfort that occurs at rest or with exertion and causes severe activity limitation.
  2. *Myocardial infarction (MI)* occurs when myocardial tissue is abruptly and severely deprived of oxygen. When blood flow is quickly reduced by 80% to 90%, ischemia can lead to injury and necrosis of myocardial tissue if blood flow is not restored.
     - There are two types of MI: non–ST-segment elevation MI (NSTEMI) and ST elevation MI (STEMI).
       - NSTEMI: indicates myocardial ischemia
       - STEMI: indicates myocardial necrosis. STEMI is attributable to rupture of the fibrous atherosclerotic plaque, leading to platelet aggregation and thrombus formation at the site of rupture (Rogers, 2023). The thrombus causes an abrupt 100% occlusion to the coronary artery, is a medical emergency, and requires immediate revascularization of the blocked coronary artery.
     - Infarction is a dynamic process that does not occur instantly. Rather, it evolves over a period of several hours.

Interprofessional Collaborative Care
Recognize Cues: Assessment

- If symptoms of coronary artery disease (CAD) are present, delay collecting historical data until interventions for symptom relief.
- Rapid assessment of the patient with chest pain or other presenting symptoms is crucial.

A

- Assess for signs and symptoms of angina and MI.
  1. Quality, onset, duration, and alleviating and aggravating factors related to chest pain. Assess for associated symptoms, such as jaw pain, back pain, nausea and vomiting, palpitations, extreme fatigue, sudden and severe dyspnea, diaphoresis, dizziness, or weakness. (See Key Features: Angina and Myocardial Infarction.)
  2. Vital signs (VS), including heart rhythm and SpO_2
  3. Distal peripheral pulses and skin temperature
  4. Heart sounds, noting S_3 gallop (indicator of heart failure)
  5. Assess breath sounds for heart failure (HF is a serious complication of MI)
  6. Fear and anxiety, denial, or depression
  7. Elevated serum troponin levels
  8. 12-lead ECG changes:
     - ST depression or elevation or T-wave inversion
     - ST elevation or abnormal Q wave in two or more contiguous leads
  9. Results of echocardiography, exercise test (stress test), thallium scan, contrast-enhanced cardiovascular magnetic resonance (CMR), CT coronary angiography, and cardiac catheterization, if performed

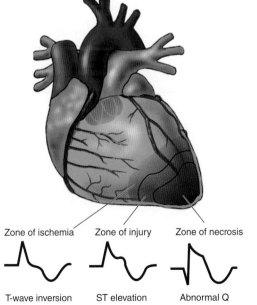

Zone of ischemia   Zone of injury   Zone of necrosis

T-wave inversion   ST elevation   Abnormal Q

Electrocardiographic changes and patterns associated with myocardial infarction.

KEY FEATURES

Angina and Myocardial Infarction

Angina	Myocardial Infarction

• Substernal chest discomfort:
  • Radiating to the left arm
  • Precipitated by exertion or stress (or rest in vasospastic angina)
  • Relieved by nitroglycerin or rest
  • Lasting less than 15 minutes
• Few, if any, associated symptoms
	• Pain or discomfort
	  • Substernal chest pain/pressure radiating to the left arm
	  • Pain or discomfort in jaw, back, shoulder, or abdomen
	  • Occurring without cause, usually in the morning
	  • Relieved only by opioids
	  • Lasting 30 minutes or more
	• Frequent associated symptoms:
	  • Nausea/vomiting
	  • Diaphoresis
	  • Dyspnea
	  • Feelings of fear and anxiety
	  • Dysrhythmias
	  • Fatigue
	  • Palpitations
	  • Epigastric distress
	  • Anxiety
	  • Dizziness
	  • Disorientation/acute confusion
	  • Feeling "short of breath"

Analyze Cues and Prioritize Hypotheses: Analysis

- The patient with CAD may have either stable angina or ACS. If ACS is suspected or cannot be completely ruled out, the patient is admitted to a telemetry unit for continuous monitoring or to a critical care unit if hemodynamically unstable.
- The priority collaborative problems for most patients with ACS include:
  1. Acute *pain* due to an imbalance between myocardial oxygen supply and demand
  2. Decreased myocardial tissue *perfusion* due to interruption of arterial blood flow

3. Potential for dysrhythmias due to ischemia and ventricular irritability

4. Potential for heart failure due to left ventricular dysfunction

Generate Solutions and Take Actions: Planning and Implementation
Managing Acute Pain

- Manage pain to improve oxygen supply to the myocardium and decrease myocardial oxygen demand.

  1. Nitroglycerin may be prescribed to dilate peripheral veins, reducing oxygen demand.

  2. Morphine may be prescribed for persistent cardiac *pain*. Morphine decreases pain, decreases myocardial oxygen demand, relaxes smooth muscle, and reduces circulating catecholamines.

  3. If hypoxemia is present, oxygen may be prescribed at a flow of 2 to 4 L/min to maintain an arterial oxygen saturation of 90% or higher. The use of oxygen in the absence of hypoxemia has been shown to increase coronary vascular resistance, decrease coronary blood flow, and increase mortality.

✚ NURSING SAFETY PRIORITY
Critical Rescue

If the patient is experiencing an MI, prepare the patient for transfer to a specialized unit, where close monitoring and appropriate management can be provided. If the patient is at home or in the community, call 911 for transfer to the closest emergency department.

Increasing Myocardial Tissue Perfusion

- Because MI is a dynamic process, restoring **perfusion** to the injured area (usually within 4 to 6 hours for NSTEMI and 60 to 90 minutes for STEMI) often limits the amount of extension and improves left ventricular function.

  1. Administer and monitor patient response to drug therapy.
     - *Aspirin* (chewed to hasten absorption) reduces platelet aggregation and prevents clot extension in coronary arteries.
     - $P2Y_{12}$ *platelet inhibitors*, such as clopidogrel or ticagrelor, may be prescribed with an initial loading dose followed by a daily dose for up to 12 months after diagnosis. These oral agents work to prevent platelets from aggregating (clumping) together to form clots.

- *Glycoprotein (GP) IIb/IIIa inhibitors,* such as eptifibatide or tirofiban, may be administered IV to prevent fibrinogen from attaching to activated platelets at the site of a thrombus. These medications are used in unstable angina and NSTEMI.
- Once-a-day beta-adrenergic blocking agents (metoprolol XL or carvedilol CR) reduce HR and oxygen demand, decrease sympathetic stimulation of the compromised myocardium, and prevent life-threatening dysrhythmias.

 NURSING SAFETY PRIORITY

Drug Alert

Dual antiplatelet therapy (DAPT) is suggested for all patients with ACS, incorporating aspirin with a $P2Y_{12}$ receptor blocker, such as clopidogrel or ticagrelor (Lincoff & Cutlip, 2023). The major side effect for *each* of these agents is bleeding. Observe for bleeding tendencies, such as nosebleeds or blood in the stool. Medications will need to be discontinued if evidence of bleeding occurs. Teach patients signs of bleeding and when to contact the health care provider.

NURSING SAFETY PRIORITY

Drug Alert

Do not give beta-blockers if the pulse is below 50 or the systolic blood pressure is below 100 mm Hg without first checking with the primary health care provider. The beta-blocking agent may lead to persistent bradycardia or further reduction of systolic BP, leading to poor peripheral and coronary perfusion.

- Angiotensin-converting enzyme inhibitor (ACEI) or angiotensin receptor blocker may be given to prevent ventricular remodeling and development of HF.
- For patients with angina, a calcium channel blocker may be prescribed to promote vasodilation and perfusion.
- Statin therapy reduces the risk of developing recurrent MI, mortality, and stroke.
2. Support reperfusion therapy so that it occurs within 30 minutes of arrival to the hospital or emergency department.
   - Thrombolytic therapy using a fibrinolytic such as tissue plasminogen activator (tPA), alteplase, reteplase, or tenecteplase dissolves thrombi in coronary arteries.

🖊 NURSING SAFETY PRIORITY

Drug Alert

During and after thrombolytic administration, immediately report any indications of bleeding to the primary health care provider or Rapid Response Team. Observe for signs of bleeding by:
- Documenting the patient's neurologic status (in case of intracranial bleeding)
- Observing all IV sites for bleeding and patency
- Monitoring clotting studies
- Observing for signs of internal bleeding (monitor hemoglobin, hematocrit, HR, and BP)
- Testing stools, urine, and emesis for occult blood

- Percutaneous coronary intervention (PCI) typically involves placement of a stent to open the clotted coronary artery.
- PCI, an invasive but technically nonsurgical technique, is performed to provide symptom reduction for patients with chest discomfort within 90 minutes of a diagnosis of AMI unless there are specific contraindications.
- Other nonsurgical techniques used to ensure patency of the vessel are stent placement, laser angioplasty, and atherectomy.

✚ NURSING SAFETY PRIORITY

Critical Rescue

After PCI, monitor for potential problems, including acute closure of the vessel (causes chest pain and potential ST elevation on 12-lead ECG), bleeding from the insertion (sheath) site, and reaction to the contrast medium used in angiography. Also monitor for and document hypotension, hypokalemia, and dysrhythmias. Document and report any of these findings to the health care provider or Rapid Response Team immediately!

Identifying and Managing Dysrhythmias (see Dysrhythmias, Cardiac)
- *Dysrhythmias are the leading cause of prehospital death in most patients with ACS.* Even in the early period of hospitalization, most patients with ACS experience some abnormal cardiac rhythm.
  1. Monitor ECG.
  2. Evaluate hemodynamic status with dysrhythmia onset.

Monitoring for and Managing Heart Failure (see Heart Failure)

- Decreased cardiac output due to heart failure is a relatively common complication after an MI, resulting from left ventricular dysfunction, rupture of the intraventricular septum, papillary muscle rupture with valvular dysfunction, or right ventricular infarction.
- Hemodynamic monitoring may be required. This type of monitoring can vary from noninvasive to highly invasive. (See Hemodynamic Monitoring.)
- Monitor for cardiogenic shock. (See Critical Rescue below.)

✚ NURSING SAFETY PRIORITY

Critical Rescue

Monitor for, report, and document manifestations of cardiogenic shock immediately. These signs and symptoms include:
- Tachycardia
- Hypotension
- Systolic BP less than 90 mm Hg or 30 mm Hg less than the patient's baseline
- Urine output of less than 0.5 to 1 mL/kg/hr
- Cold, clammy skin with poor peripheral pulses
- Agitation, restlessness, or confusion
- Pulmonary congestion
- Tachypnea
- Continuing chest discomfort

Early detection is essential because undiagnosed cardiogenic shock has a high mortality rate!

Coronary Artery Bypass Graft Surgery

- Coronary artery bypass graft (CABG) surgery is indicated when other treatments are deemed unlikely to succeed or have been unsuccessful in managing CAD and ACS. This procedure is performed while the patient is under general anesthesia and undergoing cardiopulmonary bypass (CPB) surgery. CABG can be done as a traditional open-heart technique or as a minimally invasive surgical (MIS) approach.
- CPB is used to provide oxygenation, circulation, and hypothermia during induced cardiac arrest. Blood is diverted from the heart to the bypass machine, where it is heparinized, oxygenated, and returned to the circulation through a cannula placed in the ascending aortic arch or femoral artery.
- After traditional surgery, the patient is transported to a post–open heart surgery unit. They will require highly skilled nursing care from a nurse qualified to provide post–cardiac surgery care, including routine postoperative care.

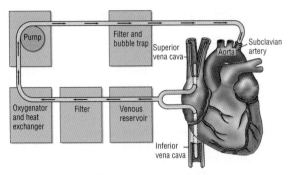

Heart lung bypass circuitry.

! NURSING SAFETY PRIORITY

Action Alert

Bleeding after CABG surgery occurs to a limited extent in all patients. Measure mediastinal and pleural chest tube drainage at least hourly. Report drainage amounts over 150 mL/hr to the surgeon. Patients with internal mammary artery (IMA) grafts may have more chest drainage than those with saphenous vein grafts (from the leg).

- Care following CABG includes:
  1. Preventing surgical site infections.
     - Sternal wound infections develop between 5 days and several weeks after surgery in a small number of patients and are responsible for increased costs and longer hospital stays. Be alert for mediastinitis (infection of the mediastinum) by observing for:
       - Fever continuing beyond the first 4 days after CABG
       - Instability (bogginess) of the sternum
       - Redness/hyperpigmentation, induration, swelling, or drainage from suture sites
       - An increased white blood cell count
       - Closely monitoring for dysrhythmias
  2. Monitoring for, reporting, and documenting other complications of CABG, including:
     - Fluid and electrolyte imbalance
     - Hypotension
     - Hypothermia
     - Hypertension
     - Bleeding
     - Cardiac tamponade
     - Decreased level of consciousness
     - Anginal pain

> **! NURSING SAFETY PRIORITY**
>
> *Action Alert*
>
> After a CABG, check the patient's neurologic status every 30 to 60 minutes until the patient awakens from anesthesia. Then check every 2 to 4 hours or per agency policy.

Care Coordination and Transition Management

* Patients who have experienced a myocardial infarction (MI), angina, or coronary artery bypass graft (CABG) surgery are usually discharged to home or to a transitional care setting with drug therapy and specific activity prescriptions.
  1. Teach the patient and family about:
     * The pathophysiology of CAD, angina, and MI
     * Risk factor modification:
       * Smoking cessation
       * Dietary changes (limiting fat and sodium intake)
       * BP control
       * Blood glucose control
     * Gradual increase in physical and sexual activity, according to cardiac rehabilitation protocol
     * Cardiac drugs: dose effects, adverse effects, and rationale for use
     * Occupational considerations, if any
     * Complementary and integrative therapies such as progressive relaxation, guided imagery, music therapy, and pet therapy

> **⊘ NURSING SAFETY PRIORITY**
>
> *Drug Alert*
>
> Use of sublingual or spray nitroglycerin (NTG) deserves special attention. *Teach the patient to carry NTG at all times.* Keep the tablets in a glass, light-resistant container. The drug should be replaced every 3 to 5 months before it loses its potency or stops producing a tingling sensation when placed under the tongue.

  2. Teach patients to seek medical assistance if they experience:
     * A heart rate that remains less than 50 after arising
     * Wheezing or difficulty breathing

A

- Weight gain of 3 pounds in 1 week, or 1 to 2 pounds overnight
- Persistent increase in nitroglycerin use
- Dizziness, faintness, or shortness of breath with activity

3. Patients should call for emergency transportation to the hospital if they experience the following:
   - Chest discomfort that is not relieved with nitroglycerin
   - Chest or epigastric discomfort with weakness, nausea, or fainting
   - Other associated symptoms that are particular to the patient, such as fatigue or nausea

4. Other important discharge plans include:
   - Teaching for drug adherence and provider follow-up
   - Referring the patient and caregiver for continued cardiac rehabilitation

Evaluate Outcomes: Evaluation

- Evaluate the care of the patient with CAD based on the identified priority patient problems. The expected outcomes are that the patient will:
  1. State that pain is alleviated
  2. Have adequate myocardial perfusion
  3. Be free of complications such as dysrhythmias and heart failure

See Chapter 32 in the main text for more information on acute coronary syndrome.

ACUTE RESPIRATORY DISTRESS SYNDROME

- Acute respiratory distress syndrome (ARDS) is acute respiratory failure with these features:
  1. Hypoxemia that persists even when 100% oxygen is given (refractory hypoxemia)
  2. Decreased pulmonary compliance
  3. Dyspnea
  4. Noncardiac-associated bilateral pulmonary edema
  5. Dense pulmonary infiltrates on x-ray (ground-glass appearance)
- Often ARDS occurs after an acute lung injury in people who have no pulmonary disease. These lung injuries may be related to other conditions such as sepsis, burns, pancreatitis, trauma, and transfusion.
  1. Despite different causes in ARDS, the trigger is a systemic inflammatory response. As a result, ARDS symptoms are similar regardless of the cause.
  2. The main site of injury in the lung is the alveolar-capillary membrane, which normally is permeable only to small molecules. When injured, this membrane becomes more permeable

to large molecules, which allows debris, proteins, and fluid into the alveoli.

3. Lung tissue normally remains relatively dry, but in patients with ARDS, lung fluid increases and contains more proteins. In ARDS associated with COVID-19, the thick exudate inhibits gas exchange.

Interprofessional Collaborative Care
Recognize Cues: Assessment

- The nursing priority in the prevention of ARDS is early recognition of patients at high risk for the syndrome.
    1. Because patients who aspirate gastric contents are at great risk, closely assess and monitor those receiving tube feedings (because the tube keeps the gastric sphincter open) and those with problems that impair swallowing and gag reflexes.
    2. To help prevent ARDS, follow meticulous infection control guidelines, including handwashing, invasive catheter and wound care, and Contact Precautions. Teach assistive personnel the importance of always adhering to infection control guidelines.
    3. Assess breathing patterns. Assess for difficulty breathing (hyperpnea, noisy respirations, cyanosis, pallor/ash gray appearance, and retraction intercostally or substernally).
    4. Abnormal lung sounds are **not** always heard on auscultation because the edema occurs first in the interstitial spaces and not in the airways.
    5. Assess vital signs frequently for hypotension, tachycardia, and dysrhythmias.
    6. The diagnosis of ARDS is established by a lowered partial pressure of arterial oxygen (Pao_2) value (decreased *gas exchange* and oxygenation), determined by arterial blood gas (ABG) measurements.

Take Actions: Interventions

- General management of the patient with ARDS focuses on the three phases of ARDS. Timing of the phases varies from patient to patient.
    1. *Exudative phase.* This phase includes early changes of dyspnea and tachypnea, resulting from the alveoli becoming fluid filled and from pulmonary shunting and atelectasis. Early interventions focus on supporting the patient and providing oxygen.

A

2. *Fibrosing alveolitis phase.* Increased lung injury leads to pulmonary hypertension and fibrosis. The body attempts to repair the damage, and increasing lung involvement reduces **gas exchange** and oxygenation. Multiple organ dysfunction syndrome (MODS) can occur. Interventions focus on delivering adequate oxygen, preventing complications, and supporting the lungs.

3. *Resolution phase.* Usually occurring after 14 days, resolution of the injury can occur; if not, the patient either dies or has chronic disease. Fibrosis may or may not occur. Patients surviving ARDS often have neuropsychologic deficits.

- Management includes:
  1. Endotracheal intubation and mechanical ventilation with positive end-expiratory pressure (PEEP) or continuous positive airway pressure (CPAP)
  2. Positioning: Prone positioning has been shown to reduce mortality in moderate to severe ARDS patients on low-tidal-volume ventilation (Malhotra, 2023). Routine turning every 2 hours can improve perfusion.
  3. Antibiotics to manage identified infections
  4. Conservative IV fluid volume administration to prevent excess lung tissue fluid while managing hypotension and inadequate perfusion
  5. Enteral nutrition or parenteral nutrition as soon as possible to prevent malnutrition, loss of respiratory muscle function, and reduced immune response

✚ **NURSING SAFETY PRIORITY**

Critical Rescue

For the patient requiring emergency intubation and ventilation, call for help or notify the Rapid Response Team, and secure the code (or "crash") cart, airway equipment box, and suction equipment (often already on the code cart). Maintain a patent airway through positioning (head tilt, chin lift) and the insertion of an oral or nasopharyngeal airway until the patient is intubated. Delivering manual breaths with a bag-valve-mask may also be required.

🏹 *See Chapter 26 in the main text for more information on acute respiratory distress syndrome.*

ADRENAL GLAND HYPOFUNCTION

- Decreased production of these adrenocortical steroids occurs as a result of:
  1. Inadequate secretion of adrenocorticotropic hormone (ACTH) (hypopituitarism)
  2. Dysfunction of the hypothalamic-pituitary control mechanisms
  3. Direct problems of adrenal gland tissue (such as adrenal tumors)
     - Acute adrenal insufficiency or *addisonian crisis* is a life-threatening event in which the need for cortisol and aldosterone is greater than the body's supply (Rogers, 2023).
       - It often occurs in response to a stressful event such as surgery, trauma, and severe infection when the adrenal hormone output is already reduced.
       - Acute adrenal insufficiency is an emergency and is managed in an acute care setting. Without appropriate management, death ensues (Nieman, 2022b).

Interprofessional Collaborative Care
Recognize Cues: Assessment

- Obtain patient information about:
  1. Change in activity level or lethargy and fatigue
  2. Increased salt craving or intake (occurs with adrenal hypofunction)
  3. GI problems, such as anorexia, nausea and vomiting, diarrhea, and abdominal pain
  4. Unplanned weight loss
  5. History of radiation to the abdomen or head
  6. Past or current medical problems (e.g., tuberculosis, previous intracranial surgery)
  7. History of or exposure to COVID-19
  8. Past and current drugs, especially steroids, anticoagulants, opioids, or cancer drugs
- Assess for:
  1. Hypoglycemia (e.g., sweating, headaches, tachycardia, and tremors)
  2. Fluid depletion (postural hypotension and dehydration)
  3. *Hyperkalemia* (elevated blood potassium levels), which can cause dysrhythmias with an irregular heart rate and result in cardiac arrest
  4. Hyponatremia, which can lead to hypotension and decreased cognition

KEY FEATURES

Adrenal Insufficiency

Neuromuscular Symptoms	**Integumentary Symptoms**
• Muscle weakness	• Vitiligo
• Fatigue	• Hyperpigmentation
• Joint and/or muscle pain	
	Cardiovascular Symptoms
Gastrointestinal Symptoms	• Anemia
• Anorexia	• Hypotension
• Nausea, vomiting	• Hyponatremia
• Abdominal pain	• Hyperkalemia
• Constipation or diarrhea	• Hypercalcemia
• Weight loss	
• Salt craving	

- Diagnosis is based on signs and symptoms and:
  1. Laboratory findings of low salivary cortisol levels, low fasting blood glucose, low sodium, elevated potassium, and increased blood urea nitrogen (BUN) levels
  2. Low urinary 17-hydroxycorticosteroid and 17-ketosteroid levels
  3. Magnetic resonance imaging (MRI) or CT scans of brain, abdomen, and pelvis
  4. ACTH stimulation (provocative) test

Take Actions: Interventions

- Nursing interventions focus on promoting fluid balance, monitoring for fluid deficit, and preventing hypoglycemia. Because hyperkalemia can cause dysrhythmias with an irregular heart rate and result in cardiac arrest, assessing cardiac function is a nursing priority.
  1. Cortisol and aldosterone deficiencies are corrected by hormone replacement therapy.
     - For oral cortisol therapy, divided doses are usually given, with two-thirds given in the morning and one-third at 6:00 p.m. This divided dose mimics the normal release of this hormone.
  2. Nursing interventions include:
     - Weighing the patient daily and recording intake and output
     - Assessing vital signs every 1 to 4 hours

- Checking for dysrhythmias or postural hypotension
- Monitoring glucose levels
- Monitoring laboratory values to identify hemoconcentration (e.g., increased hematocrit, blood urea nitrogen [BUN])

> ### 🖊 NURSING SAFETY PRIORITY
> #### *Drug Alert*
>
> Prednisone and prednisolone are sound-alike drugs, and care is needed not to confuse them. Although they are both corticosteroids, they are not interchangeable, because prednisolone is several times more potent than prednisone.

See Chapter 54 in the main text for more information on adrenal gland hypofunction.

ALKALOSIS

- In patients with alkalosis, the acid-base balance of the blood is disturbed and has an excess of bases, especially bicarbonate (HCO_3^-). The amount of bases is greater than normal compared with the amount of the acids. Alkalosis is a *decrease* in the free hydrogen ion level of the blood and is reflected by an arterial blood pH *above* 7.45.
- Alkalosis is not a disease; it is a condition caused by a metabolic problem, a respiratory problem, or both.
- Alkalosis can result from an actual or relative increase in the amount of bases. In an actual base excess, alkalosis occurs when base (usually bicarbonate) is either overproduced or undereliminated.

Metabolic Alkalosis
- Common causes include:
  1. Increase of base (especially bicarbonate)
     - Excessive use of antacids or bicarbonate
     - Multiple transfusions of blood products
     - IV administration of bicarbonate
  2. Acid loss
     - Prolonged vomiting
     - Continuous nasogastric suctioning
     - Dehydration from excessive diuretic use
     - Hypercortisolism
     - Hyperaldosteronism
- The hallmark of metabolic acidosis is an ABG result with an elevated pH and an elevated bicarbonate level, along with normal oxygen and carbon dioxide levels.

Respiratory Alkalosis
- Common causes:
  1. Excessive loss of CO_2 though hyperventilation
     - Hyperventilation can occur in response to anxiety, fear, or improper settings on mechanical ventilation. Hyperventilation can also occur from direct stimulation of the central respiratory centers because of fever, central nervous system lesions, and salicylates.
- The hallmark of respiratory alkalosis is an ABG result with an elevated pH coupled with a low carbon dioxide level. Usually the oxygen and bicarbonate levels are normal.

Interprofessional Collaborative Care
Recognize Cues: Assessment
- Symptoms of problems with *acid-base balance* regulation are the same for metabolic and respiratory alkalosis. Many symptoms are the result of the low calcium levels (hypocalcemia) and low potassium levels (hypokalemia) that usually occur with alkalosis. These problems change the function of the nervous, neuromuscular, cardiac, and respiratory systems. See Key Features: Alkalosis.

 KEY FEATURES

Alkalosis

Central Nervous System Signs and Symptoms
- Increased activity
- Anxiety, irritability, tetany, seizures
- Positive Chvostek sign
- Positive Trousseau sign
- Paresthesias

Neuromuscular Signs and Symptoms
- Hyperreflexia
- Muscle cramping and twitching
- Skeletal muscle weakness

Cardiovascular Signs and Symptoms
- Increased heart rate
- Normal or low BP

Respiratory Signs and Symptoms
- Hyperventilation in respiratory alkalosis (often the cause of the acidosis)
- Decreased respiratory effort associated with skeletal muscle weakness

- Assessment findings include:
  1. CNS changes: caused by overexcitement of the nervous system
     - Dizziness, agitation, confusion, and hyperreflexia, which can progress to seizures
     - Positive Chvostek sign and positive Trousseau sign
  2. Neuromuscular changes: related to hypocalcemia and hypokalemia
     - Skeletal muscle weakness, muscle cramping and twitching, hyperreflexia, tetany
  3. Cardiovascular changes: occur because alkalosis increases myocardial irritability, especially when combined with hypokalemia
     - Thready pulse, increased heart rate, possible hypotension
  4. Respiratory changes, especially increases in the rate of breathing, are the main causes of respiratory alkalosis.

Take Actions: Interventions
- Management focuses on:
  1. Preventing further loss of hydrogen, potassium, calcium, and chloride ions
  2. Restoring fluid balance
  3. Monitoring changes in patient assessment
  4. Treating the cause of the alkalosis
  5. Providing patient safety
- Nursing care priority is prevention of injury from falls. The patient with alkalosis has hypotension and muscle weakness, which increase the risk for falls, especially among older adults.

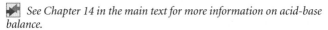 *See Chapter 14 in the main text for more information on acid-base balance.*

ALLERGY AND ALLERGIC RESPONSES (HYPERSENSITIVITIES)

- Allergy or hypersensitivity is an overactive *immunity* reaction with excessive *inflammation*.
- Allergy occurs in response to the presence of an antigen (foreign protein or allergen) to which the patient has been previously exposed.
- Hypersensitivity reactions are classified into four basic types, determined by differences in timing, pathophysiology, and symptoms:
  1. Type I: Anaphylactic Response
     - Results from the increased production of immunoglobulin E (IgE)

- Examples include allergies to latex, bee venom, peanuts, shellfish, and certain drugs.
- Symptoms can be life-threatening with angioedema or anaphylaxis, or relatively mild with rhinosinusitis.

2. Type II: Cytotoxic Mediated Response
   - Results when the body makes autoantibodies directed against self cells that have some form of foreign protein attached to them
   - Examples include drug-induced hemolytic anemia and hemolytic transfusion reactions (when a patient receives the wrong blood type during a transfusion).

3. Type III: Immune Complex Reaction
   - Results from excess antigens causing immune complexes to form in the blood. These circulating complexes then lodge in small blood vessels of the kidneys, skin, and joints. The complexes trigger inflammation, and tissue or vessel damage results.
   - Most immune complex disorders (autoimmune disorders) are caused by type III reactions. Rheumatoid arthritis is a common example.

4. Type IV: Hypersensitivity Reaction
   - Results when sensitized T cells (from a previous exposure) respond to an antigen by releasing chemical mediators and triggering macrophages to destroy the antigen
   - Common examples include contact dermatitis such as poison ivy skin rashes or metal-induced skin irritations, stem cell or solid organ rejections, positive tuberculosis (TB) skin test, and sarcoidosis.

See Chapter 17 in the main text for more information on allergy and allergic responses.

⊞ ALZHEIMER'S DISEASE: COGNITION CONCEPT EXEMPLAR

Overview
- Alzheimer's disease (AD) is the most common type of dementia that affects people older than 65 years.
- AD is characterized by neurofibrillary tangles, amyloid-rich or neuritic plaques, and vascular degeneration.
- The exact cause of AD is unknown. It is well established that *age, gender, and genetics are the most important risk factors.*

Interprofessional Collaborative Care
Recognize Cues: Assessment
- The most important information to be obtained is the onset, duration, progression, and course of the symptoms. Question both the patient and the family.

1. Assess for changes in memory or increasing forgetfulness and about the ability to perform ADLs. *One of the first symptoms of AD is short-term memory impairment.*

 KEY FEATURES

Alzheimer's Disease

Early Stage
- Independent in ADLs
- May deny presence of symptoms
- Forgets names; misplaces household items
- Has short-term memory loss and difficulty recalling new information
- Shows subtle changes in personality and behavior
- Loses initiative and is less engaged in social relationships
- Has mild impaired **cognition** and problems with judgment
- Demonstrates decreased performance, especially when stressed
- Unable to travel alone to new destinations
- Often has decreased sense of smell

Moderate Stage
- Has impairment of all cognitive functions
- Demonstrates problems with handling or unable to handle money and finances
- Is disoriented to time, place, and event
- Is possibly depressed and/or agitated
- Increasingly dependent in ADLs
- Has visuospatial deficits: has difficulty driving and gets lost
- Has speech and language deficits: less talkative, decreased use of vocabulary, increasingly nonfluent, and eventually aphasic
- Incontinent of urine and stool
- Has episodes of wandering; trouble sleeping

Late Stage (Severe)
- Completely incapacitated; bedridden
- Totally dependent in ADLs
- Has loss of **mobility** and verbal skills
- May have seizures and tremors
- Has agnosia (loss of facial recognition)

2. Assess for changes in driving ability, ability to handle routine financial transactions, and language and communication skills.
   - Alterations in communication abilities, such as **apraxia** (inability to use words or objects correctly), **aphasia** (inability

to speak or understand), **anomia** (inability to find words), and **agnosia** (loss of sensory comprehension, including facial recognition), are due to dysfunction of the temporal and parietal lobes.

3. Document any changes in personality and behavior.

Laboratory and Imaging Assessment
- The most sensitive diagnostic tool to detect biomarkers for the disease is amyloid positron emissions tomography (PET) imaging.
- A variety of laboratory or imaging tests are performed to rule out other treatable causes of dementia or delirium, such as electrolyte derangements, metabolic derangements (glucose), and stroke.

Analyze Cues and Prioritize Hypotheses: Analysis
- The priority collaborative problems for patients with AD include:
  1. Decreased memory and *cognition* due to neuronal changes in the brain
  2. Potential for injury or falls due to wandering or inability to ambulate independently
  3. Potential for elder abuse by caregivers due to the patient's prolonged progression of disability and the patient's increasing care needs
  4. Potential need for symptom management at end of life

Generate Solutions and Take Actions: Planning and Implementation
- The priority for interprofessional care is safety! Chronic confusion and physical deficits place the patient with AD at a high risk for injury, accidents, and elder abuse.

Managing Memory and Cognitive Dysfunction
- Collaborate with the health care team to provide a structured and consistent environment.
  1. Provide a safe environment with adequate lighting and remove items that can obstruct walking.

! NURSING SAFETY PRIORITY
Action Alert

When a patient with Alzheimer's disease is in a new setting or environment, collaborate with the staff and admitting department to select a room that is in the quietest area of the unit and away from obvious exits, if possible. A private room may be needed if the patient has a history of agitation or wandering. The television should remain off unless the patient turns it on or requests that it be turned on.

2. Implement fall precautions in the acute care setting.
3. Arrange the patient's schedule to provide as much uninterrupted sleep at night as possible. Fatigue increases confusion and behavioral problems such as agitation and aggression.
4. Establish a daily routine.
5. Place familiar objects, pictures, clocks, and single-date calendars in easy view of the patient.
6. Use orientation and validation therapy; acknowledge the patient's feelings and concerns.
7. Support the use of cognitive stimulation and memory training.
8. Collaborate with physical and occupational therapists to assist the patient to maintain independence in ADLs as long as possible through the use of assistive devices (grab bars in the bathroom) and exercise programs.
9. Attract the patient's attention before conversing; then use short, clear sentences.
10. Administer drug therapy as prescribed:
    - Cholinesterase inhibitors are approved for symptomatic treatment of AD.
    - Memantine is indicated for advanced AD and has been shown in some patients to slow the pace of deterioration (Burchum & Rosenthal, 2022).

Preventing Injuries or Falls

- The risk for injury can be related to falls, impaired mobility, wandering, or elder abuse.
  1. Ensure that the patient always wears an identification bracelet or badge that cannot be removed by the patient.
  2. Ensure that alarms or other barriers to outside doors are working properly at all times.
  3. Check on the patient often, and provide a variety of structured activities, such as walks, games, puzzles, music, or art, to manage restlessness.

Preventing Elder Abuse

- Teach family caregivers to be aware of their own health and stress levels.
  1. Signs of stress include:
     - Anger, social withdrawal, anxiety, depression, lack of concentration, sleepiness, irritability, and physical health problems.
  2. When signs of stress and strain occur, caregivers should be referred to their primary health care provider or should seek one independently.
- Encourage the family to maintain its own social network and to obtain respite care periodically.

- Assist the family to identify and develop strategies to cope with the long-term consequences of the disease, including recognition of the role of religion and spirituality in caregiving.
- Advise the family to seek legal counsel regarding the patient's competency and the need to obtain guardianship or durable power of attorney.
- Refer the family to a local support group affiliated with the Alzheimer's Association.

PATIENT AND FAMILY EDUCATION
Reducing Family/Informal Caregiver Stress

- Maintain realistic expectations for the person with Alzheimer's disease (AD).
- Try to find the positive aspects of each incident or situation.
- Use humor with the person who has AD.
- Use the resources of the Alzheimer's Association in the United States (or Alzheimer's Society of Canada), including attending local support group meetings and using the AD toll-free hotline when needed.
- Explore alternative care settings early in the disease process for possible use later.
- Establish an advance directive with the AD patient early in the disease process.
- Set aside time each day, if possible, for rest or recreation away from the patient.
- Seek respite care periodically for longer periods of time.
- Take care of yourself by watching your diet, exercising, and getting plenty of rest.
- Be realistic about what you or the patient with AD can do, and accept help from family, friends, and community resources.
- Use relaxation techniques, including meditation and massage.

Managing Symptoms at End of Life (EOL)
- As AD progresses, patients and families need assistance with advance care planning for each stage.
- Patients in the late stage usually require 24-hour total care.
- Assist families in EOL decisions that include hospice or palliative care.

Care Coordination and Transition Management
- When possible, the patient should be assigned to a case manager who can assess the patient's need for health care resources and facilitate appropriate placement throughout the continuum of care.

- The patient is usually cared for in the home until late in the disease process.

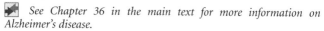 *See Chapter 36 in the main text for more information on Alzheimer's disease.*

✳ AMPUTATION: PERFUSION CONCEPT EXEMPLAR

Overview
- An **amputation** is the removal of a part of the body. Amputations may be elective or traumatic. Most are *elective* and are related to complications of peripheral arterial disease (PAD), which result in decreased *perfusion* to distal areas of the lower extremity. Traumatic amputations most often result from accidents or war.

👤 PATIENT-CENTERED CARE: VETERAN HEALTH
Traumatic Amputations

> The number of traumatic amputations has increased during recent wars as a result of improvised explosive devices (IEDs), bombs, and motor vehicle crashes (e.g., in Iraq and Afghanistan). Multiple limbs or parts of limbs are amputated as a result of these events. Thousands of veterans have multiple limb trauma and have had to adjust to major changes in their lifestyles. Many veterans have multiple amputations that affect *mobility* and ADL function. Additionally, many veteran amputees have comorbid physical and mental health problems, including traumatic brain injury (TBI) and posttraumatic stress disorder (PTSD) (Elliott et al., 2021).

Lower Extremity (LE) Amputation
- Loss of the great toe is significant because it affects balance, gait, and push-off ability during walking.
- Midfoot amputations (e.g., Syme amputation) remove most of the foot but retain the intact ankle so that weight bearing can be accomplished without the use of prosthesis and with reduced pain.
- Other lower extremity amputations are below-knee amputation (BKA), above-knee amputation (AKA), hip disarticulation, or removal of the hip joint, and hemipelvectomy (removal of half of the pelvis with the leg).
- The higher the level of amputation, the more energy is required for *mobility*.

Upper Extremity (UE) Amputation
- Rare and more incapacitating than amputations of lower extremities.

- Early replacement with a prosthetic device is vital for the patient with UE amputation.

Complications of Elective or Traumatic Amputation Include:

- Hemorrhage leading to hypovolemic shock
- Infection
- Phantom limb *pain*
- Neuroma
- Flexion contractures

Interprofessional Collaborative Care

Recognize Cues: Assessment

- Assess:
  1. Neurovascular status of extremity to be amputated
     - Examine skin color, temperature, sensation, capillary refill, and pulses.
     - Compare findings with those of the unaffected extremity.
     - Check and document the presence of discoloration, edema, ulcerations, hair distribution, and any necrosis.
  2. Psychosocial responses
     - Preparation for a planned amputation
     - Expectations of how the loss of a body part may affect employment, social relationships, and recreational activities
     - Current self-concept and self-image
     - Willingness and motivation to withstand prolonged rehabilitation after the amputation
  3. Patient and family coping abilities
  4. Patient's religious, spiritual, and cultural beliefs
  5. Diagnostic assessment may include:
     - Ankle brachial index (ABI). Normal ABI is 0.9 or higher.
       - ABI is calculated by dividing ankle systolic pressure by brachial systolic pressure.
     - Blood flow by Doppler ultrasonography or laser Doppler flowmetry or use of transcutaneous oxygen pressure ($TcPO_2$)

Analyze Cues and Prioritize Hypotheses: Analysis

- The collaborative problems for patients with amputations include:
  1. Potential for decreased tissue *perfusion* in residual limb due to soft tissue damage, edema, and/or bleeding
  2. Acute and/or persistent *pain* related to soft-tissue damage, muscle spasm, and edema
  3. Decreased *mobility* due to pain, muscle spasm, soft tissue damage, and/or lack of balance due to a missing body part
  4. Decreased self-esteem due to one or more ADL deficits, disturbed self-concept, and body image, and/or lack of support systems

Generate Solutions and Take Actions: Planning and Implementation

Monitoring for Decreased Tissue Perfusion

- Monitor for signs indicating that there is sufficient tissue perfusion:
  1. The skin at the end of the residual limb should be pink in a light-skinned person and not discolored in a dark-skinned patient, have a brisk capillary refill, and be warm.
  2. Perform neurovascular checks, including mobility, sensory perception, and assessment of the closest proximal pulse for strength and comparing it with that in the other extremity.

✚ NURSING SAFETY PRIORITY

Critical Rescue

If the patient has impaired perfusion, notify the surgeon or Rapid Response Team immediately to communicate your assessment findings! If the patient's BP drops and the pulse increases, suspect covert (hidden) bleeding and notify the surgeon. To check for the presence of overt (obvious) bleeding, be sure to lift the residual limb and feel under the pressure dressing for dampness or drainage. If bleeding occurs, apply direct pressure and notify the Rapid Response Team or primary health care provider immediately. Continue to monitor the patient until help arrives.

✚ NURSING SAFETY PRIORITY

Critical Rescue

For prehospital care with any traumatic amputation:
- Call 911.
- Assess the patient for airway or breathing problems.
- Apply direct pressure to amputation site with layers of dry gauze or other cloth.
- Elevate the extremity above the patient's heart to decrease the bleeding.
- Wrap the completely severed digit or limb in a dry, sterile gauze or clean cloth.
- Put the digit or limb in a watertight, sealed plastic bag.
- Place the bag in ice water—never directly on ice. Use one part ice and three parts water.
- Be sure that the amputated part goes with the patient to the hospital.

Managing Acute and/or Persistent Pain

- Pain management for surgical pain may start with opioids, then transition to nonsteroidal antiinflammatory drugs (NSAIDs).
- Phantom limb pain (PLP) is managed with calcitonin, beta-blocking agents, antiepileptic, and antispasmodic drugs.

> ### ! NURSING SAFETY PRIORITY
> #### *Action Alert*
>
> If the patient reports PLP, recognize that the ***pain*** is real and should be managed promptly and completely! It is *not* therapeutic to remind the patient that the limb cannot be hurting because it is missing. To prevent increased pain, handle the residual limb carefully when assessing the site or changing the dressing.

Promoting Mobility

- Coordinate with the physical and/or occupational therapists to begin exercises as soon as possible after surgery.
- For patients with above- or below-the-knee amputations, teach range-of-motion (ROM) exercises for prevention of flexion contractures, particularly of the hip and knee.
- Ensure that a trapeze and an overhead frame are used to aid in strengthening the upper extremities and in allowing the patient to move independently in bed.
- For above- and below-the-knee amputations, teach the patient how to push the residual limb down toward the bed while supporting it on a soft pillow at first.
- Follow primary health care provider and agency policy for elevation of a lower leg residual limb on a pillow while the patient is in a supine position.
- Coordinate with a certified prosthetist-orthotist (CPO) for appropriate postoperative planning.
- Instruct the patient being fitted for a leg prosthesis to bring a sturdy pair of shoes to the fitting.
- After surgery, apply the prescribed device, such as an air splint or elastic bandage, to shape and shrink the residual limb in preparation for the prosthesis. If elastic bandages are used, reapply the bandages in a figure-eight wrap every 4 to 6 hours or more often if they become loose.

Promoting Self-Esteem

- If possible, arrange for the patient to meet with a rehabilitated amputee who is about the same age.
- Assess the patient's verbal and nonverbal references to the affected area, and determine the patient's preference for terminology (e.g., *stump*).
- Ask the patient to describe personal feelings about any changes in body image and self-esteem.
- Check whether the patient looks at the area during a dressing change.
- Document behavior that indicates acceptance or nonacceptance of the amputation.

Care Coordination and Transition Management

- The patient is discharged directly to home or to a skilled facility or rehabilitation facility, depending on the extent of the amputation.
  1. Help the patient and family set realistic desired outcomes and take one day at a time.
  2. Teach the patient or family to care for the limb after it has healed by cleaning it each day with the rest of the body during bathing with soap and water.
  3. Teach the patient and family to inspect the limb every day for signs of inflammation or skin breakdown.
  4. Teach the patient and family about available resources and support from organizations such as the Amputee Coalition (www.amputee-coalition.org) and the Amputation Foundation (www.amputationfoundation.org).
  5. Refer to specialty veteran organizations and support groups if the individual has served in the armed forces.

Evaluate Outcomes: Evaluation

- Evaluate the care of the patient with one or more amputations based on the identified priority patient problems. The expected outcomes include that the patient will:
  1. Have adequate *perfusion* to the residual limb
  2. State that *pain* is controlled to between a 2 and 3 or as acceptable to the patient on a 0-10 pain intensity assessment scale
  3. Perform *mobility* skills independently and not experience complications of decreased mobility
  4. Have a positive self-esteem and lifestyle adaptation to live a productive, high-quality life

See Chapter 44 in the main text for more information on amputation.

AMYOTROPHIC LATERAL SCLEROSIS (ALS)

- Amyotrophic lateral sclerosis (ALS) is a chronic, neurological disease of unknown cause.
- ALS causes progressive muscle weakness and wasting, leading to paralysis of respiratory muscles.
- As the disease progresses, flaccid quadriplegia develops. Increased risk for pneumonia and respiratory failure result from paralysis of breathing muscles, including the diaphragm.
- Treatment is symptomatic, as there is no cure for ALS and the disease is 100% fatal. Treatment is directed toward the following: preventing complications of immobility, promoting comfort, providing ongoing support and counseling to the patient and

family, and informing the patient about the need for advance directives, such as a living will and durable power of attorney.
- The drug riluzole is associated with increased survival time, but there is no cure.

🐟 *See Chapter 37 in the main text for more information on amyotrophic lateral sclerosis.*

ANAPHYLAXIS

- Anaphylaxis is the most life-threatening example of a type I hypersensitivity reaction.
- It occurs rapidly and systemically, affecting many organs within seconds to minutes of allergen exposure.
- Drugs and dyes are common allergens in acute care settings, and food and insect bites/stings are common causes in community settings.
- Anaphylaxis episodes vary in severity and can be fatal. The major factor in fatal outcomes for anaphylaxis is a delay in the administration of epinephrine (Hayden, 2019).

Interprofessional Collaborative Care
Recognize Cues: Assessment
- Assessment findings include:
  1. History of anaphylactic response and documentation of allergen
  2. Subjective feelings of uneasiness, apprehension, weakness, and impending doom
  3. Generalized itching, urticaria (hives)
  4. Erythema/hyperpigmentation and angioedema (diffuse swelling) of the eyes, lips, or tongue
  5. Bronchoconstriction, mucosal edema, and excess mucous production
  6. Crackles, wheezing, and reduced breath sounds on auscultation
  7. Laryngeal edema (hoarseness and stridor)
  8. Respiratory failure with hypoxemia
  9. Rapid, weak, irregular pulse
  10. Dysrhythmias
  11. Increasing anxiety and confusion

➕ **NURSING SAFETY PRIORITY**

Critical Rescue

Closely monitor any patient receiving a drug that is associated with anaphylaxis to recognize symptoms early. If you suspect anaphylaxis, respond by immediately notifying the Rapid Response Team. Many deaths associated with anaphylaxis occur from dysrhythmias, shock, and cardiopulmonary arrest that are related to treatment delay.

Take Actions: Interventions

- Emergency respiratory management
    1. Immediately assess the respiratory status, airway, and oxygen saturation of patients who show any symptoms of an anaphylactic reaction.
    2. If the airway is compromised in any way, call the Rapid Response Team and establish or stabilize the airway.
    3. Immediately discontinue the IV drug or infusing solution of a patient having an anaphylactic reaction. Do not discontinue the IV, but change the IV tubing and hang normal saline.
    4. Anticipate the following:
        - Epinephrine is the first-line drug for anaphylaxis.
        - Place the patient in a recumbent position with legs and feet elevated.
        - Apply oxygen therapy using a high-flow, nonrebreather face mask at 90% to 100%.
        - If bronchospasm is present, administer albuterol via nebulizer or inhaler.
        - Corticosteroids are added to emergency interventions, but they are not effective immediately.
    5. Document all drugs administered, and observe patient responses to drugs.

 See Chapter 17 in the main text for more information on anaphylaxis.

ANEMIA

- Anemia is a reduction in the number of red blood cells (RBCs), the amount of hemoglobin, or the hematocrit (percentage of packed RBCs per deciliter of blood).
- Anemia is a clinical indicator, not a specific disease, and occurs with many health problems. The many causes of anemia include dietary problems, genetic disorders, bone marrow disease, or excessive bleeding. GI bleeding is a common reason for anemia in adults.
- For men a hemoglobin level of less than 14 g/dL (8.7 mmol/L) indicates anemia.
- For women a hemoglobin level of less than 12 g/dL (7.4 mmol/L) indicates anemia.

KEY FEATURES
Anemia

Skin Signs and Symptoms
- Cool to the touch
- Intolerance of cool temperatures
- Pallor/ash gray skin

Cardiovascular Signs and Symptoms
- Tachycardia

Respiratory Signs and Symptoms
- Breathless on exertion
- Decreased oxygen saturation levels

Gastrointestinal Signs and Symptoms
- Anorexia
- Diarrhea
- Glossitis
- Nausea
- Weight loss

Neurologic Signs and Symptoms
- Fatigue
- Numbness in hands and feet
- Reduced energy levels

Types of Anemia

- *Iron-deficiency anemia*— can occur from a diet inadequate in iron intake, poor absorption of iron in the GI tract, and blood loss. The most common type of anemia.
  1. Management: Increase the oral intake of iron from food sources (e.g., red meat, organ meat, egg yolks, kidney beans, leafy green vegetables, and raisins). If iron losses are mild, oral iron supplements are started until the hemoglobin level returns to normal.
- *Vitamin B_{12} deficiency*—also known as cobalamin deficiency. Risks include vegan diets or other diets lacking proteins, small bowel resection, chronic diarrhea, diverticula, tapeworm, or overgrowth of intestinal bacteria.
  1. Management: Teach patients to increase their intake of foods rich in vitamin B_{12} (animal proteins, fish, eggs, nuts, dairy products, dried beans, citrus fruit, and leafy green vegetables). Vitamin supplements may be prescribed when anemia is severe.

- *Pernicious anemia*—results from failure to absorb vitamin B_{12}. It is caused by a deficiency of **intrinsic factor** (a substance normally secreted by the gastric mucosa), which is needed for the intestinal absorption of vitamin B_{12}. Pernicious anemia is a type of autoimmune disorder.
  1. Management: Patients are given vitamin B_{12} injections weekly at first and then monthly for the rest of their lives. Oral B_{12} preparations and nasal spray or sublingual cobalamin preparations may be used to maintain vitamin levels after the patient's deficiency has first been corrected by the traditional injection method.
- *Folate (folic acid) deficiency*—results from poor diet intake (especially a diet lacking green leafy vegetables and citrus fruits, beans, and nuts) or malabsorption syndromes and some drugs, including anticonvulsants and oral contraceptives.
  1. Management: Prevention is the best strategy. A diet rich in foods containing folic acid, as well as scheduled folic acid replacement therapy, can be used.

PATIENT-CENTERED CARE: OLDER ADULT HEALTH

Risk for Anemia

Older patients may have poor diets or chewing difficulties that place them at risk for anemias that result from vitamin B_{12} deficiency. Ask about a family history of anemia. B_{12} deficiency anemia often occurs in older adults due to a decrease in gastric secretions and intrinsic factor (Touhy & Jett, 2023). Because symptoms are vague, the disorder can easily be overlooked.

- *Aplastic anemia*—a deficiency of circulating red blood cells (RBCs) because of impaired **cellular regulation** of the bone marrow, which then fails to produce these cells. Often caused by long-term exposure to toxic agents, drugs, ionizing radiation, or infection, but many times the cause is unknown. The disease also may follow a viral infection. The most common hereditary form of the disease is Fanconi's anemia.
  1. Management: Varies based on cause. Short-term management may include blood transfusions along with discontinuing the responsible drug. Immunosuppressive therapy may be used if the disease course is similar to that of an autoimmune problem.
- *Glucose-6-phosphate dehydrogenase (G6PD) deficiency,* an X-linked recessive deficiency of an enzyme needed for RBC glucose metabolism

A

1. Management: Prevention is the most important strategy. Patients who belong to the high-risk groups, especially men, should be tested for this problem before receiving drugs that can cause the hemolytic reaction.
- *Acquired autoimmune hemolytic anemia* occurs when antibodies attack and destroy one's own RBCs, including warm and cold antibody anemias.
  1. Management: Steroid therapy to suppress *immunity* is temporarily effective in many patients. Rituximab is the first-line therapy for steroid-refractory warm autoimmune hemolytic anemia (wAIHA), and as first- and second-line treatment for cold agglutinin disease (Murakhovskaya, 2020). Splenectomy may be considered if steroid therapy fails.

See Chapter 34 in the main text for more information on anemia.

ANEURYSMS OF THE CENTRAL ARTERIES

- An aneurysm is a permanent, localized dilation of an artery that enlarges the artery to at least two times its normal diameter.
  1. It can be *fusiform,* affecting the entire circumference of the artery; or *saccular,* affecting only a portion of the artery as an outpouching.
  2. *True* aneurysms are those caused by weakened medial arterial layers (stretching of the inner and outer layers) from acquired or congenital problems, while *false* aneurysms result from vessel injury or trauma to all three arterial layers.
  3. *Dissecting aneurysms* differ from aneurysms in that they are formed when blood accumulates in the wall of an artery.
- Aneurysms can cause symptoms by exerting pressure on surrounding structures or by rupturing. Rupture is the most frequent complication and is life-threatening because abrupt and massive hemorrhagic shock results.
- Atherosclerosis is the most common cause of aneurysms, with hypertension, hyperlipidemia, and cigarette smoking being contributing factors. Age, gender, genetics, or family history also may play a role (Rogers, 2023)

Interprofessional Collaborative Care
Recognize Cues: Assessment
- Most patients with abdominal or thoracic aneurysms are asymptomatic.

- Signs and symptoms of abdominal aortic aneurysms:
  1. Abdominal, flank, or back pain that is usually steady, with a gnawing quality, is unaffected by movement, and may last for hours or days
  2. Prominent pulsation in the upper abdomen (Do not palpate)
  3. Abdominal or femoral bruit (Auscultate for bruit. Do NOT palpate as there is a risk for rupture!)

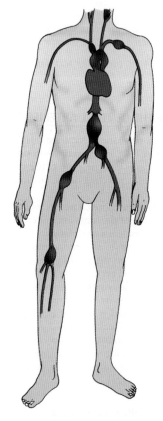

Common anatomic sites of arterial aneurysms.

- Signs and symptoms of thoracic aneurysms:
  1. Back pain
  2. Shortness of breath
  3. Hoarseness
  4. Difficulty swallowing
- Assess for abdominal or thoracic aortic rupture:
  1. Pain that is described as tearing, ripping, and stabbing and located in the chest, back, and abdomen
  2. Symptoms of hypovolemic hemorrhagic shock: hypotension, tachycardia, diaphoresis, absent or faint peripheral pulses, and decreased mentation
  3. Nausea, vomiting, and apprehension

Take Actions: Interventions
- Patients with hypertension are treated with antihypertensive drugs to decrease the rate of enlargement and the risk for early rupture.
- Teach the patient the importance of keeping scheduled appointments to monitor the size of the aneurysm with ultrasound or CT.
- Review with the patient the signs and symptoms of aneurysms that need to be reported promptly.

Surgical Management
- The repair of the abdominal aortic aneurysm with endovascular stent grafts is the procedure of choice for almost all patients on an elective or emergent basis. Stents are inserted percutaneously (through the skin), avoiding abdominal incisions, and therefore decreasing the risk for a prolonged postoperative recovery. Postoperative care is similar to care required after an arteriogram (angiogram). Complications of stent repair include:
  1. Conversion to open surgical repair
  2. Bleeding
  3. Aneurysm rupture
  4. Peripheral embolization
  5. Misplacement of the stent graft
  6. Endoleak
  7. Infection
- Surgical removal of the aneurysm is used when the aneurysm ruptures or when endovascular graft placement is not possible. The excised portion of the aorta is replaced with a graft.

> **! NURSING SAFETY PRIORITY**
>
> *Action Alert*
>
> Teach patients receiving treatment for hypertension about the importance of continuing to take prescribed drugs. Instruct them about the signs and symptoms that must promptly be reported to the primary health care provider, which include:
> * Abdominal fullness or pain
> * Chest or back pain
> * Shortness of breath
> * Difficulty swallowing or hoarseness

ANEURYSMS OF THE PERIPHERAL ARTERIES

* An aneurysm is a permanent, localized dilation of an artery that enlarges the artery to at least two times its normal diameter. Refer to *Aneurysms of Central Arteries.*
* While uncommon, the typical peripheral arterial aneurysm is at the femoral or popliteal artery.
* Monitor patients for lower limb ischemia, such as a decreased pulse, cool skin, and pain.
* These aneurysms are managed with vascular surgery, using a synthetic graft or autogenous saphenous vein graft repair (bypass).
* Report the sudden development of pain or discoloration of the extremity immediately to the surgeon. It may indicate thrombo-embolism preprocedure or graft occlusion postprocedure!

See Chapter 30 in the main text for more information on aneurysms in the central and peripheral arteries.

ANGIOEDEMA

* Angioedema is a severe type I hypersensitivity reaction that involves the blood vessels and all layers of the skin, mucous membranes, and subcutaneous tissues in the affected area (Abbas et al., 2022).
* It is most often seen in the lips, face, tongue, larynx, and neck.
* Exposure to any ingested drug or chemical can cause the problem. The most common drugs associated with angioedema are angiotensin-converting enzyme inhibitors (ACEIs) and NSAIDs, including aspirin (Simon, 2022).

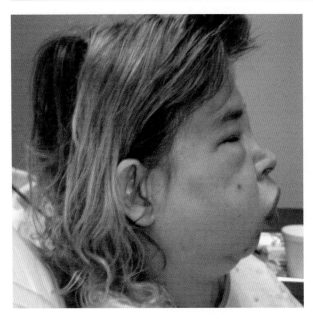

A

Angioedema of the face, lips, and mouth.

Interprofessional Collaborative Care
Recognize Cues: Assessment

- Ask the patient for a list of all drugs taken on a regular basis, especially drugs for BP control. Although it would be helpful to have more information, intervention is critically important because laryngeal edema can cause patients to lose their airway.
- Airway and breathing
    1. Problems that indicate a need for immediate intervention are the inability to swallow, the feeling of a lump in the throat, or stridor.
    2. Anticipate that the patient will be anxious, particularly if the patient is hypoxic.
- Other signs and symptoms
    1. The patient with angioedema (with or without laryngeal edema) has deep, firm swelling of the face, lips, tongue, and

neck. The patient may have difficulty speaking or drinking because the lips are so stiff from swelling. The face can be so distorted that friends and relatives may not recognize the patient. Often nasal swelling interferes with breathing through the nose.

Take Actions: Interventions
- Interventions focus on stopping the reaction and ensuring an adequate airway. Prompt intervention can reverse angioedema before laryngeal edema forms and intubation is needed.
  1. Administer oxygen to maintain gas exchange.
  2. Establish intravenous access, and administer drugs as prescribed to interfere with the immune and inflammatory response, including corticosteroids and epinephrine.
  3. Severe angioedema of the face or mouth is an acute emergency. If laryngeal edema forms and intubation is not possible, an emergency tracheostomy is needed.
  4. Stay with the patient and reassure that proper treatment is occurring.
  5. With successful management, the patient is discharged to resume usual activities.
  6. Determine the cause of the angioedema, and teach the patient to avoid the offending agent.

See Chapter 17 in the main text for more information on angioedema.

APPENDICITIS
- Appendicitis is an acute *inflammation* of the vermiform appendix that occurs most often among young adults.
- Inflammation of the appendix occurs when the lumen of the appendix is obstructed.
- Inflammation leads to *infection* as bacteria invade the wall of the appendix.

Interprofessional Collaborative Care
Recognize Cues: Assessment
- Assessment findings include:
  1. Abdominal pain in the right lower quadrant (McBurney's point), although pain can be anywhere in the abdomen or flank

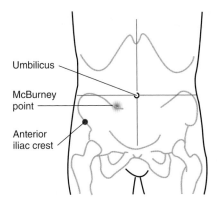

Umbilicus

McBurney point

Anterior iliac crest

McBurney's point is located midway between the anterior iliac crest and the umbilicus in the right lower quadrant. This is the classic area for localized tenderness during the later stages of appendicitis.

2. Abdominal pain that increases with cough or movement and is relieved by flexion of the right hip or knees suggests a perforated appendix with peritonitis.
3. Nausea and vomiting
4. Abdominal muscle rigidity or rebound tenderness may indicate perforation and peritonitis.
5. Increased WBC count with neutrophilia; increased segmented neutrophils
6. Ultrasound or CT scan showing an enlarged appendix

Take Actions: Interventions
• All patients with suspected or confirmed appendicitis are hospitalized, and most have surgery to remove the inflamed appendix.
1. Provide routine preoperative care; keep the patient NPO to prepare for the probability of surgery and avoid making the *inflammation* worse.
2. An appendectomy may be performed as a traditional procedure through external skin incision (laparoscopy or open procedure).
3. Provide routine postoperative care with an anticipated length of stay of less than 24 hours for uncomplicated procedures and 3 to 5 days when perforation or peritonitis is present.
4. Administer analgesics and antibiotics as prescribed to patients with a complicated appendicitis presentation and surgery.

> ## ❗ NURSING SAFETY PRIORITY
> ### *Action Alert*
>
> For the patient with suspected appendicitis, administer IV fluids as pre-scribed to maintain *fluid and electrolyte balance* and replace fluid vol-ume. If tolerated, advise the patient to maintain a semi-Fowler's position so that abdominal drainage can be contained in the lower abdomen. Once the diagnosis of appendicitis is confirmed and surgery is scheduled, administer opioid analgesics and antibiotics as prescribed. *The patient with suspected or confirmed appendicitis should not receive laxatives or enemas, which can cause perforation of the appendix. Do not apply heat to the abdomen be-cause this may increase circulation to the appendix and result in increased* **inflammation** *and perforation!*

 See Chapter 49 in the main text for more information on appen-dicitis.

ARTERIOSCLEROSIS AND ATHEROSCLEROSIS

- Arteriosclerosis is a thickening or hardening of the arterial wall often associated with aging.
- Atherosclerosis, a type of arteriosclerosis, involves the formation of a plaque within the arterial wall and is the leading cardiovas-cular disease.
- The exact pathophysiologic mechanism of atherosclerosis is unknown but is thought to occur with inflammation of the vessel.
- After the vessel becomes inflamed, a fatty streak appears on the intimal surface of an artery and, over time, develops into a fibrous plaque that obstructs the blood flow of the artery.
- When plaque ruptures, the exposed underlying tissue causes platelet adhesion and rapid thrombus formation. The thrombus may suddenly block a blood vessel, resulting in ischemia and in-farction (e.g., MI, ischemic stroke, arterial occlusion).
- The rate of progression of plaque formation and rupture is thought to be influenced by genetic factors, diabetes and other chronic conditions, and lifestyle (e.g., smoking, dietary intake of fat, sedentary habits).

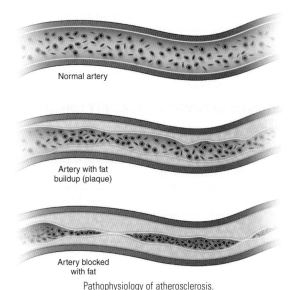

Normal artery

Artery with fat
buildup (plaque)

Artery blocked
with fat

Pathophysiology of atherosclerosis.

Interprofessional Collaborative Care
Recognize Cues: Assessment
- Assess:
  1. Risk for cardiovascular disease, using history and standard tools
  2. BP in both arms, and note any differences
  3. Pulses at all major sites, and note any bruits and diminishment or absence
  4. Presence of prolonged capillary refill or cool extremities
  5. Serum cholesterol (total, low-density lipoprotein [LDL], protective high-density lipoprotein [HDL]) and triglyceride levels

Take Actions: Interventions
- Interventions include:
  1. Teaching the patient to adopt dietary habits to reduce risk, including limiting saturated fat to 5% to 6% of calories and emphasizing the intake of vegetables, fruit, and whole grains. DASH or Mediterranean diets are examples of guideline diets.
  2. Developing and reinforcing the plan for regular activity, with at least 40 minutes three to four times weekly that is moderate to vigorous (Grundy et al., 2018)
  3. Administering drug therapy as prescribed:
     - Cholesterol-lowering drugs, usually a statin

4. Using best practices to assist patients to stop smoking and informing nonsmokers to avoid secondhand smoke
5. Planning for follow-up and ongoing care with primary care provider at least annually

 See Chapter 30 in the main text for more information on arteriosclerosis and atherosclerosis.

ARTHRITIS, RHEUMATOID: IMMUNITY CONCEPT EXEMPLAR

Overview
- Rheumatoid arthritis (RA) is a chronic, progressive, systemic inflammatory autoimmune disease process that affects primarily the synovial joints. *Systemic* means that this disease can affect any or all parts of the body while affecting many joints.
- Onset may be acute and severe or slow and insidious, and the pattern of illness progression includes remissions and exacerbations.
- Permanent joint changes may be avoided or mitigated when RA is diagnosed early. Early aggressive treatment to suppress synovitis may lead to a remission.

Interprofessional Collaborative Care
Recognize Cues: Assessment
- Assess for disease signs and symptoms. See Key Features: Rheumatoid Arthritis.

KEY FEATURES
Rheumatoid Arthritis

Early Signs and Symptoms (Early Disease)	Late Signs and Symptoms (Advanced Disease)
Joint • **Inflammation**	**Joint** • Deformities (e.g., swan neck or ulnar deviation) • Moderate to severe **pain** and morning stiffness
Systemic • Low-grade fever • Fatigue • Weakness • Anorexia • Paresthesias	**Systemic** • Osteoporosis • Severe fatigue • Anemia • Weight loss • Subcutaneous nodules • Peripheral neuropathy • Vasculitis • Pericarditis • Fibrotic lung disease • Sjögren syndrome • Kidney disease

✚ NURSING SAFETY PRIORITY

Critical Rescue

Cervical RA may result in subluxation (partial joint dislocation), especially of the first and second vertebrae. This complication may be life-threatening because branches of the phrenic nerve that supply the diaphragm are restricted, and respiratory function may be compromised. The patient is also in danger of becoming quadriparetic (weak in all extremities) or quadriplegic (paralyzed in all extremities). If cervical pain (may radiate down one arm) or loss of range of motion is present in the cervical spine, keep the neck straight in a neutral position to prevent permanent damage to the spinal cord or spinal nerves. *Notify the Rapid Response Team and primary health care provider immediately about these neurologic changes!*

- Assess for psychosocial issues.
  1. Fear of becoming disabled and dependent, uncertainty about the disease process, altered body image, devaluation of self, frustration, and depression are common.
  2. Body changes may cause poor self-esteem and body image.
  3. The patient may grieve, experience degrees of depression, or have feelings of helplessness caused by a loss of control over a disease that can "consume" the body.
- Assess laboratory data.
  1. Laboratory tests help support a diagnosis of RA, but no single test or group of tests can confirm the diagnosis.
  2. *Anticyclic citrullinated peptide (anti-CCP)* is a very specific and sensitive laboratory test used in detecting early RA. The presence of anti-CCP is also a marker for aggressive and erosive late-stage disease.
- Other diagnostic assessments
  1. Joint x-rays
  2. Bone scan or joint scan
  3. Arthrocentesis is a procedure to aspirate a sample of the synovial fluid to relieve pressure and analyze the fluid for inflammatory cells and immune complexes,

Analyze Cues and Prioritize Hypotheses: Analysis
- The priority collaborative problems for patients with RA include:
  1. Chronic *inflammation* and *pain* due to systemic autoimmune disease process
  2. Potential for decreased *mobility* related to joint deformity, muscle atrophy, and fatigue
  3. Potential for decreased self-esteem image related to joint deformity

Generate Solutions and Take Actions: Planning and Implementation

- Patients who have RA are managed in the community under the supervision of a qualified primary health care provider. The goal of management is that the disease goes into remission and its progression slows to decrease pain, prevent joint destruction, and increase mobility. When patients with RA are admitted to the inpatient acute care or long-term care facility, it is usually for health problems other than for complications of arthritis.

Managing Chronic Inflammation and Pain

- The removal of inflamed synovium, or *synovectomy*, may be needed for joints such as the knee or elbow.
- Total joint arthroplasty (TJA) may be indicated when other measures fail to relieve pain.
- Drug therapy used to treat RA:
  1. *NSAIDs* are sometimes used for RA to help promote comfort and decrease inflammation.
  2. First-line disease-modifying antirheumatic drugs *(DMARDs)* are used to slow the progression of RA:
     - Methotrexate (MTX), an immunosuppressive medication, in a low, once-a-week dose is the mainstay of therapy for RA because it is effective and relatively inexpensive.
     - Hydroxychloroquine
  3. Biological response modifiers (BRMs), sometimes called biologics, are one of the newest and most effective classes of DMARDs.
     - Common examples include etanercept and infliximab.
     - Do not give BRMs if the patient has a serious infection, TB, or MS because BRMs may exacerbate these health problems.
     - Teach patients to avoid crowds and people with infections because serious infections, especially respiratory infections, can lead to hospitalization or cause death.
  4. Janus kinase (JAK) inhibitors are the newest class of DMARDs.
     - Examples include tofacitinib and baricitinib.
  5. Glucocorticoids (steroids)—usually prednisone—are given for their fast-acting antiinflammatory and immunosuppressive effects.

Nonpharmacologic Management

- Nonpharmacologic pain-relief measures include rest, positioning, ice, and heat
- Plasmapheresis (or plasma exchange) to remove the antibodies causing the disease
- Complementary and integrative health measures to relieve pain, such as hypnosis, acupuncture, magnet therapy, imagery, or music therapy

- Stress management to reduce pain perception
- Nutrition to meet caloric and protein goals

Promoting Mobility
- Identify assistive devices to allow the patient as much independence as possible.
- Teach the patient to use larger muscle groups to perform tasks usually performed by fine muscle groups (e.g., use the flat of the hand to squeeze toothpaste tubes instead of the fingers).
- Refer the patient to an occupational or physical therapist or the Arthritis Foundation for special assistive and adaptive devices.
- Collaborate with the health care team to alleviate or manage factors that contribute to fatigue and immobility:
  1. Anemia
     - Administer iron, folic acid, vitamin supplements, or a combination of these.
     - Assess the patient for drug-related GI bleeding, such as that caused by NSAID therapy, by testing the stool for occult blood.
  2. Muscle atrophy
     - Collaborate with a physical therapist to develop and help the patient implement a personalized daily exercise program.
     - Encourage the patient to maintain independence in ADLs, and set priorities in the care and assistance the patient needs.
  3. Inadequate rest
     - Arrange for a quiet environment.
     - Encourage the patient to develop a bedtime routine for sleep hygiene, such as drinking a warm beverage before bedtime.
- Teach principles of energy conservation.
  1. Pacing activities
  2. Setting priorities
  3. Planning rest periods

Enhancing Self-Esteem
- Identify factors to enhance self-esteem when dysfunction or joint deformity occurs.
- Determine the patient's perception of role and social changes, and identify sources of support for role changes and to avoid isolation.
- Communicate acceptance of the patient; establish a trusting relationship.

Care Coordination and Transition Management

- Remind patients to avoid crowds and other possible sources of infection when they are taking drugs that decrease immunity.
- Assist the patient and family to identify structural changes needed in the home before discharge.
- Instruct patients with arthritic pain to use multiple modalities for pain relief, including ice/heat, rest, positioning, complementary and alternative therapies, and medications as prescribed.
- Teach the patient to consult with the primary health care provider before trying any over-the-counter (OTC) or home remedies.
- Teach joint protection measures related to splinting, positioning, and function.
- Review the prescribed exercise program.
- Encourage patients with arthritis and connective tissue diseases to discuss their chronic illness and to identify coping strategies that have previously been successful.
- Refer the patient to a nutritionist, counselor, home health nurse, rehabilitation therapist, financial counselor, and local and state support groups as needed.

See Chapter 43 in the main text for more information on arthritis, rheumatoid.

ASTHMA

- One of the most common lower respiratory disorders that reduces *gas exchange* is asthma, which can lead to severe lower airway obstruction and death. **Asthma** is a chronic disease in which reversible airway obstruction occurs intermittently, reducing airflow.
  1. Airway obstruction occurs in two ways:
     - Inflammation: obstructs the airway lumens (or the hollow insides)
     - Airway tissue sensitivity (hyperresponsiveness): obstructs airways by constricting bronchial smooth muscle and causing a narrowing of the airway from the outside. It can occur with exercise, an upper respiratory illness, or for unknown reasons.
  2. Airway inflammation and sensitivity can trigger bronchiolar constriction, and many adults with asthma have both problems (Rogers, 2023).
  3. Although asthma may be classified into different types based on the events known to trigger the attacks, the effect on **gas exchange** is the same.
  4. Asthma can occur at any age. About half of adults with asthma also had the disease in childhood.

Interprofessional Collaborative Care

Recognize Cues: Assessment

- Obtain the patient's personal history.
  1. Episodes of dyspnea, chest tightness, coughing, wheezing, and increased mucous production
  2. Specific patterns of dyspnea appearance (at night, with exercise, seasonally, or in association with other specific activities or environments)
  3. Other allergic symptoms, such as rhinitis, skin rash, or pruritus, and whether other family members have asthma or respiratory problems
- Signs and symptoms during an attack include:
  1. Audible wheeze (at first, louder on exhalation)
  2. Increased respiratory rate
  3. Coughing
  4. Inability to complete a sentence of more than five words
  5. Decreased oxygen saturation
  6. Pallor or cyanosis of oral mucous membranes and nail beds
  7. Tachycardia
  8. Changes in level of consciousness
  9. Use of accessory muscles (muscle retraction at the sternum, the suprasternal notch, and between the ribs)
- Physical changes from frequent asthma attacks include:
  1. Increased anteroposterior (AP) chest diameter; occurs with chronic asthma
  2. Increased space between the ribs
- Laboratory assessment data changes during an asthma attack:
  1. Decreased Pao_2
  2. Decreased $Paco_2$ (early in attack)
  3. Elevated $Paco_2$ (later in attack)
- Laboratory assessment data changes from allergic asthma:
  1. Elevated serum eosinophil count
  2. Elevated immunoglobulin E (IgE) levels
  3. Sputum-containing eosinophils, mucous plugs, and shed epithelial cells (Curschmann spirals)
- Diagnostic assessment:
  1. Pulmonary function tests (PFTs) measured using spirometry, especially:
     - Forced vital capacity (FVC) (volume of air exhaled from full inhalation to full exhalation)
     - Forced expiratory volume in the first second (FEV_1) (volume of air blown out as hard and fast as possible during the first second of the most forceful exhalation after the greatest full inhalation)

- Peak expiratory flow (PEF) (fastest airflow rate reached at any time during exhalation)
2. Chest x-ray

Take Actions: Interventions
- The goals of asthma therapy are to improve airflow and *gas exchange*, relieve symptoms, and prevent episodes by making the patient an active partner in the management plan.
  1. Teach the patient to keep a symptom and intervention diary to learn triggers of asthma symptoms, early cues for impending attacks, and personal response to drugs.
  2. Stress the importance of proper use of the asthma action plan for any severity of asthma.
  3. Drug therapy focuses on the prevention of asthma attacks (control therapy) and on stopping attacks that have already started (with reliever or rescue drugs).
     - Bronchodilators cause bronchiolar smooth muscle relaxation and include beta$_2$ agonists, cholinergic antagonists, and methylxanthines.
     - Short-acting bronchodilators provide rapid but short-term relief. They are most useful when administered as an asthma attack begins. One example is albuterol.
     - Long-acting beta$_2$ agonists (LABAs) are delivered by inhaler directly to the site of action, the bronchioles. They need time to build up an effect, but the effects are longer lasting. Examples include formoterol and salmeterol. These drugs can prevent an attack but cannot stop an acute attack.

 NURSING SAFETY PRIORITY
Drug Alert

LABAs should never be prescribed as the *only* drug therapy for asthma and are not to be used during an acute asthma attack or bronchospasm. Teach the patient to use these control drugs daily as prescribed, even when no symptoms are present, and to use a SABA to relieve acute symptoms. Any patient using these drugs must be monitored closely.

- Cholinergic antagonists (anticholinergic drugs) are similar to atropine and block the parasympathetic nervous system, causing bronchodilation and decreased pulmonary secretions. Most are used by inhaler. A common example is ipratropium.

- Xanthines are rarely used and only when other types of management are ineffective.
- Antiinflammatory agents decrease airway inflammation. The inhaled forms have fewer systemic side effects than those taken systemically. *All of the antiinflammatory drugs, whether inhaled or taken orally, are controller drugs only.*
- Corticosteroids: inhaled corticosteroids (ICSs) can be helpful in controlling asthma symptoms. Common examples include fluticasone and budesonide.
- Cromolyns: inhalation agents that are useful as *controller* asthma therapy when taken on a scheduled basis. A common example is cromolyn sodium.
- Leukotriene modifiers: oral drugs that work in several ways to control asthma when taken on a scheduled basis. A common example is montelukast.
- Monoclonal antibodies: newer drugs specifically for the management of eosinophilic asthma. Examples include benralizumab, mepolizumab, and reslizumab.

✚ NURSING SAFETY PRIORITY
Critical Rescue

Teach patients to always carry the rescue short-acting beta agonist drug inhaler with them and to ensure that there is enough drug remaining in the inhaler to provide a quick dose when needed.

---

4. Regular exercise, including aerobic exercise, is a recommended part of asthma therapy.
    - Teach patients to examine the conditions that trigger an attack and adjust the exercise routine as needed.
    - Some patients may need to premedicate with inhaled SABAs before beginning activity.
5. Supplemental oxygen by mask or cannula is often used during an acute asthma attack.
6. *Status asthmaticus* is a severe, life-threatening acute episode of airway obstruction that intensifies once it begins and often does not respond to usual therapy.
    - Assess for signs and symptoms, including:
        - Extremely labored breathing and wheezing
        - Use of accessory muscles
        - Distention of neck veins

- Immediate interventions include:
  - IV fluids
  - Systemic bronchodilators, steroids, epinephrine, and oxygen are given immediately to reverse the condition.
- Prepare for emergency intubation. Sudden absence of wheezing can indicate a complete airway obstruction and may require a tracheotomy.

 See Chapter 24 in the main text for more information on asthma.

✳ ATRIAL FIBRILLATION: PERFUSION CONCEPT EXEMPLAR

Overview
- **Atrial fibrillation (AF)** is the most common dysrhythmia seen in clinical practice. In patients with AF, multiple rapid impulses from many atrial foci depolarize the atria in a totally disorganized manner at a rate of 350 to 600 times per minute; ventricular response is usually 120 to 200 beats/min. The result is a chaotic rhythm with no clear P waves, no atrial contractions, loss of atrial kick, and an irregular ventricular response. The atria merely quiver in fibrillation (commonly called *A fib*).

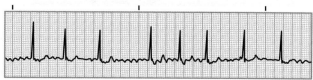

Atrial fibrillation. Note wavy baseline with atrial electrical activity and irregular ventricular rhythm.

Interprofessional Collaborative Care
Recognize Cues: Assessment
- Determine history of cardiovascular disease, such as hypertension, heart failure, or acute coronary syndrome.
- Determine characteristics of the heart rate and rhythm.
- Assess for signs of poor perfusion:
  1. Fatigue or weakness
  2. Shortness of breath
  3. Dizziness
  4. Anxiety
  5. Syncope
  6. Palpitations
  7. Chest *pain*
  8. Hypotension
- Definitive diagnosis occurs with a 12-lead ECG.

Analyze Cues and Prioritize Hypotheses: Analysis

- The priority collaborative problems for most patients with atrial fibrillation are:
  1. Potential for embolus formation due to irregular cardiac rhythm
  2. Potential for heart failure due to altered conduction pattern

Generate Solutions and Take Actions: Planning and Implementation

- Interventions for AF depend on the severity of the problem and the patient's response. Be sure to individualize care based on the patient's values and preferences, your clinical expertise, and best current evidence.

Preventing Embolus Formation

- The purpose of collaborative care is to restore regular blood flow through the atrium when possible. Correcting the rhythm and controlling the rate of the rhythm restore blood flow, which helps prevent embolus formation and increases cardiac output.

❗ NURSING SAFETY PRIORITY

Action Alert

The loss of coordinated atrial contractions in AF can lead to pooling of blood, resulting in ***clotting***. *The patient is at high risk for pulmonary embolism!* Thrombi may form within the right atrium and then move through the right ventricle to the lungs. If pulmonary embolism is suspected, remain with the patient and monitor for shortness of breath, chest pain, and/or hypotension. Initiate the Rapid Response Team and notify the provider.

In addition, the patient is at risk for systemic emboli, particularly an embolic stroke, which may cause severe neurologic impairment or death. Monitor patients carefully for signs of stroke. Initiate the Rapid Response team if stroke is suspected to facilitate a timely diagnosis.

Patients with AF who have valvular disease are particularly at risk for venous thromboembolism (VTE). In VTE, the patient may report lower extremity pain and swelling. Anticipate ultrasound of vasculature and initiation of systemic anticoagulation.

- Administer drugs as prescribed to slow conduction:
  1. Calcium channel blockers such as diltiazem
  2. Amiodarone
  3. Dronedarone: better tolerated than amiodarone, yet should be avoided in patients with heart failure because it can cause an exacerbation of cardiac symptoms; with permanent AF,

it increases the risk of stroke, myocardial infarction or cardio-vascular death

4. Beta blockers, such as metoprolol and esmolol
5. Digoxin for patients with heart failure and AF

- Administer drugs as prescribed to control rhythm, such as:
  1. Flecainide
  2. Dofetilide
  3. Propafenone
  4. Ibutilide
- Anticipate continuous cardiac monitoring and frequent 12-lead ECGs with new-onset AF.
- Administer prescribed anticoagulation therapy:
  1. Warfarin
  2. Direct oral anticoagulants (DOACs), such as dabigatran, riva-roxaban, apixaban, or edoxaban, may be given on a long-term basis to prevent strokes associated with nonvalvular AF. Be-cause these drugs achieve a steady state, there is no need for laboratory test monitoring.

PATIENT-CENTERED CARE: HEALTH EQUITY

Anticoagulation Therapy

Atrial fibrillation is the most common arrhythmia in the United States and is associated with an increased risk of stroke. The key to decreasing the stroke risk is the use of long-term anticoagulant therapy. Evidence indicates clear racial and ethnic disparities exist regarding the use of anticoagulants. Black patients are significantly less likely to receive direct oral anticoagulants (DOACs) (Essien et al., 2018).

This data indicates that disparities exist regarding the use of anticoagu-lants due to access to care. A novel approach is needed to eliminate barriers associated with anticoagulation therapy, as well as the need to facilitate equitable initiation of anticoagulation (Essien & Litam, 2021). It is important for the nurse to teach all patients about the importance of prescribed anti-coagulation, as well as to ensure access to medications upon discharge.

- Monitor for bleeding with anticoagulation therapy.
  1. Warfarin is monitored with international normalized ratio (INR) to achieve a goal of two to three times normal; these values increase bleeding risk.
  2. DOACs do not require serum monitoring. Idarucizumab is the reversal agent for dabigatran and andexanet alfa is approved for the reversal of rivaroxaban and apixaban

(Garcia & Crowther, 2022). Reversal agents are used only in the event of life-threatening bleeding.

 See Chapter 30 in the main text for more on patients receiving anticoagulant therapy.

🔒 NURSING SAFETY PRIORITY
Drug Alert

Teach patients taking any type of anticoagulant drug to report bruising, bleeding nose or gums, or other signs of bleeding to their primary health care provider immediately.

Preventing Heart Failure
- Promote cardiac output by restoration of normal conduction or by achieving a ventricular rate of 60 to 90 beats per minute.
  1. Nonsurgical interventions
     - Antidysrhythmic drugs described earlier
     - Electrical cardioversion: a *synchronized* countershock that may be performed to restore normal conduction in a hospitalized patient with *new-onset* AF.
     - Left atrial appendage closure to reduce the area for clot formation and subsequent emboli when the patient is not able to safely take anticoagulants
     - Radiofrequency catheter ablation (RCA), an invasive procedure that may be used to destroy an irritable focus in atrial or ventricular conduction
     - Biventricular pacemaker/defibrillator placement
  2. Surgical interventions
     - Surgical maze procedure: an open-chest surgical technique often performed with coronary artery bypass grafting (CABG). The surgical MAZE procedure is being replaced by catheter procedures using a minimally invasive form.
     - The *catheter* maze procedure is done by inserting a catheter through a leg vein into the atria and dragging a heated ablating catheter along the atria to create lines (scars) of conduction block. Patients having this minimally invasive form of the procedure have fewer complications, less pain, and a quicker recovery than those with the open surgical maze procedure.

Care Coordination and Transition Management
- Teach self-management of prescribed medication therapy, including antidysrhythmic and anticoagulant agents.

- Provide emotional support; it is common for patients with AF to experience anxiety.
- Evaluate the need for home health care or care coordination to promote ongoing access to services, including laboratory testing of INR or pacemaker testing.
- Remind patients to report any signs of a change in heart rhythm, such as a significant decrease in pulse rate, a rate more than 100 beats/min, or increased rhythm irregularity.

See Chapter 28 in the main text for more information on atrial fibrillation.

BLINDNESS

See *Visual Impairment (Reduced Vision)*.

BREAST, FIBROCYSTIC CHANGES (FCC) AND CYSTS

- Fibrocystic changes of the breast include a range of changes involving the lobules, ducts, and stromal tissues of the breast. This condition most often occurs in premenopausal women between 20 and 50 years of age and is thought to be caused by an imbalance in the normal estrogen-to-progesterone ratio.

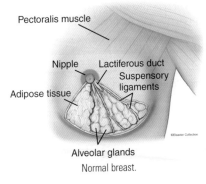

Normal breast.

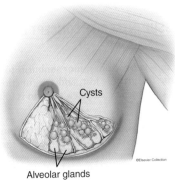

Breast with fibrocystic changes. (© Elsevier Collection.)

- Because fibrocystic changes affect at least half of women over the life span, they are referred to as fibrocystic changes (FCC) rather than fibrocystic disease.

- Typical symptoms include breast *pain* and firm, hard, tender lumps or swelling in the breasts, particularly before a women's menstrual period.

Interprofessional Collaborative Care
- Management of FCC focuses on the symptoms of the condition:
  1. Teach supportive measures, such as the use of mild analgesics or the limiting of salt intake before menses to help decrease swelling. Reduction of caffeine can also help to reduce symptoms.
  2. Wearing a supportive bra can reduce pain by decreasing tension on the ligaments.
  3. Local application of ice or heat may provide temporary relief of *pain*.
  4. If severe symptoms persist, hormonal drugs, such as oral contraceptives or selective estrogen receptor modulators (SERMs), may be prescribed to suppress oversecretion of estrogen.

 NURSING SAFETY PRIORITY

Drug Alert

Explain to women the benefits and risks associated with hormonal drug therapy for FCC. Risks include an increased chance of thrombotic events (e.g., stroke or blood clots) and the risk of development of uterine cancer. Teach them to seek medical attention immediately if any signs or symptoms of these complications occur.

See Chapter 62 in the main text for more information on breast disorders.

BURNS: TISSUE INTEGRITY CONCEPT EXEMPLAR

Overview
- Burns range in severity from minor sunburns to life-threatening trauma. *Tissue integrity* is lost, and the function of numerous body systems can be changed when the skin is injured.

Severity of Burn Injury
- The severity of a burn is determined by how much of the body surface area is involved. The quickest method for calculating the size of a burn injury in adult patients whose weights are in normal proportion to their heights is the *rule of nines*. With this method, the body is divided into areas that are multiples of 9%. It is useful when used for initial assessment at the injury site, as well as upon presentation to the emergency department. More accurate evaluations using other methods are made in a burn unit.

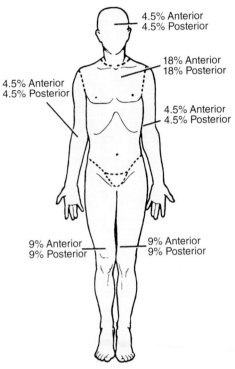

4.5% Anterior
4.5% Posterior

18% Anterior
18% Posterior

4.5% Anterior
4.5% Posterior

4.5% Anterior
4.5% Posterior

9% Anterior
9% Posterior

9% Anterior
9% Posterior

Rule of nines for estimating burn percentage.

Burn Classification
- Burns can be classified by depth of destruction. The amount of **tissue integrity** loss is related to the agent causing the burn, the temperature of the heat source, and how long the skin is exposed to it.
- Two primary systems of classification exist:
  1. Degree of burn (first, second, third, or fourth degree)
  2. Degree of thickness (superficial or deep, with thickness designations)

Burn Etiology
- There are six types of burns, representing the different mechanisms of injury. These include chemical burns, contact burns, electrical burn injuries, fire burns (including flash and flame burns), radiation burns, and scalds.

Classification of Burn Depth

	Damage	Appearance	Edema	Blistering	Pain	Eschar	Method of healing	Healing Time
Superficial								
Superficial first-degree burns	Above basal layer of epidermis	Dry Pink to red	No	No	Yes	No	Injured epidermis peels away; reveals new epidermis	About a week
Superficial second-degree burns (superficial partial-thickness)	Into dermis	Moist Red Blanching Blistering	Mild to moderate	Yes	Yes (very)	No	Re-epithelialization from skin adnexa	About 2 weeks
Deep								
Deep second-degree burns (deep partial-thickness)	Deeper into dermis	Less moist Less blanching Less painful	Moderate	Rare	Some	Yes, soft and dry	Scar deposition, contraction, limited re-epithelialization; may need grafting	2–6 weeks
Third-degree burns (full-thickness)	Entire thickness of skin destroyed, into fat	Any color (black, red, yellow, brown, white) Dry	Severe	No	No	Yes, hard and inelastic	Contraction and scar deposition; requires grafting	Weeks to months
Fourth-degree burns	Damage extends into muscle, tendon, bone	Black	Severe	No	No	Yes	Need specialized care; grafting does not work	Weeks to months, if at all

Data from Rice, P., & Orgill, D. (2021). Assessment and classification of burn injury. In Jeschke, M. (Ed.). Available at www.uptodate.com; and U.S. Department of Health and Human Services. (2019). Burn triage and treatment. Available at https://chemm.hhs.gov/burns.htm.

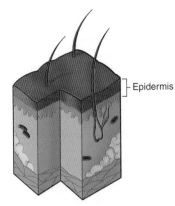

Superficial burns damage only the top layer of the skin—the epidermis. Healing occurs in 3-6 days.

Epidermis

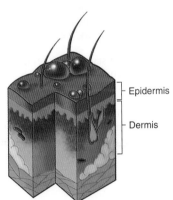

Superficial partial-thickness burns are those in which the entire epidermis and variable portions of the dermis layer of skin are destroyed. Uncomplicated healing occurs in 10-21 days.

Epidermis

Dermis

Deep partial-thickness burns extend into the deeper layers of the dermis. Healing occurs in 2-6 weeks.

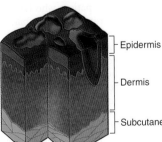

Full-thickness burns reach through the entire dermis and sometimes into the subcutaneous fat. The skin cannot heal on its own.

Epidermis

Dermis

Subcutaneous tissue

Tissues involved in burns of various depths.

Interprofessional Collaborative Care

- Burn care takes place in three phases: emergent (resuscitation), acute (healing), and rehabilitative (restorative).
  1. The **emergent (resuscitation)** phase of a burn injury begins at the onset of injury and continues for about 24 to 48 hours. The priorities of care during the emergent phase include:
     - Securing the airway
     - Supporting circulation and *perfusion*
     - Maintaining body temperature
     - Keeping the patient comfortable with analgesics
     - Providing emotional support
  2. The **acute (healing)** phase of burn injury begins about 36 to 48 hours after injury, when the fluid shift resolves, and lasts until wound closure is complete. During this phase, the nurse coordinates interprofessional care that is directed toward continued assessment and maintenance of the cardiovascular and respiratory systems, as well as toward nutritional status, burn wound care to preserve *tissue integrity*, *pain* control, and psychosocial interventions.
  3. Although rehabilitation efforts are started at the time of admission, the technical **rehabilitative (restorative)** phase begins with wound closure and ends when patients achieve their highest level of functioning. The emphasis is on the psychosocial adjustment of the patient, the prevention of scars and contractures, and the resumption of preburn activity, including resuming work, family, and social roles. This phase may take years or even last a lifetime, depending on the degree and impact of the burn(s).

Recognize Cues: Assessment

- Knowledge of circumstances surrounding the burn injury is valuable in planning the management of a patient who has experienced a burn. Obtain information directly from the patient, or ask those who witnessed the event to provide context.
- Assess signs and symptoms, including:
  1. Respiratory assessment: This is the most critical to prevent life-threatening complications for those with inhalation injuries. Even if you think the burn is minor, inspect the mouth, nose, and pharynx. *Continuous airway assessment is a nursing priority!*
  2. Skin assessment: Assess the skin to determine the extent and depth of burn injury. The size of the injury is first estimated in comparison with the *TBSA*. For example, a burn that involves 40% of the TBSA is a 40% burn.

⟫ BEST PRACTICE FOR PATIENT SAFETY AND QUALITY CARE

Nursing Burn Care Priorities by Phase

B

Phase of Burn Injury	Nursing Priorities
Emergent (Resuscitation)	• Determine extent of burn(s) and any other injuries. • Prevent or address respiratory compromise, shock, and hypovolemia. • Perform initial wound assessment. • Provide initial burn management interventions, such as burn care, fluid resuscitation, and ventilation, based on the extent of injury.
Acute (Healing)	• Prevent infection; intervene immediately if symptoms arise. • Continue wound care. • Prevent local and systemic complications associated with the burn injury. • Provide ongoing nutritional and metabolic support.
Rehabilitative (Restoration)	• Prevent contractures. • Continue wound care as indicated. • Support physical recovery and optimization of functional ability to the degree possible based on the extent of injury. • Provide professional emotional support. • In conjunction with the primary health care provider, refer to members of the interprofessional team as indicated (e.g., mental health provider, physical and/or occupational therapy).

NURSING SAFETY PRIORITY

Critical Rescue

Monitor the patient's respiratory efforts closely to recognize possible airway involvement, even if you think a burn injury is minor. If the patient has or develops a brassy cough, drooling, difficulty swallowing, or audible breath sounds on exhalation, respond immediately by positioning the patient upright, applying oxygen, and notifying the Rapid Response Team.

Analyze Cues and Prioritize Hypothesis: Analysis

- The priority collaborative problems for patients with burns include:
  1. Potential for impaired *gas exchange* due to smoke inhalation or burn injury sequelae
  2. Potential for life-threatening complications due to impaired *fluid and electrolyte balance* associated with severe burns
  3. Compromised *tissue integrity* due to burn injury
  4. Potential for *infection* due to reduced *tissue integrity*
  5. *Pain* related to burn injury

Generate Solutions and Take Actions: Planning and Implementation

- Nurses play an important role in teaching strategies to prevent burn injuries.
  1. Instruct people to assess water temperature before bathing or showering. Hot water heaters should be set below 120°F (49°C).
  2. Stress the importance of never adding a flammable substance (e.g., gasoline, kerosene, alcohol, lighter fluid, charcoal starter) to an open flame.
  3. Suggest the use of sunscreen agents and protective clothing to avoid sunburn.
  4. Teach people to reduce the risk for house fires by never smoking in bed and by avoiding smoking when drinking alcohol or when taking drugs that induce sleep.
  5. Keep matches and lighters out of the reach of children or people who are cognitively impaired.
  6. Remind patients using home oxygen not to smoke or have open flames in a room where oxygen is in use.

Promoting Gas Exchange

- Nonsurgical management for patients seeking burn care on an ambulatory basis includes:
  1. Airway maintenance: Although most patients treated on an ambulatory basis will not have airway compromise, tailor interventions to your respiratory assessment findings. For any patient suspected of an inhalation injury, be prepared to

administer oxygen and keep emergency airway equipment near the bedside. This equipment includes oxygen, masks, cannulas, manual resuscitation bags, laryngoscope, endotracheal tubes, and equipment for tracheostomy.

Preventing Life-Threatening Complications

- For patients with severe burn injury, preventing complex life-threatening complications is a priority problem of critical importance. Two of these types of potential complications include impaired *fluid and electrolyte balance* and shock (Carey et al., 2021).
  1. Fluid volume and perfusion are restored through IV fluid therapy and drug therapy.
  2. There are various formulas for calculating IV fluid needs, but the most used one for adult patients is the Parkland formula, also known as the Baxter formula. The formula calls for the fluid requirement in the first 24 hours postburn to be **4 mL/kg of body weight for each percent of total body surface area (TBSA) burned**.

⟫ BEST PRACTICE FOR PATIENT SAFETY AND QUALITY CARE

Fluid Resuscitation for the Patient With Severe Burns

- Initiate and maintain at least one large-bore IV line in an area of intact skin (if possible).
- Coordinate with health care providers to determine the appropriate fluid type and total volume to be infused during the first 24 hours postburn.
- Administer one-half of the total 24-hour prescribed volume within the first 8 hours postburn and the remaining volume over the next 16 hours.
- Assess IV access site, infusion rate, and infused volume at least hourly.
- Monitor these parameters at least hourly:
  - Breath sounds
  - Voice quality (if not intubated)
  - Oxygen saturation
  - End-tidal carbon dioxide levels
  - Blood pressure, pulse, respiratory rate
  - Urine volume and color, hourly output; laboratory values indicating specific gravity and signs of protein
  - Signs of fluid overload (dependent edema, engorged neck veins, rapid or thready pulse, lung crackles or wheezes)

▶▶ **BEST PRACTICE FOR PATIENT SAFETY AND QUALITY CARE**

Parkland Formula Calculation Example

Calculate the fluid needs for a patient weighing 154 lb with a 50% total burned surface area (TBSA) burn using the Parkland formula:

4 mL/kg of body weight for each percent of TBSA burned

1. Convert lb to kg (1 kg = 2.2 lb).
   - 154 lb divided by 2.2 = 70 kg
2. Multiply 70 kg by 4 mL.
   - 70 kg × 4 mL = 280
3. Multiply 280 by 50 (TBSA) = 14,000 mL of fluid is to be given over the first 24 hours

A total of 14,000 mL of fluid will be given over the first 24 hours postburn; half of this requirement—7000 mL—will be given in the first 8 hours postburn, with 7000 mL more to be given over the following 16 hours.

3. Monitor urine output: The goal is 0.5 mL/kg of hourly output (about 30 mL/hr).
4. Monitor vital signs, distal pulses, capillary refill, and skin color and turgor hourly to assess volume status.

Preserving Tissue Integrity and Preventing Infection
- Nonsurgical burn wound management involves removing exudates and necrotic tissue, cleaning the area, stimulating granulation and revascularization, and applying dressings.
- Priority nursing interventions include assessing the burn(s), providing wound care, and preventing infection and other complications.
- Surgical management of burn wounds involves excision and wound covering. Surgical excision is performed early in the postburn period.
  1. Autograft: skin replacement using the patient's own tissue
  2. Allograft: use of tissue from someone other than the patient to apply to the burn
  3. Xenograft: use of tissue from a nonhuman species to apply to the burn

Managing Pain
- **Pain** associated with burn injuries can be acute, persistent, or absent. When pain is present, the causes are multifactorial.
  1. Drug therapy for pain is chosen based on the causative agent and tailored to the degree of discomfort the patient is experiencing.

2. A superficial or partial-thickness burn may be very painful initially, whereas a patient with severe burns may not feel pain until much later, after stabilization, when dressings are being changed or mobility is attempted.
3. Schedule dressing changes after recent doses of pain medication.

B

 NURSING SAFETY PRIORITY

Drug Alert

Administer opioid medication for pain only by the IV route during the resuscitation phase to prevent delayed rapid absorption, which can lead to lethal blood levels of the drugs.

Care Coordination and Transition Management

· Discharge planning for the patient with a burn injury begins at admission to the hospital or burn center.

 HOME HEALTH CARE

Needs to Address Prior to the Discharge of the Patient With a Burn Injury

Prior to discharge, assess for these needs as indicated, based on the patient's status. One, more, or all may be necessary.
• Financial resources to cover ongoing treatment needs
• Psychological referral
• Patient and family teaching regarding wound care and infection control
• Physical, occupational, and/or speech therapy referral
• Rehabilitation referral
• Home assessment (on-site visit)
• Medical equipment
• Available community resources
• Reentry programs for school or work environment
• Long-term care placement
• Auditory testing
• Prosthetic rehabilitation

Evaluate Outcomes: Evaluation

· Evaluate the care of the patient with a burn injury on the basis of the identified priority patient problems. The expected outcomes include that the patient will:
1. Maintain appropriate *gas exchange*
2. Avoid development of life-threatening complications due to impaired *fluid and electrolyte balance* associated with severe burns

3. Have as much **tissue integrity** preserved as possible
4. Avoid development of **infection** due to reduced **tissue integrity**
5. Have pain adequately managed

See Chapter 21 in the main text for more information on burns. For severe burn care, consult a critical care nursing text.

CANCER

- **Cancer**, also called **malignancy**, is a type of abnormal cell growth in which cellular regulation is lost, resulting in new tissues that serve no useful function, are harmful to the function of normal cells and organs, and can lead to death if left untreated.
- *Benign tumor cells* are normal cells growing in the wrong place or at the wrong time.
    1. Examples include moles, skin tags, endometriosis, and nasal polyps.
- Cancer (malignant) cells are abnormal, serve no useful function, and are harmful to normal body tissues.
- Carcinogenesis, oncogenesis, and malignant transformation are different terms for cancer development, which is the process of changing a normal cell into a cancer cell.
    1. The original cancer cells or tumor caused by carcinogenesis is called the **primary tumor**. It is usually identified by the tissue from which it arose *(parent tissue)*, as in breast cancer or lung cancer.
    2. *Metastasis* occurs when cancer cells move from the primary location by breaking off from the original group and establishing remote colonies. These additional tumors are called **metastatic** or **secondary tumors**. *Even though the tumor is now in another organ, it is still a cancer from the original altered tissue.*

Staging of Cancer—TNM Classification

Primary Tumor (T)	
T_x	Primary tumor cannot be assessed
T_0	No evidence of primary tumor
T_{is}	Carcinoma in situ
T_1, T_2, T_3, T_4	Increasing size and/or local extent of the primary tumor
Regional Lymph Nodes (N)	
N_x	Regional lymph nodes cannot be assessed
N_0	No regional lymph node metastasis
N_1, N_2, N_3	Increasing involvement of regional lymph nodes
Distant Metastasis (M)	
M_x	Presence of distant metastasis cannot be assessed
M_0	No distant metastasis
M_1	Distant metastasis

- Systems of grading and staging have been developed to help standardize cancer diagnosis, prognosis, and treatment.
  1. Grading of a tumor classifies the cellular aspects of the cancer.
  2. Ploidy classifies the number and structure of tumor chromosomes as normal or abnormal.
  3. Staging classifies the clinical aspects of the cancer. The *tumor, node, metastasis (TNM)* system is used to describe the anatomic extent of cancers. The TNM staging systems have specific prognostic value for each solid tumor type.

Personal Factors and Cancer Development

- Personal factors, including ***immunity***, age, and genetic risk, also affect whether an adult is likely to develop cancer.
  1. Immunity protects the body from foreign invaders. Cancer incidence increases among patients with reduced ***immunity,*** such as:
     - Adults older than age 60: Advanced age is the single most important risk factor for cancer (ACS, 2022a; CCS, 2021)
     - Organ transplant recipients
     - Patients with stage HIV-III disease (AIDS)
  2. Genetic testing for cancer predisposition is available to confirm or rule out an adult's genetic risk for some specific cancer types.
     - These tests do not diagnose the presence of cancer; they only provide risk information.

Cancer Prevention

- Primary cancer prevention: The use of strategies to prevent the actual occurrence of cancer
  1. *Avoidance of known or potential carcinogens* is an effective prevention strategy when a cause of cancer is known and avoidance is easily accomplished.
     - For example, teach adults to use skin protection during sun exposure to avoid skin cancer. Most lung cancer can be avoided by not using tobacco and eliminating exposure to loose asbestos particles.
  2. *Modifying associated factors* appears to help reduce cancer risk.
     - Absolute causes are not known for many cancers, but some conditions appear to increase risk. Examples are the increased incidence of cancer among adults who consume alcohol; the association of a diet high in fat and low in fiber with colon cancer, breast cancer, and ovarian cancer; and a greater incidence of cervical cancer among women who have multiple sexual partners (ACS, 2022a).

3. *Removal of "at-risk" tissues* reduces cancer risk for an adult who has a known high risk for developing a specific type of cancer.

4. *Vaccination* is a newer method of primary cancer prevention. Currently, the only vaccines approved for prevention of cancer are related to prevention of infection from several forms of the human papillomavirus (HPV).

5. *Chemoprevention* is a strategy that uses drugs, chemicals, natural nutrients, or other substances to disrupt one or more steps important to cancer development.

- Secondary cancer prevention: The use of screening strategies to detect cancer early, at a time when cure or control is more likely.

1. Regular screening for cancer does not reduce cancer incidence but can greatly reduce some types of cancer deaths.

2. Examples of recommended screenings include (ACS, 2021a):
   - The choice of annual mammography for women 40 to 44 years of age, annual mammography for women 45 to 54 years of age, and annual or biennial mammography for women older than 55 years
   - Annual fecal occult blood test or colonoscopy for adults starting at age 45
   - Cervical screening starting at age 25

Interprofessional Collaborative Care
Recognize Cues: Assessment
- Impact of Cancer on Physical Function:

1. **Impaired Immunity and Clotting**: Impaired immunity and blood-producing functions can occur when cancer starts in or invades the bone marrow, where blood cells are formed.

2. **Altered GI Function**: Tumors of the GI tract increase the metabolic rate and the need for nutrients; however, many patients develop disease- and treatment-related appetite loss and alterations in taste, which have a negative impact on nutrition and lead to weight loss.

3. **Altered Peripheral Nerve Function**: Although tumors in the spine can change peripheral nerve function, the more common cause is chemotherapy. Neurotoxic chemotherapy agents injure peripheral nerves, leading to peripheral neuropathy with reduced sensory perception.

4. **Motor and Sensory Deficits**: Motor and *sensory perception* deficits occur when cancers invade bone or the brain or compress nerves. In patients with bone metastasis, the primary cancer started in another organ (e.g., lung, prostate, breast).

5. **Cancer Pain:** The patient with cancer may have *pain*, especially persistent (chronic) pain. Pain does not always accompany cancer, but it can be a major problem.

6. **Altered Respiratory and Cardiac Function:** Cancer can disrupt respiratory function, capacity, and ***gas exchange*** and may result in death. Tumors that grow in the airways cause obstruction. If lung tissue is involved, lung capacity is decreased, leading to dyspnea and hypoxemia. Cancer cells thicken the alveolar membrane and damage lung blood vessels, both of which impair ***gas exchange***.

Take Actions: Interventions

- Cancer treatment can include surgery, radiation, chemotherapy, immunotherapy, targeted therapy, and hormonal therapy

Surgical Management

- Surgery often plays a part in the diagnosis and/or management of cancer. Surgery is only one part of a comprehensive treatment approach for cancer therapy. Surgery is used for prophylaxis, diagnosis, cure, control, palliation, and tissue reconstruction.
  1. *Prophylactic surgery* removes potentially cancerous tissue as a means of preventing cancer development.
  2. *Diagnostic surgery* (e.g., excisional biopsy) is the removal of all or part of a suspected lesion for examination and testing to confirm or rule out a cancer diagnosis.
  3. *Curative surgery* removes all cancer tissue.
  4. *Debulking surgery* removes part of the tumor if removal of the entire mass is not possible.
  5. *Palliative surgery* focuses on providing symptom relief and improving the quality of life but is not curative.
  6. *Reconstructive* or restorative *surgery* increases function, enhances appearance, or both.

Nonsurgical Management

- ***Radiation Therapy:*** Radiation therapy uses high-energy radiation to kill cancer cells, with the intent to cure or relieve symptoms (palliative). The goal of radiation is to kill the cancer cells while having minimal damaging effects on the surrounding normal tissue.
  1. External beam or teletherapy is radiation delivered from a source outside of the patient. Because the source is external, the patient is not radioactive and there is no hazard to others.
  2. *Brachytherapy*, also known as internal radiation therapy. The radiation source (seeds, ribbons, or capsules) comes into direct, continuous contact with the tumor for a specific time

period. *With all types of brachytherapy, the radiation source is within the patient. Therefore, the patient emits radiation for a period of time and is a potential hazard to others.*

3. Radiation therapy has both short- and long-term effects, depending upon the area(s) radiated.
   - Changes to the skin, known as *radiation dermatitis*, are the most common side effect of radiotherapy and can range from redness/hyperpigmentation and rash to skin desquamation (Gosselin et al., 2020).
   - Radiation damage to normal tissues during therapy can start inflammatory responses that lead to tissue fibrosis and scarring. These effects may appear years after radiation treatment.

! NURSING SAFETY PRIORITY

Action Alert

When a nurse is caring for a patient undergoing radiation treatment, there are precautions that the nurse needs to take. Using the general guidelines below, the nurse reduces exposure to ionizing radiation.

- *Time* is length of exposure to the radiation field. Try to coordinate care to limit time directly at the radiation source.
- *Distance* is how far from the radiation source you remain. The farther away from the radiation source, the less exposure.
- *Shielding* is using a material (such as a lead apron) to avoid exposure.

From Center for Nuclear Science and Technology Information. (2021). *Protecting against exposure.* https://www.ans.org/nuclear/radiation/exposure/.

! NURSING SAFETY PRIORITY

Action Alert

Ingested isotopes enter body fluids and eventually are eliminated in waste products. These wastes are radioactive, and you must ensure that they are not directly touched by anyone. Handle the wastes according to guidelines established by the institution. During a patient's hospitalization for radiation, pregnant women and children are not allowed to visit the patient. After the isotope has been completely eliminated from the body, neither the patient nor the body wastes are radioactive.

BEST PRACTICE FOR PATIENT SAFETY AND QUALITY CARE

Care of the Patient With Sealed Implants of Radioactive Sources

- Assign the patient to a private room with a private bath.
- Place a "Caution: Radioactive Material" sign on the door of the patient's room.
- If portable lead shields are used, place them between the patient and the door.
- Keep the door to the patient's room closed as much as possible.
- Wear a dosimeter film badge at all times while caring for patients with radioactive implants. The badge offers no protection but measures a person's exposure to radiation. Each person caring for the patient should have a separate dosimeter to calculate individual radiation exposure.
- Wear a lead apron while providing care. Always keep the front of the apron facing the source of radiation (do not turn your back toward the patient).
- If you are attempting to conceive, do not perform direct patient care regardless of whether you are male or female.
- Nurses who are pregnant should not care for these patients; do not allow women who are pregnant or children younger than 16 years to visit.
- Never touch the radioactive source with bare hands. In the rare instance that it is dislodged, use a long-handled forceps to retrieve it. Deposit the radioactive source in the lead container kept in the patient's room.
- After the source is removed, dispose of dressings and linens in the usual manner. Other equipment can be removed from the room at any time without special precautions and does not pose a hazard to other people.

- *Systemic Therapy:* Systemic therapy refers to the use of antineo-plastic (chemotherapy) drugs that are used to kill cancer cells and disrupt their cellular regulation.
  1. *Chemotherapy:* The treatment of cancer with chemical agents is used to cure and increase survival time. This killing effect on cancer cells is related to the ability of chemotherapy to damage DNA and interfere with cell division.
     - Chemotherapy is to be given only by registered nurses who have completed an approved chemotherapy program and have demonstrated competence in administering these agents. However, responsibility for monitoring the patient

Acute and Late Site-Specific Effects of Radiation Therapy

Acute Effects

Brain
- Alopecia and dermatitis of the scalp
- Ear and external auditory canal irritation
- Cerebral edema and increased intracranial pressure
- Nausea and vomiting
- Blurry vision

Head and Neck
- Oral mucositis
- Taste changes
- Oral candidiasis, herpes, or other infections
- Acute xerostomia
- Dental caries
- Esophagitis and pharyngitis

Breast and Chest Wall
- Skin reactions
- Esophagitis

Chest and Lung
- Esophagitis and pharyngitis
- Taste changes
- Pneumonia
- Cough

Abdomen and Pelvis
- Anorexia
- Nausea and vomiting
- Diarrhea
- Cystitis or proctitis
- Vaginal dryness/vaginitis
- Sexual and fertility problems

Eye
- Conjunctival edema and tearing

Late Effects

Subcutaneous and Soft Tissue
- Radiation-induced fibrosis

Central Nervous System
- Brain necrosis
- Leukoencephalopathy
- Cognitive and emotional dysfunction
- Pituitary and hypothalamic dysfunction
- Spinal cord myelopathies

Head and Neck
- Xerostomia and dental caries
- Trismus
- Osteoradionecrosis
- Hypothyroidism

Lung
- Pulmonary fibrosis

Heart
- Pericarditis
- Cardiomyopathy
- Coronary artery disease

Breast/Chest Wall
- Atrophy, fibrosis of breast tissue
- Lymphedema

Abdomen and Pelvis
- Small and large bowel injury
- Diarrhea

C

during chemotherapy administration rests with all nurses providing patient care.

- A serious complication of IV infusion is **extravasation**, which occurs when drug leaks into the surrounding tissues (also called *infiltration*).

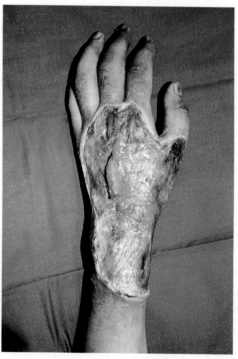

Appearance of tissue damage and loss after chemotherapy extravasation. (From Weinzweig, J., & Weinzweig, N. (2005). *The mutilated hand.* St. Louis: Mosby.)

- Many anticancer drugs are available currently as oral agents.
  - A big misperception by patients and nononcology nurses is that oral anticancer drugs are less toxic than IV chemotherapy. This is *not* true. *Oral anticancer drugs are just as toxic to the patient taking the drug and to the person handling the drug as are IV chemotherapy agents.*
- The chemotherapy drug categories are in the following drug table.

Common Examples of Drug Therapy

Chemotherapy Drugs

Common Chemotherapy Classifications	Nursing Implications
Antimetabolites act as "counterfeit" metabolites that fool cancer cells into using the antimetabolites in cellular reactions.	
• Azacitidine • Capecitabine (oral) • Cytarabine • Decitabine • 5-Fluorouracil	• Risk of neutropenia is high. • Patients must be screened for fever and infection at regular intervals. • Growth factors may be prescribed. • Patient will be prone to diarrhea and mucositis; aggressive hydration and oral hygiene are crucial to prevent complications.
Antitumor antibiotics damage the cell's DNA and interrupt DNA or RNA synthesis.	
• Bleomycin • Doxorubicin • Doxorubicin liposomal	• There is a lifetime maximum dosage for these agents. • Cardiac and pulmonary toxicity can occur. • Monitoring of ejection fraction (EF) or pulmonary function tests (PFTs) at regular intervals is required. • These agents are vesicants and can cause severe tissue damage with extravasation.
Antimitotics interfere with the formation and actions of microtubules so that cells cannot complete mitosis during cell division.	
• Docetaxel • Paclitaxel • Vinblastine • Vincristine	• May cause peripheral neuropathy. Ensure patient safety during ambulation. • Patients may experience extreme constipation, and an aggressive bowel regimen may be required. • Ensure that patients are using pharmacologic and nonpharmacologic interventions to manage bowel changes.
Alkylating agents prevent proper DNA and ribonucleic acid (RNA) synthesis, which inhibits cell division.	
• Carboplatin • Cisplatin • Cyclophosphamide • Dacarbazine	• May cause peripheral neuropathy. Ensure patient safety during ambulation. • May cause renal failure if the patient is not adequately hydrated. Patients will need aggressive hydration before and after administration. • May cause severe nausea and vomiting. Ensure adequate control of nausea and vomiting. Patients may need alternating or around-the-clock management of nausea and vomiting.

C

Continued

💊 Common Examples of Drug Therapy—cont'd

Chemotherapy Drugs

Common Chemotherapy Classifications	Nursing Implications
Topoisomerase inhibitors—When drugs disrupt the topoisomerase enzyme, proper DNA maintenance is prevented, resulting in increased DNA breakage and eventual cell death.	
• Irinotecan • Topotecan	• May cause significant diarrhea. • Ensure adequate hydration and also use of antidiarrheals. • Occasionally, atropine may be required to maintain control of diarrhea.

Data from the U.S. Food and Drug Administration website at https://www.accessdata.fda.gov/scripts/cder/daf/index.cfm.

- Temporary and permanent damage can occur to normal tissues from chemotherapy because it is systemic and exerts its effects on all cells. These adverse effects include:
  1. Irritation and damage at the site of administration. Many chemotherapeutic agents are given intravenously.
  2. Bone marrow suppression: anemia, reduced immunity (reduced white blood cells [WBCs] and low neutrophils [neutropenia]), and thrombocytopenia with associated fatigue, immunosuppression, and bleeding and clotting abnormalities
  3. Chemotherapy-induced nausea and vomiting (CIN); antiemetics are available to relieve nausea and vomiting.
  4. Mucositis (sores in mucous membranes)
  5. Alopecia (hair loss)
  6. Changes in cognitive function, which are usually temporary and resolve but may persist with permanent anatomic changes to the brain
  7. Chemotherapy-induced peripheral neuropathy (loss of sensory perception or motor function of peripheral nerves)

➕ NURSING SAFETY PRIORITY

Critical Rescue

Monitor patients with reduced **immunity** to recognize signs of infection. When any temperature elevation (above 100.4°F or 38°C) is present, respond by reporting this to the primary health care provider immediately and implement standard infection protocols. When IV antiinfective drugs are started, the neutropenic patient is admitted to the hospital. The patient with neutropenia does *not* pose an infection risk to other people; however, other people can be an infection risk to the patient.

▶ BEST PRACTICE FOR PATIENT SAFETY AND QUALITY CARE

Care of the Patient With Myelosuppression and Neutropenia

- Place the patient in a private room whenever possible.
- Use good handwashing technique or alcohol-based hand rubs before touching the patient or any of the patient's belongings.
- Ensure that the patient's room and bathroom are cleaned at least once a day.
- Monitor vital signs, including temperature, every 4 hours.
- Inspect the patient's skin and mucous membranes for the presence of fissures and abscesses per facility policy.
- Inspect IV sites for indications of infection.
- Change wound dressings daily or as ordered.
- Use strict aseptic technique for all invasive procedures.
- Promptly notify the primary health care provider if any area appears infected, and obtain order for culture, per protocol.
- Encourage activity at a level appropriate for the patient's current health status.
- Keep frequently used equipment in the room for use with this patient only.
- Visitors with signs or symptoms of illness should be restricted.
- Monitor the white blood cell count daily.
- Avoid the use of indwelling urinary catheters if possible. Provide perineal hygiene per protocol and at least daily.
- Follow agency policy for restriction of fresh flowers and potted plants in the patient's room.

▨ PATIENT AND FAMILY EDUCATION

Prevention of Infection

During the times your white blood cell counts are low:
- Avoid crowds and other large gatherings of people who might be ill.
- Do not share personal toiletries.
- If possible, bathe daily. If total bathing is not possible, wash the armpits and entire perineal area twice a day with an antimicrobial soap.
- Wash your hands thoroughly with an antimicrobial soap before you eat and drink, after touching a pet, after shaking hands with anyone, as soon as you come home from any outing, and after using the toilet.
- Do not drink perishable liquids that have been standing at room temperature for longer than an hour.

Continued

PATIENT AND FAMILY EDUCATION—cont'd

Prevention of Infection

- Use food safety when preparing meals.
- Wash fresh fruits and vegetables prior to eating.
- Do not change pet litter boxes or clean up after pets. Wear gloves if necessary.
- Take your temperature at least once a day and whenever you do not feel well.
- Report any of these indicators of infection to your oncologist immediately:
  - Temperature greater than 100.4°F (38°C)
  - Persistent cough (with or without sputum)
  - Pus or foul-smelling drainage from any open skin area or normal body opening
  - Presence of a boil or abscess
  - Urine that is cloudy or foul smelling or that causes burning on urination
- Take all drugs as prescribed.
- Wear gardening gloves when working in the garden or with houseplants.
- Wear a condom when having sex. If you are a female having sex with a male partner, ensure that he wears a condom.

- *Immunotherapy* is the use of the body's own defense system to attack foreign cells. Although this treatment is generally well tolerated, it still can have some significant and life-threatening complications.
  1. **Immune-related adverse events (irAEs)** occur when the stimulation of the immune system affects healthy cells as well. When healthy cells are targeted instead of cancerous cells, a patient experiences an exacerbation of an inflammatory response caused by the immune system activation.
- *Monoclonal antibody therapy* combines actions from immunotherapy and targeted therapy to help treat specific cancers. Monoclonal antibodies bind to their target antigens, which are often specific cell surface membrane proteins (Abramson, 2019). Binding prevents the protein from performing its functions; monoclonal antibodies therefore change *cellular regulation* and prevent cancer cell division.
  1. Infusion-related reactions, or hypersensitivity reactions (HSRs), may occur in patients receiving monoclonal antibodies.

2. Nursing assessment is key for early recognition of a potentially life-threatening infusion-related reaction. Infusion reactions usually occur during the infusion and typically develop within 30 minutes to 2 hours of initiation of the drug (LaCasce et al., 2022).

3. Monoclonal antibody infusion-related reactions include fever, chills, rigors, rash, headache, hypotension, shortness of breath, bronchospasm, nausea, vomiting, and abdominal pain. Side effects can vary from mild to life-threatening (LaCasce et al., 2022).

- *Targeted therapies* block the growth and spread of cancer by interfering with the specific cellular growth pathways or molecules involved in the *cellular regulation* of growth and progression of cancer cells.
  1. Targeted therapies work by acting directly on the cancerous cell, and they have less of an impact on normal cells that do not have this pathway.
  2. Side effects and management of the patient vary from drug to drug, and these targeted agents usually do not have systemic side effects, as chemotherapy does.
  3. Targeted therapy agents are classified based on their action.

- *Endocrine therapy:* Some hormones cause hormone-sensitive tumors to grow more rapidly. Decreasing the amount of these hormones that reaches hormone-sensitive tumors can slow cancer growth. Breast cancer is one example of a cancer that can be hormonally driven.
  1. *Side effects* of endocrine therapy include fatigue, arthralgias, joint stiffness and/or bone pain, hot flashes, and sexual dysfunction. Long-term side effects include osteoporosis, increased cardiovascular risks, and risk of thrombotic events.

- *Colony-stimulating factors:* Colony-stimulating factors (CSFs) are used as supportive therapy during chemotherapy by enhancing recovery of bone marrow function after treatment-induced myelosuppression. These are also referred to as *growth factors*.
  1. Bone pain is a common side effect in patients receiving colony-stimulating factors. Usually acetaminophen or ibuprofen will control the pain, but occasionally an opioid prescription is required.

Oncologic Emergencies

- **Sepsis and Disseminated Intravascular Coagulation (DIC):** *Sepsis,* or *septicemia,* is a condition in which organisms enter the bloodstream and cause severe infection. This infection can result in septic shock, a life-threatening condition. Adults with cancer who have low WBCs (neutropenia) and impaired immunity from cancer therapy are at risk for infection and sepsis.
  1. Often a low-grade fever (100.4°F or 38°C) is the only sign of infection.

2. *Disseminated intravascular coagulation* (DIC) is a problem with the blood-*clotting* process. DIC is triggered by many severe illnesses, including cancer. In patients with cancer DIC often is caused by sepsis from a variety of organisms (bacterial, fungal, viral, or parasitic).

3. Extensive, abnormal clotting occurs throughout the small blood vessels of patients with DIC. This widespread clotting depletes circulating clotting factors and platelets. As this happens, extensive bleeding occurs. Bleeding from many sites is the most common problem; it ranges from oozing to fatal hemorrhage.

✚ NURSING SAFETY PRIORITY

Critical Rescue

DIC is a life-threatening problem with a high mortality rate, even when proper treatment is initiated. Identify patients at greatest risk for sepsis and DIC. Prevention of sepsis and DIC is a priority nursing intervention. Practice strict adherence to aseptic technique during invasive procedures and during contact with nonintact skin and mucous membranes. Teach patients and families the early indicators of infection and to seek prompt assistance.

- **Syndrome of Inappropriate Antidiuretic Hormone:** In healthy adults, antidiuretic hormone (ADH) is secreted by the posterior pituitary gland only when more fluid (water) is needed in the body, such as when plasma volume is decreased. Certain conditions induce ADH secretion when not needed by the body, which leads to syndrome of inappropriate antidiuretic hormone (SIADH).

1. Cancer is a common cause of SIADH, especially small cell lung cancer (SCLC). SIADH also may occur with other cancers, including head and neck, melanoma, GI, prostate, and hematologic malignancies, especially when metastatic tumors are present in the brain.

✚ NURSING SAFETY PRIORITY

Critical Rescue

Monitor patients at least every 2 hours to recognize signs and symptoms of increasing fluid overload (bounding pulse, increasing neck vein distention [jugular venous distention (JVD)], presence of crackles in lungs, increasing peripheral edema, reduced urine output) because pulmonary edema can occur very quickly and lead to death. When symptoms indicate that the fluid overload from SIADH either is not responding to therapy or is becoming worse, respond by notifying the primary health care provider immediately.

- **Spinal Cord Compression**: Spinal cord compression (SCC) is an oncologic emergency that requires immediate intervention to relieve pain and prevent neurologic damage. Damage from SCC occurs either when a tumor directly enters the spinal cord or spinal column or when the vertebrae collapse from tumor degradation of the bone. Tumors metastasizing from the lung, prostate, breast, and colon account for most SCC.
  1. Back pain is a common first symptom and occurs before other problems or nerve deficits. Other symptoms include weakness, loss of sensation, urinary retention, and constipation.
- **Hypercalcemia:** Hypercalcemia (increased serum calcium level) occurs frequently in patients with cancer. It is a metabolic emergency and can lead to death. Multiple myeloma and metastatic cancer to the bone, for example, carry a risk for hypercalcemia (Bohnenkamp & Bass, 2021).
  1. Early symptoms of hypercalcemia are nonspecific. Common symptoms include fatigue, loss of appetite, nausea, vomiting, constipation, and increased urine output. Additional symptoms include skeletal pain, kidney stones, abdominal discomfort, and altered cognition that can range from lethargy to coma
- **Superior Vena Cava Syndrome**: The superior vena cava (SVC), which returns all blood from the head, neck, and upper extremities to the heart, has thin walls, and compression or obstruction by tumor growth or by clots in the vessel leads to congestion of the blood. Compression of the SVC is painful and can be life-threatening.
  1. Early signs and symptoms include edema of the face, especially around the eyes (periorbital edema) on arising in the morning, and tightness of the collar. As the compression worsens, the patient develops engorged blood vessels and erythema/hyperpigmentation of the upper body, edema in the arms and hands, and dyspnea. The development of stridor (a high-pitched crowing sound) indicates narrowing of the pharynx or larynx and is an alarming sign of rapid SVCS progression. Symptoms are more apparent when the patient is in the supine position.
- **Tumor Lysis Syndrome (TLS)**: Large numbers of tumor cells are destroyed rapidly. The intracellular contents of damaged cancer cells, including potassium and purines (DNA components), are released into the bloodstream faster than the body can eliminate them. Severe or untreated TLS can cause acute kidney injury (AKI) and death.
  1. Early symptoms of TLS stem from electrolyte imbalances and can include lethargy, nausea, vomiting, anorexia, flank pain, muscle weakness, cramps, seizures, and altered mental status.
  2. Hydration prevents and manages TLS by increasing the kidney flow rates, preventing uric acid buildup in the kidneys, and diluting the serum potassium levels.

Survivorship

- With new treatments, patients are living longer with cancer. What used to be a death sentence is now being considered a chronic disease.
- Survivors have unique physical and psychosocial needs, including long-term effects from treatment. Follow-up care and considerations for survivors includes:
  1. Routine imaging, blood work, and follow-up care with the primary health care provider.
  2. Chemotherapy can lead to cardiac and pulmonary toxicity, infertility, menopause, and peripheral neuropathy, as well as an increased risk of secondary malignancies.
  3. If lymph nodes were removed during surgery, the risk of lymphedema is lifelong.
  4. Radiation can cause fibrosis and permanent skin changes in the radiation path.

 See Chapter 18 in the main text for more information on cancer.

Common Cancer Sites

Common cancer sites include breast cancer, cervical cancer, colorectal cancer, endometrial cancer, head and neck cancer, lung cancer, ovarian cancer, pancreatic cancer, prostate cancer, and skin cancer. These specific cancer locations are discussed in the next sections along with care unique to that type and location of cancer.

BREAST CANCER: CELLULAR REGULATION
✳ CONCEPT EXEMPLAR

Overview

- There are two broad categories of breast cancer: noninvasive and invasive. As long as the cancer remains within the mammary duct, it is referred to as *noninvasive*. The more common type of breast cancer is classified as *invasive*; this type grows into surrounding breast tissue.
  1. Noninvasive (In Situ) Breast Cancers
     - Ductal carcinoma in situ (DCIS): contained within the duct; does not invade the fatty breast tissue
     - Lobular carcinoma in situ (LCIS): contained within the milk-producing glands of the breast
  2. Invasive Breast Cancers
     - Invasive ductal carcinoma: invades through the ducts into the surrounding breast tissue; most common invasive cancer
     - Inflammatory breast cancer: rare but highly aggressive invasive cancer characterized by diffuse edema and erythema/hyperpigmentation

3. Others Types of Breast Cancer
   - Paget's disease: rare cancer that occurs in or around the nipple
   - Triple negative breast cancer (TNBC): lacks expression of the estrogen receptor (ER), progesterone receptor (PR), and human epidermal growth factor receptor 2 (HER2) (Anders & Carey, 2023). This type of breast cancer grows rapidly and is often found in women with a *BRCA* mutation who are premenopausal.

Interprofessional Collaborative Care
Recognize Cues: Assessment
- Ask about the woman's gynecologic and obstetric (if any) history, including:
  1. Age at menarche
  2. Age at menopause
  3. Symptoms of menopause
  4. Age at first child's birth (or nulliparity—having no children)
  5. Number of children and pregnancies, including miscarriages or terminations

---

▷▷ BEST PRACTICE FOR PATIENT SAFETY AND QUALITY CARE

Assessing a Breast Mass

- Identify the location of the mass by using the "face of the clock" method.
- Describe the shape, size, and consistency of the mass.
- Assess whether the mass is fixed or movable.
- Note any skin changes around the mass, such as dimpling of the skin, increased vascularity, nipple retraction, nipple inversion, or skin ulceration.
- Assess the adjacent lymph nodes, both axillary and supraclavicular nodes.
- Ask patients if they experience **pain** or soreness in the area around the mass.

Analyze Cues and Prioritize Hypotheses: Analysis
- The priority collaborative problems for patients with breast cancer include:
  1. Potential for cancer metastasis due to lack of, or inadequate, treatment
  2. Potential for impaired coping due to breast cancer diagnosis and treatment

Generate Solutions and Take Actions: Planning and Implementation
Decreasing the Risk for Metastasis

- Once cancer is diagnosed, the extent and location of breast cancer and metastases (if applicable) determine the overall treatment strategy.

  1. The management of early-stage breast cancer is surgery.
  2. Adjuvant therapy for breast cancer consists of systemic chemotherapy, radiation therapy, or a combination of both.
  3. Chemotherapy is recommended for treatment of invasive breast cancer after surgery (adjuvant chemotherapy). It may also be given before surgery to reduce the size of the tumor (neoadjuvant chemotherapy) and is most effective when combinations of more than one drug are used.
  4. Radiation therapy is administered after breast-conserving surgery to kill breast cancer cells that may remain near the site of the original tumor.

Breast-conserving Surgery

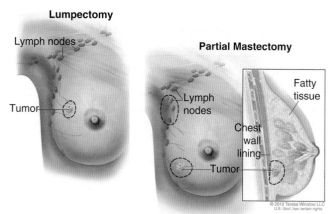

Breast-conserving surgery. Dotted lines show the area containing the tumor that is removed and some of the lymph nodes that may be removed.

Surgical treatment for breast cancer. (©2010 Terese Winslow. U.S. Govt. has certain rights.)

Total (Simple) Mastectomy

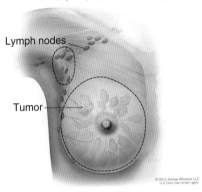

Total (simple) mastectomy. The dotted line shows where the entire breast is removed. Some lymph nodes under the arm may also be removed.

Modified Radical Mastectomy

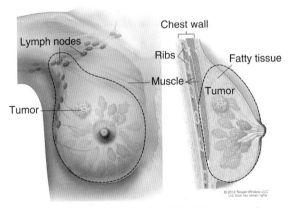

Modified radical mastectomy. The dotted line shows where the entire breast and some lymph nodes are removed. Part of the chest wall muscle may also be removed.

! NURSING SAFETY PRIORITY

Action Alert

To decrease the chance of surgical site *infection*, carefully observe the surgical wound after breast surgery for signs of swelling and infection throughout recovery. Assess the incision and flap of the postmastectomy patient for signs of bleeding, infection, and poor tissue perfusion. Drainage tubes are usually removed about 1 to 3 weeks after hospital discharge when the patient returns for an office visit. The drainage amount should be less than 30 mL in a 24-hour period. Inform the patient that tube removal may cause temporary *pain*. Provide or suggest analgesia before the tubes are removed. Document all findings, and report any abnormalities to the surgeon immediately.

Enhancing Coping Strategies
- Teach women ways to minimize surgical area deformity and enhance body image, such as the use of a breast prosthesis or the option of breast reconstruction.
- Address the reactions of family and significant others to the diagnosis of breast cancer; provide support and education.
- Helping patients diagnosed with breast cancer to be an active participant in their care, find resources to help them cope, and gain support with the physical and emotional changes is a priority for the nurse and members of the interprofessional team.

Evaluate Outcomes: Evaluation
- Evaluate the care of the patient with breast cancer based on the identified priority patient problems. The expected outcomes include that the patient:
  1. Has no recurrence or metastasis of breast cancer after completion of treatment; if metastasis occurs, have optimal palliative and end-of-life care
  2. Reports adequately coping with the uncertainty of having breast cancer and its treatment

See Chapter 62 in the main text for more information on breast cancer.

CERVICAL CANCER

- Most cases of cervical cancer are caused by certain types of human papillomavirus (HPV). The high-risk HPV types 16 and 18 are responsible for 50% of cervical cancers (World Health Organization [WHO], 2022). They impair the tumor-suppressor gene. The unrestricted tissue growth can spread, becoming invasive and metastatic (Rogers, 2023).

Risk Factors for Cervical Cancer

Women at higher risk for cervical cancer include those who:
- Are immunocompromised (e.g., have HIV, or are taking immunosuppressant drugs for an autoimmune condition)
- Are daughters of women who took diethylstilbestrol (DES; a hormone to prevent miscarriage) between 1940 and 1971
- Became sexually active at a young age
- Do not eat a diet high in fruits and vegetables
- Smoke tobacco
- Have a family history of cervical cancer
- Have infection with human papillomavirus (HPV) and/or chlamydia
- Have obesity
- Have many sexual partners, or one partner who is high risk
- Have used oral contraceptives (OCs) for a long length of time (risk diminishes when OCs are discontinued)
- Have had multiple full-term pregnancies
- Had a first full-term pregnancy earlier than age 20

Data from American Cancer Society. (2020). *Risk factors for cervical cancer.* https://www.cancer.org/cancer/cervical-cancer/causes-risks-prevention/risk-factors.html; Katz, A. (2019). Obesity-related cancer in women: A clinical review. *American Journal of Nursing, 119*(8), 34-40; Centers for Disease Control and Prevention. (2022). *Obesity and cancer.* https://www.cdc.gov/cancer/obesity/.

- Girls and young women should be immunized with one of the HPV vaccines:
  1. *Gardasil* (available in Canada)—available for ages 9 through 26
  2. *Gardasil 9* (available in the United States and Canada)—available for ages 9 to 26; can be given up until the age of 45
  3. *Cervarix* (available in Canada)—available for ages 9 through 25

Interprofessional Collaborative Care
Recognize Cues: Assessment
- Cervical cancer can be detected at early stages, when cure is most likely, through a periodic pelvic examination and Pap test. Diagnosis is made by cytological examination of the Pap smear.

- Ask the patient about vaginal bleeding. Cervical cancer may manifest as spotting between menstrual periods or after sexual intercourse.
- The classic symptom of invasive cancer is painless vaginal bleeding. As the cancer grows, bleeding increases in frequency, duration, and amount, and it may become continuous.

Take Actions: Interventions

- *Radiation therapy* can be used to treat certain stages of cervical cancer, or cervical cancer that has spread to other organs. Brachytherapy and external beam radiation therapy are the two types used.
- The choice of surgical management approach is dependent upon the patient's overall health, desire for future childbearing, tumor size and stage, cancer cell type, degree of lymph node involvement, and patient preference.
- Surgical management procedures include:
  1. *Loop electrosurgical excision procedure (LEEP):* Spotting (very scant bleeding) can occur after the procedure.
  2. *Laser surgery:* A small amount of bleeding can occur, and the woman may have slight vaginal discharge.
  3. *Cryosurgery:* The patient will have heavy, watery brown discharge for several weeks after the procedure.

PATIENT AND FAMILY EDUCATION

Care After Local Cervical Ablation Therapies

- Refrain from sexual intercourse.
- Do not use tampons.
- Do not douche.
- Take showers rather than tub baths.
- Avoid lifting heavy objects.
- Report any heavy vaginal bleeding, foul-smelling drainage, or fever.

---

  4. A *conization,* in which a cone-shaped area of cervix is removed surgically, can remove affected tissue while preserving fertility.
  5. For women who may wish to become pregnant in the future, a *radical trachelectomy* can be done. Going through the vagina or abdomen (sometimes laparoscopically), the cervix and upper part of the vagina are removed, leaving the body of the uterus intact (ACS, 2020b).
  6. A *hysterectomy* may be performed as treatment of microinvasive cancer if the woman does not wish to become pregnant in the future.

See Chapter 63 in the main text for more information on cervical cancer.

COLORECTAL CANCER

- Colorectal cancer (CRC) is cancer of the colon or rectum. Patients often consider a diagnosis of cancer as a "death sentence," but colon cancer is highly curable for many patients, especially if diagnosed early.

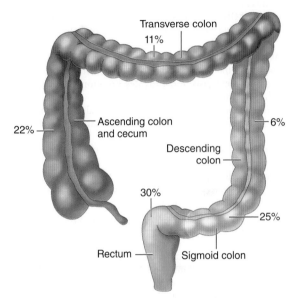

Incidence of cancer in relation to colorectal anatomy.

- Risk factors include:
  1. Age (older than 50 years)
  2. Genetic predisposition
  3. Personal or family history of cancer, and/or diseases that predispose the patient to cancer, such as familial adenomatous polyposis (FAP), Crohn's disease, and ulcerative colitis.

Interprofessional Collaborative Care
Recognize Cues: Assessment

- Assess for:
  1. Changes in bowel elimination habits, such as constipation or change in shape of stool
  2. Rectal bleeding and stool characteristics
  3. Anemia (low hemoglobin level and hematocrit; stool positive for occult blood)

4. Unintentional weight loss (late sign)
5. Abdominal fullness (late sign)

- Diagnostic assessment includes:
  1. Fecal occult blood test (FOBT)
  2. Carcinoembryonic antigen (CEA) blood test
  3. Colonoscopy (definitive test for the diagnosis of colorectal cancer)
  4. CT or MRI of the abdomen with additional views for evaluation of metastasis (pelvis, thorax, and brain)

Take Actions: Interventions

- Nonsurgical management reduces the potential for cancer recurrence and metastasis and provides symptom management and psychosocial support.
- Surgical management with tumor removal is the primary approach to treatment. The most common surgeries performed include:
  1. **Colon resection** (removal of part of the colon and regional lymph nodes) with reanastomosis
  2. **Partial colectomy** with a colostomy (temporary or permanent) or total colectomy with an ileostomy/ileoanal pull-through, and abdominoperineal (AP) resection
  3. **Colostomy** is the surgical creation of an opening (stoma) of the colon onto the surface of the abdomen to allow passage of stool.
     - The patient who has a colostomy may return from surgery with a clear ostomy pouch system in place. A clear pouch allows the health care team to observe the stoma. If no pouch system is in place, a petrolatum gauze dressing is usually placed over the stoma to keep it moist. This is covered with a dry, sterile dressing. In collaboration with the certified wound ostomy and continence nurse (CWOCN), place a pouch system as soon as possible.
     - The colostomy pouch system, also called an *appliance,* allows more convenient and suitable collection of stool than a dressing does. Pouches are available in both one- and two-piece systems and are held in place by adhesive barriers or wafers.
     - Assess the color and integrity of the stoma frequently. A healthy stoma should be reddish pink (or dark red to pink) and moist and protrude between 1 and 3 cm from the abdominal wall but most commonly about ¾ inch (2 cm).
     - During the initial postoperative period, the stoma may be slightly edematous. A small amount of bleeding at the stoma is common. These minor problems tend to resolve within 6 to 8 weeks (Stelton, 2019).

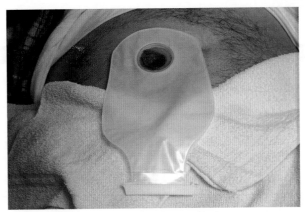

Mature colostomy stoma. (From Stromberg, H. K. [2023]. *Medical-surgical nursing: Concepts and practice* [5th ed.]. St. Louis: Elsevier.)

! **NURSING SAFETY PRIORITY**

Action Alert

Report any of these early postoperative stoma problems to the surgeon:
- Stoma ischemia and necrosis (dark red, purplish, or black color; dry)
- Continuous heavy bleeding
- Mucocutaneous separation (breakdown of the suture line securing the stoma to the abdominal wall)

- Teach the patient and family colostomy care, including:
  1. Normal appearance of a stoma, including size and how to measure size
  2. Signs and symptoms of complications
  3. The choice, use, care, and application of the appropriate appliance to cover the stoma
  4. How to protect the skin adjacent to the stoma
  5. Dietary measures to control gas and odor

See Chapter 48 in the main text for more information on colorectal cancer.

ENDOMETRIAL CANCER

- Endometrial cancer (cancer of the inner lining of the uterus) is the most common gynecologic cancer. Endometrial cancer grows slowly in most cases, and early symptoms of vaginal bleeding generally lead to prompt evaluation and treatment. As a result, this type of cancer has a generally favorable prognosis.

Risk Factors for Endometrial Cancer

- Early menarche or late menopause
- Use of estrogen after menopause
- Use of birth control pills or tamoxifen
- Use of an intrauterine device (IUD)
- Nulliparity
- History of type 2 diabetes, polycystic ovarian syndrome (PCOS), breast or ovarian cancer, or endometrial hyperplasia
- Treatment of the pelvis with radiation therapy
- Obesity; especially if BMI at age 18 was high

Interprofessional Collaborative Care
Recognize Cues: Assessment
The main symptom of endometrial cancer is abnormal uterine bleeding (AUB), especially postmenopausal.

- Ask the patient how many tampons or menstrual pads she uses each day.
- Some women also have a watery, bloody vaginal discharge, or low back, low pelvis, or abdominal *pain* (caused by pressure of the enlarged uterus).
- Ask the patient to describe the exact location and intensity of her discomfort.
- A pelvic examination performed by the health care provider may reveal the presence of a palpable uterine mass or uterine polyp. The uterus is enlarged if the cancer is advanced.
- *Transvaginal ultrasound* and *endometrial biopsy* are the gold standard diagnostic tests to determine the presence of endometrial thickening and cancer

Take Actions: Interventions
- Surgical removal and cancer staging of the tumor with adjacent lymph nodes are the most important interventions for endometrial cancer.
- Home care after surgery for endometrial cancer is the same as that after a hysterectomy.
- Cancer staging is often done using minimally invasive techniques, such as laparoscopic or robotic-assisted procedures.
- Nonsurgical interventions (radiation therapy and chemotherapy) are typically used after surgery and depend on the surgical staging.

See Chapter 63 in the main text for more information on endometrial cancer.

HEAD AND NECK CANCER

- Head and neck cancers are usually squamous cell carcinomas or slow-growing tumors that are curable when diagnosed and treated at an early stage.
- The prognosis for patients who have more advanced disease at diagnosis depends on the extent and location of the tumors.

Warning Signs of Head and Neck Cancer

- Pain
- Lump in the mouth, throat, or neck
- Difficulty swallowing
- Color changes in the mouth or tongue to red, white, gray, dark brown, or black
- Oral lesion or sore that does not heal in 2 weeks
- Persistent or unexplained oral bleeding
- Numbness of the mouth, lips, or face
- Change in the fit of dentures
- Burning sensation when drinking citrus juices or hot liquids
- Persistent, unilateral ear pain
- Hoarseness or change in voice quality
- Persistent or recurrent sore throat
- Shortness of breath
- Anorexia and weight loss

Recognize Cues: Assessment
- Assess for warning signs of head and neck cancer. Also assess:
  1. Tobacco and alcohol use
  2. History of acute or chronic laryngitis or pharyngitis
  3. Oral sores and swallowing difficulty
  4. Oral exposure to human papillomavirus (HPV)

Take Actions: Interventions
- The focus of treatment is to remove or eradicate the cancer while preserving as much function as possible. Surgery, radiation, chemotherapy, or biotherapy may be used alone or in combination, depending on the stage of the disease and the patient's general health, nutritional status, age, and personal choice.
- Treatment for laryngeal cancer may range from radiation therapy (for a small specific area or tumor) to total laryngopharyngectomy with bilateral neck dissections followed by radiation therapy, depending on the extent and location of the lesion.

- Postoperative Care
  1. Head and neck surgery often lasts 8 hours or longer, and the patient spends the immediate period after surgery in the ICU.
  2. Monitor airway patency, vital signs, hemodynamic status, and comfort levels.
  3. The first priorities after head and neck surgery are airway maintenance and ensuring *gas exchange*.
  4. Stoma care after a total laryngectomy is a combination of wound care and airway care.
     - Inspect the stoma and clean the suture line with sterile saline (or a prescribed solution) to prevent secretions from forming crusts and obstructing the airway.
     - Perform suture line care every 1 to 2 hours during the first few days after surgery and then every 4 hours. The mucosa of the stoma and trachea should be bright and shiny and without crusts, similar to the appearance of the oral mucosa.
  5. Tissue "flaps" may be used to close the wound and improve appearance. Flaps are skin, subcutaneous tissue, and sometimes muscle, taken from other body areas used for reconstruction after head and neck resection.
     - The first 24 hours after surgery are critical. Evaluate all grafts and flaps hourly for the first 72 hours.
     - Monitor capillary refill, color, drainage, and Doppler activity of the major blood vessel to the area.
     - Report changes to the surgeon immediately because surgical intervention may be needed.
     - Position the patient so that the surgical flaps are not dependent.
  6. Pain after surgery should be managed while still allowing the patient to be able to participate in care. Morphine often is given IV by a patient-controlled analgesia (PCA) pump for the first 1 to 2 days after surgery.
  7. All patients are at risk for malnutrition during treatment for head and neck cancer. A nasogastric, gastrostomy, or jejunostomy tube is placed during surgery for nutritional support while the head and neck heal, and may remain in place for 7 to 10 days.
  8. The patient's voice quality and speech are altered after surgery. Collaborate with the speech-language pathologist to develop an acceptable communication method.
  9. The surgical changes in the upper respiratory tract and altered swallowing mechanisms increase the patient's risk for

aspiration. Aspiration can result in pneumonia, weight loss, and prolonged hospitalization.

- The supraglottic method of swallowing is used after a swallowing study to exaggerate the normal protective mechanisms during swallowing.

🙌 PATIENT AND FAMILY EDUCATION

The Supraglottic Method of Swallowing

1. Sit in an upright, preferably out-of-bed, position.
2. Clear your throat.
3. Take a deep breath.
4. Place ½ to 1 teaspoon of food into your mouth.
5. Hold your breath or "bear down" (Valsalva maneuver).
6. Swallow twice.
7. Release your breath and clear your throat.
8. Swallow twice again.
9. Breathe normally.

- If no complications occur, the patient is usually discharged home or to an extended-care facility within 2 weeks. At the time of discharge, the patient or a family member should be able to perform tracheostomy or stoma care and participate in nutrition, wound care, and communication methods.

✚ NURSING SAFETY PRIORITY

Critical Rescue

Assess the patient hourly for the first several days after head and neck surgery to recognize a carotid artery leak. If you suspect a leak, respond by calling the Rapid Response Team and **do not touch the area because additional pressure could cause an immediate rupture**. If the carotid artery actually ruptures because of drying or infection, immediately place constant pressure over the site and secure the airway. Maintain direct manual, continuous pressure on the carotid artery, and immediately transport the patient to the operating room for carotid resection. Do not leave the patient. Carotid artery rupture has a high risk for stroke and death.

 See Chapter 23 in the main text for more information on head and neck cancer.

LUNG CANCER

- Lung cancers occur as a result of repeated exposure to inhaled substances that cause chronic tissue irritation or *inflammation,* interfering with *cellular regulation* of cell growth. Cigarette smoking is the major risk factor and is responsible for 81% of all lung cancer deaths (ACS, 2022a).
- Risk factors for lung cancer include:
  1. Cigarette smoking (major risk factor)
  2. Nonsmokers exposed to secondhand smoke
  3. Exposure to environmental elements such as asbestos, beryllium, chromium, coal distillates, cobalt, iron oxide, mustard gas, petroleum distillates, radiation, tar, nickel, and uranium
  4. Air pollution with benzopyrenes and hydrocarbons

Warning Signals Associated With Lung Cancer

- Hoarseness
- Change in respiratory pattern
- Persistent cough or change in cough
- Blood-streaked sputum
- Rust-colored or purulent sputum
- Frank hemoptysis
- Chest pain or chest tightness
- Shoulder, arm, or chest wall pain
- Recurring episodes of pleural effusion, pneumonia, or bronchitis
- Dyspnea
- Fever associated with one or two other signs
- Wheezing
- Weight loss
- Clubbing of the fingers

Recognize Cues: Assessment

- Assess for warning signs associated with lung cancer.
- In addition to pulmonary signs and symptoms, assess for nonpulmonary signs, including:
  1. Cardiac tamponade (muffled heard sounds)
  2. Dysrhythmias
  3. Cyanosis of the lips or clubbing of the fingers
  4. Bone pain or pathologic fractures
  5. Late symptoms: fatigue, weight loss, anorexia, dysphagia, and nausea and vomiting

- Most commonly, lung lesions are first identified on chest x-rays. CT scans are then used to identify the lesions more clearly. The definitive diagnosis of lung cancer is made by examination of cancer cells from biopsy.

Take Actions: Interventions

- Interventions for the patient with lung cancer can have the purpose of curing the disease, increasing survival time, or enhancing quality of life through palliation. Both nonsurgical and surgical interventions are used to achieve these purposes.
- Nonsurgical Management
  1. Chemotherapy
  2. Immunotherapy
  3. Targeted therapy
  4. Radiation therapy
- Surgical Management
  1. Lobectomy: removal of a lobe of the lung
  2. Pneumonectomy: removal of the entire lung
     - Complications of a pneumonectomy include *empyema* (purulent material in the pleural space) and development of a bronchopleural *fistula* (an abnormal duct that develops between the bronchial tree and the pleura).
     - Positioning of the patient after pneumonectomy varies according to surgeon preference and the patient's comfort. Some surgeons want the patient placed on the nonoperative side immediately after a pneumonectomy to reduce stress on the bronchial stump incision. Others prefer to place the patient on the operative side to allow fluids to fill in the now empty space.
  3. Removal of just the tumor or lung segment
     - Postoperative care: For patients who have undergone thoracotomy (except for pneumonectomy), a closed-chest drain is required to drain air and blood that collect in the pleural space.
       - A chest tube drain placed in the pleural space allows lung reexpansion and prevents air and fluid from returning to the chest.
       - The drainage system consists of one or more chest tubes or drains, a collection container placed below the chest level, and a water seal to keep air from entering the chest.
       - The nursing care priorities for the patient with a chest tube are to ensure the integrity of the system, promote comfort, ensure chest tube patency, and prevent complications

- The bubbling of the water in the water-seal chamber indicates air drainage from the patient. Bubbling is seen when intrathoracic pressure is greater than atmospheric pressure, such as when the patient exhales, coughs, or sneezes. When the air in the pleural space has been removed, bubbling stops.
- A blocked or kinked chest tube also can cause bubbling to stop.
- Excessive bubbling in the water-seal chamber may indicate an air leak.
- The water in the water-seal chamber column normally rises 2 to 4 inches during inhalation and falls during exhalation, a process called *tidaling*.

! NURSING SAFETY PRIORITY
Action Alert

For a water-seal chest tube drainage system, 2 cm of water is the minimum needed in the water seal to prevent air from flowing backward into the patient. Check the water level every shift, and add sterile water to this chamber to the level marked on the indicator (specified by the manufacturer of the drainage system).

⟫ BEST PRACTICE FOR PATIENT SAFETY AND QUALITY CARE
Management of Chest Tube Drainage System

Patient
- Ensure that the dressing on the chest around the tube is tight and intact. Depending on agency policy and the surgeon's preference, reinforce or change loose dressings.
- Assess for difficulty breathing.
- Assess breathing effectiveness by pulse oximetry.
- Listen to breath sounds for each lung.
- Check alignment of trachea.
- Check tube insertion site for condition of the skin. Palpate area for puffiness or crackling that may indicate subcutaneous emphysema.
- Observe site for signs of infection (redness/hyperpigmentation, purulent drainage) or excessive bleeding.
- Check to see if tube "eyelets" are visible (they should not be visible).
- Assess for pain and its location and intensity, and administer drugs for pain as prescribed.
- Assist patient to deep breathe, cough, perform maximal sustained inhalations, and use incentive spirometry.
- Reposition the patient who reports a "burning" pain in the chest.

BEST PRACTICE FOR PATIENT SAFETY AND QUALITY CARE—cont'd

Management of Chest Tube Drainage System

Drainage System
- Do not "strip" the chest tube; use a hand-over-hand "milking" motion.
- Keep drainage system lower than the level of the patient's chest.
- Keep the chest tube as straight as possible from the bed to the suction unit, avoiding kinks and dependent loops. Extra tubing can be loosely coiled on the bed.
- Ensure that the chest tube is securely taped to the connector and that the connector is taped to the tubing going into the collection chamber.
- Assess bubbling in the water-seal chamber; you should see gentle bubbling on the patient's exhalation, forceful cough, or position changes.
- Assess for "tidaling" (rise and fall of water in chamber three with breathing).
- Check water level in the water-seal chamber, and keep at the level recommended by the manufacturer.
- Check water level in the suction control chamber, and keep at the level prescribed by the surgeon (unless a dry suction system is used).
- Clamp the chest tube only for brief periods to change the drainage system or when checking for air leaks.
- Check and document amount, color, and characteristics of fluid in the collection chamber as often as needed, according to the patient's condition and agency policy.
- Empty the collection chamber or change the system before the drainage makes contact with the bottom of the tube.
- When a sample of drainage is needed for culture or other laboratory test, obtain it from the chest tube; after cleaning the chest tube, use a 20-gauge (or smaller) needle and draw up a specimen into a syringe.

Immediately Notify Surgeon or Rapid Response Team for:
- Tracheal deviation
- Sudden onset or increased intensity of dyspnea
- Oxygen saturation of less than 90%
- Drainage greater than 70 mL/hr
- Visible eyelets on chest tube
- Chest tube falls out of the patient's chest (first, cover the area with dry, sterile gauze)
- Chest tube disconnects from the drainage system (first, put end of tube in a container of sterile water and keep below the level of the patient's chest)
- Drainage in tube stops (in the first 24 hours)

C

Palliation Interventions

- *Oxygen therapy* is prescribed when the patient is hypoxemic and helps relieve dyspnea and anxiety.
- *Radiation therapy* can help relieve hemoptysis, obstruction of the bronchi and great veins (superior vena cava syndrome), difficulty swallowing from esophageal compression, and pain from bone metastasis. Radiation for palliation uses higher doses for shorter periods.
- *Thoracentesis* is performed when pleural effusion is a problem for the patient with lung cancer. The excess fluid increases dyspnea, discomfort, and the risk for infection. The purpose of treatment is to remove pleural fluid and prevent its formation.
- *Dyspnea management* is needed because the patient with lung cancer tires easily and is often most comfortable resting in a semi-Fowler's position. Dyspnea is reduced with oxygen, use of a continuous morphine infusion, and positioning for comfort.
- *Pain management* is usually to help the patient be as pain free and comfortable as possible. Pharmacologic management with opioid drugs as oral, parenteral, or transdermal preparations is needed. Analgesics are most effective when given around the clock, with additional PRN analgesics used for breakthrough pain.
- *Hospice care* can be beneficial for the patient in the terminal phase of lung cancer.

See Chapter 24 in the main text for more information on lung cancer.

OVARIAN CANCER

- Ovarian cancer is the leading cause of gynecologic cancer death, and the second most common type of gynecologic cancer in the United States (Chen & Berek, 2023). Most ovarian cancers are epithelial tumors that grow on the surface of the ovaries. These tumors grow rapidly, spread quickly, and are often bilateral.
- Risk factors include:
  1. Older age
  2. Obesity
  3. Nulliparity
  4. Use of estrogen with or without progesterone after menopause
  5. Women with genetic mutations of *BCRA1* or *BCRA2*

Interprofessional Collaborative Care
Recognize Cues: Assessment

- Assess for early signs, including bloating, urinary urgency, difficulty eating or feeling full, and pelvic pain.
- Assess for unexpected weight loss and/or vaginal bleeding.

Take Actions: Interventions

- The options for treatment depend on the extent of the cancer; these options usually include surgery first, followed by chemotherapy. A total abdominal hysterectomy, bilateral salpingo-oophorectomy (BSO; removal of the ovaries and fallopian tubes), and pelvic and para-aortic lymph node dissection are usually performed.

 See Chapter 63 in the main text for more information on ovarian cancer.

PANCREATIC CANCER

- Cancer of the pancreas is difficult to diagnose early because the pancreas is hidden and surrounded by other organs. Most often, the tumor is discovered in the late stages of development and may be a well-defined mass or diffusely spread throughout the pancreas. Treatment has limited results, and 5-year survival rates are low (ACS, 2021a).
- The tumor may be a primary cancer, or it may result from metastasis from cancers of the lung, breast, thyroid, kidney, or skin.

Risk Factors Associated With Pancreatic Cancer

- Smoking and tobacco use
- Obesity
- Chronic pancreatitis
- Cirrhosis
- Older age (over 65 years)
- Genetic syndromes

Interprofessional Collaborative Care

Recognize Cues: Assessment

- Pancreatic cancer often presents in a slow and vague manner. The presenting symptoms depend somewhat on the location of the tumor. The first sign may be jaundice, which suggests late, advanced disease. Assess for key features of pancreatic cancer.

KEY FEATURES

Pancreatic Cancer

- Jaundice
- Icterus
- Clay-colored (light) stools
- Dark urine
- Abdominal *pain*: usually vague, dull, or nonspecific that radiates into the back
- Weight loss
- Anorexia
- Nausea or vomiting
- Glucose intolerance
- Splenomegaly (enlarged spleen)
- Flatulence
- Gastrointestinal bleeding
- New-onset diabetes mellitus
- Ascites (abdominal fluid)
- Leg or calf pain (from thrombophlebitis)
- Weakness and fatigue

Take Actions: Interventions

- Management of the patient with pancreatic cancer is geared toward preventing tumor spread and decreasing pain. These measures are not curative, only palliative. The cancers are often metastatic and recur despite treatment.
- Nonsurgical Management includes:
  1. Chemotherapy
  2. Radiation
  3. Targeted therapy
  4. Opioid analgesic for pain control
- Surgical Management includes:
  1. Partial pancreatectomy
  2. Radical pancreatectomy
  3. Whipple procedure (pancreaticoduodenectomy)
     - An extensive surgical procedure used most often to treat cancer of the head of the pancreas. The procedure entails removal of the proximal head of the pancreas, the duodenum, a portion of the jejunum, the stomach (partial or total *gastrectomy*), and the gallbladder, with anastomosis of the pancreatic duct (*pancreaticojejunostomy*), the common bile duct (*choledochojejunostomy*), and the stomach (*gastrojejunostomy*) to the jejunum. In addition, the surgeon may remove the spleen (**splenectomy**).

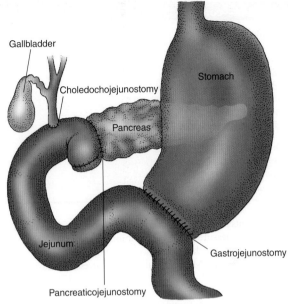

The three anastomoses that constitute the Whipple procedure: choledochojejunostomy, pancreaticojejunostomy, and gastrojejunostomy.

Potential Complications of the Whipple Procedure

Cardiovascular Complications
- Hemorrhage at anastomosis sites with hypovolemia
- Myocardial infarction
- Heart failure
- Thrombophlebitis

Pulmonary Complications
- Atelectasis
- Pneumonia
- Pulmonary embolism
- Acute respiratory distress syndrome
- Pulmonary edema

Endocrine/Renal Complications
- Unstable diabetes mellitus
- Chronic kidney disease

Continued

Potential Complications of the Whipple Procedure—cont'd

GI Complications
- Adynamic (paralytic) ileus
- Gastric retention
- Gastric ulceration
- Bowel obstruction from peritonitis
- Acute pancreatitis
- Hepatic failure
- Thrombosis to mesentery

Integumentary Complications
- Infection
- Dehiscence
- Fistulas: pancreatic, gastric, and biliary

- For patients having a surgical procedure, observe for and implement preventive measures for these common surgical complications:
  1. Diabetes (Check blood glucose often.)
  2. Hemorrhage (Monitor pulse, blood pressure, skin color, and mental status [e.g., level of consciousness (LOC)].)
  3. Wound infection (Monitor temperature and assess wounds for redness/hyperpigmentation and induration [hardness].)
  4. Bowel obstruction (Check bowel sounds and stools.)
  5. Intraabdominal abscess (Monitor temperature and patient's report of severe pain.)
- Immediately after surgery the patient is NPO and usually has a nasogastric tube (NGT) to decompress the stomach.
  1. Assess the tubes and drainage devices for tension or kinking, and maintain them in a dependent position.
  2. Monitor the drainage for color, consistency, and amount. The drainage should be serosanguineous.
  3. Place the patient in the semi-Fowler's position to reduce tension on the suture line and to optimize lung expansion.
  4. Observe for fistula formation and excoriation (Drainage of pancreatic fluids is corrosive and irritating to the skin; internal leakage causes peritonitis.)
- The stage of progression of pancreatic cancer and available home care resources determine whether the patient can be discharged to home or whether additional care is needed in a skilled nursing facility or with a hospice provider.

See Chapter 51 in the main text for more information on pancreatic cancer.

PROSTATE CANCER: CELLULAR REGULATION CONCEPT ✳ EXEMPLAR

Overview
- Prostate cancer is the most diagnosed non-skin cancer in men in the United States (Rogers, 2023).
- Men older than 65 years have the greatest risk for the disease (Rogers, 2023), with the average age of diagnosis at 66 (ACS, 2022a).
- Of all malignancies, prostate cancer is one of the slowest growing, and it metastasizes (spreads) in a predictable pattern.
- Common sites of metastasis are the nearby lymph nodes, bones, lungs, and liver.

Interprofessional Collaborative Care
Recognize Cues: Assessment
- Assess for risk, signs, and symptoms of prostate cancer, including:
  1. Changes in elimination, such as difficulty starting urination, frequent bladder infections, urinary retention, frequency, hematuria, or nocturia
  2. Pain during intercourse
  3. Pain in the pelvis, hips, spine, and legs (associated with advanced prostate cancer)
- Diagnostic assessment for cancer and metastasis may include:
  1. Digital rectal exam (DRE)
  2. Prostate-specific antigen (PSA) analysis. *Because other prostate problems also increase the PSA level, it is not specifically diagnostic for cancer.* Levels greater than 4 ng/mL have been noted in more than 80% of men with prostate cancer (Pagana et al., 2022).
  3. Transrectal ultrasound of the prostate; if cancer is suspected, a biopsy can be performed.

❗ NURSING SAFETY PRIORITY

Action Alert

After a transrectal ultrasound with biopsy, instruct the patient about possible complications, although rare, including hematuria with clots, signs of **infection**, and perineal pain. Teach the patient to report fever, chills, bloody urine, and any difficulty voiding. Advise him to avoid strenuous physical activity and to drink plenty of fluids, especially in the first 24 hours after the procedure. Teach him that a small amount of bleeding turning the urine pink is expected during this time. However, bright red bleeding should be reported to the health care provider immediately.

Analyze Cues and Prioritize Hypotheses: Analysis

- The priority collaborative problem for the patient with prostate cancer is:
  1. Potential for cancer metastasis due to lack of, or inadequate, treatment

Generate Solutions and Take Actions: Planning and Implementation
Preventing Metastasis

- Active Surveillance: Because prostate cancer is slow growing with late metastasis, older men who are asymptomatic may choose observation without immediate active treatment, an option known as *active surveillance (AS)*.
  1. The average time from diagnosis to start of treatment is up to 10 years.
  2. During the AS period, men are monitored at regular intervals through DRE and PSA testing.

Nonsurgical Management
- Nonsurgical Management includes:
  1. Radiation Therapy
     - *External beam radiation therapy (EBRT)* comes from a source outside the body. Patients are usually treated 5 days a week for a minimum of several weeks.
     - *Low-dose brachytherapy* is a type of internal radiation that is delivered by implanting low-dose radiation "seeds" (the size of a grain of rice) directly into the prostate gland. This treatment involves transrectal ultrasound, CT scans, or MRI, which are used to guide implantation of the seeds. These procedures are usually done on an ambulatory care basis under spinal or general anesthesia, and are the most cost-effective treatment for early-stage prostate cancer.
  2. Drug Therapy: may consist of either hormone therapy (androgen deprivation therapy [ADT]) or chemotherapy
     - Hormone therapy: *luteinizing hormone-releasing hormone (LHRH) agonists* such as leuprolide, goserelin, histrelin, and triptorelin stimulate the pituitary gland to release the luteinizing hormone (LH); once LH is depleted, testosterone production in testes decreases.
     - *Androgen receptor blockers (also known as anti-androgen drugs)* block the body's and tumor's ability to use the available androgens. Examples include flutamide, bicalutamide, and nilutamide.

NURSING SAFETY PRIORITY
Drug Alert

Teach patients taking LHRH agonists that side effects include "hot flashes," which usually decrease as treatment progresses. The subsequent reduction in testosterone may contribute to erectile dysfunction and decreased libido. Some men also develop **gynecomastia** (abnormal enlargement of the breasts in men). These drugs can also increase the patient's risk for osteoporosis and fractures. Teach the patient to take calcium and vitamin D, and to engage in regular weight-bearing exercise. Bisphosphonates can be prescribed to prevent bone fractures.

Surgical Management
- Surgery is the most common intervention for a cure.
  1. Minimally invasive surgery (MIS) or, less commonly, an open surgical technique for radical prostatectomy (prostate removal) can be performed.
  2. Bilateral orchiectomy (removal of both testicles) is another palliative surgery that slows the spread of cancer by removing the main source of testosterone.

BEST PRACTICE FOR PATIENT SAFETY AND QUALITY CARE
Care of the Patient After an Open Radical Prostatectomy

- Encourage the patient to use patient-controlled analgesia (PCA) as needed.
- Help the patient to get out of bed into a chair on the night of surgery and to ambulate by the next day.
- Maintain the sequential compression device until the patient begins to ambulate.
- Monitor the patient for venous thromboembolism and pulmonary embolus.
- Keep an accurate record of intake and output, including drainage from a Jackson-Pratt or other drainage device.
- Keep the urinary meatus clean using soap and water.
- Avoid rectal procedures or treatments.
- Emphasize the importance of not straining during a bowel movement. Teach the patient to avoid suppositories or enemas.
- Remind the patient about the importance of follow-up appointments with the surgeon and oncologist to monitor progress.
- For patients who had an open procedure, teach them how to care for the urinary catheter at home; the catheter will be in place for 1 to 2 weeks.

Care Coordination and Transition Management

- Collaborate with the case manager to coordinate the efforts of various primary health care providers and possibly a home care nurse.
- Include Health Teaching about:
  1. Indwelling urinary catheter care if recovering from an open procedure
  2. Restrictions for activity or weight lifting; these may be as brief as 2 to 3 days for minimally invasive procedures or as long as 6 weeks for open surgical procedures
  3. Teach the patient to avoid straining at defecation until surgical sites have healed.
  4. Refer patients with ED or urinary incontinence to a urologist or other specialist.

Evaluate Outcomes: Evaluation

- Evaluate the care of the patient with prostate cancer based on the identified priority patient problem.
- The primary expected outcome is that the patient with prostate cancer is expected to remain free of metastases or recurrence of disease, if possible.

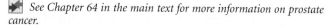 *See Chapter 64 in the main text for more information on prostate cancer.*

SKIN CANCER

- Overexposure to sunlight is the major cause of skin cancer, although other factors also are associated.
- The most common precancerous lesions are:
  1. Actinic (solar) keratoses—premalignant lesions of the cells of the epidermis. These appear as pink, reddish, or reddish-brown scaly macules or papules.

- The most common skin cancers are:
  1. Squamous cell carcinoma—cancer of the epidermis
  2. Basal cell carcinoma—arising from the basal cell layer of the epidermis; the most common skin cancer worldwide (Rogers, 2023)
  3. Melanoma-pigmented cancers, arising in the melanin-producing epidermal cells

C

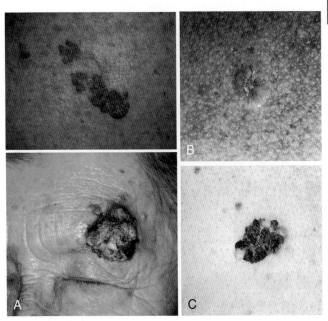

(A) Varying presentations of squamous cell carcinoma. **(B)** Basal cell carcinoma, **(C)** Melanoma. (B from Bolognia, J.L., Jorizzo, J.L., & Schaffer, J.V. [2012]. *Dermatology* [3rd ed.]. St. Louis: Saunders.)

Interprofessional Collaborative Care

- The patient with skin cancer, depending on the degree of cancer and associated health concerns, may be treated in the hospital, ambulatory surgical, or outpatient setting.

Recognize Cues: Assessment

* Assess for:
  1. Family history of skin cancer
  2. Past surgery for removal of skin growths
  3. Recent changes in size, color, or sensation of any mole, birthmark, wart, or scar
  4. Assess for geographical region, occupational exposure (arsenic, coal tar, pitch, radioactive waste, radium), or recreational activities in relation to sun exposure

Take Actions: Interventions

* Treatment is determined by the size and severity of the malignancy, the location of the lesion, and the age and general health of the patient.
  1. Prepare patients for self-management by teaching steps to avoid skin cancer, particularly avoiding exposure to sun and examining one's body for changes in spots, moles, scars, and other lesions.
  2. Advise patients to seek medical advice if they notice changes in skin, particularly changes in color, rapid growth, swelling around a lesion, or new bleeding or draining near a lesion.

See Chapter 21 in the main text for more information on skin cancer.

UROTHELIAL (BLADDER) CANCER

* Urothelial cancers are malignant tumors of the *urothelium,* which is the lining of transitional cells in the kidney, renal pelvis, ureters, urinary bladder, and urethra. Most urothelial cancers occur in the bladder, and the term *bladder cancer* describes this condition. Urothelial cancer is also known as transitional cell carcinoma (TCC).
  1. Tumors confined to the bladder mucosa are treated by simple excision.
  2. Tumors that are deeper but not into the muscle layer are treated with excision plus **intravesical** (inside the bladder) chemotherapy.
  3. Cancer that has spread deeper into the bladder muscle layer is treated with more extensive surgery, often a **radical cystectomy**

(removal of the bladder and surrounding tissue) with urinary diversion.
4. Chemotherapy and radiation therapy are used in addition to surgery.

Interprofessional Collaborative Care
Recognize Cues: Assessment
- Examine the urine for color and clarity. Blood in the urine is often the first indication of bladder cancer. It may be gross or microscopic and is usually painless and intermittent. Dysuria, frequency, and urgency occur when infection or obstruction is also present.
- Cystoscopy is usually performed to evaluate painless hematuria. A biopsy of a visible bladder tumor can be performed during cystoscopy.

Take Actions: Interventions
- Therapy for the patient with bladder cancer usually begins with surgical removal of the tumor for diagnosis and staging of disease.
  1. For tumors extending beyond the mucosa, surgery is followed by intravesical chemotherapy or immunotherapy.
  2. High-grade or recurrent tumors are treated with more radical surgery plus intravesical chemotherapy, radiotherapy, or both.
  3. The type of surgery for bladder cancer depends on the type and stage of the cancer and the patient's general health.
     - Transurethral resection of the bladder tumor (TURBT) or partial cystectomy is performed for small, early, superficial tumors, and only a portion of the bladder is removed.
     - When the entire bladder must be removed (complete cystectomy), the ureters are diverted into a collecting reservoir.
     - With an ileal conduit, the ureters are surgically placed in the ileum, and urine is collected in a pouch on the skin around the stoma.
     - More often, a continent reservoir known as a "neobladder" is created from an intestinal graft to store urine and replace the surgically removed bladder.
     - With cutaneous ureterostomy or ureteroureterostomy, the ureter opening is brought out onto the skin. The cutaneous ureterostomies may be located on either side of the abdomen or side by side.
     - Different types of drains and nephrostomy catheters are used, sometimes on a temporary basis, to drain urine from the kidney. Some are totally internal, with no drainage to the outside. Others may drain exclusively to the outside,

and urine is collected in a pouch or bag. For this type of drainage system, urine output remains constant. Decreased or no drainage is cause for concern and is reported to the surgeon or nephrologist, as is leakage around the catheter.

❗ NURSING SAFETY PRIORITY

Action Alert

Infection is common in patients who have a neobladder. Teach patients and family members the symptoms of infection and the importance of reporting them immediately to the surgeon.

Instruct the patient and family about any changes in self-care activities related to the urinary diversion. In collaboration with the enterostomal therapist, demonstrate external pouch application, local skin care, pouch care, methods of adhesion, and drainage mechanisms. If a Kock pouch has been created, teach the patient how to use a catheter to drain the pouch. For all instruction, observe at least one return demonstration or "teach-back" session by the patient or the caregiver. Ideally the patient assumes responsibility for self-care before discharge.

See Chapter 58 in the main text for more information on urothelial (bladder) cancer.

CARDIAC TAMPONADE

- Acute cardiac tamponade may occur when small volumes (20 to 30 mL) of fluid accumulate in the pericardium.
- It is a medical emergency and requires prompt confirmation with an echocardiogram and primary health care provider intervention.

Interprofessional Collaborative Care

- Signs and symptoms of cardiac tamponade include:
  1. Paradoxical pulse *(pulsus paradoxus)*
  2. Jugular venous distention
  3. Tachycardia
  4. Muffled heart sounds
  5. Hypotension
- Anticipate emergent interventions of IV fluid administration and *pericardiocentesis,* or insertion of a long large-bore needle by the provider into the pericardium to remove fluid.

See Chapter 29 in the main text for more information on cardiac tamponade.

CARDIOMYOPATHY

- Cardiomyopathy is a subacute or chronic heart muscle disease.
- Cardiomyopathy is divided into four categories on the basis of abnormalities in structure and function.
  1. *Dilated cardiomyopathy* (DCM), the most common type, involves extensive damage to the myofibrils and interference with myocardial metabolism; both ventricles are dilated and systolic function is impaired.
  2. *Hypertrophic cardiomyopathy* (HCM) is characterized by asymmetric ventricular hypertrophy and disarray of the myocardial fibers, resulting in a stiff left ventricle and diastolic filling abnormalities. HCM is transmitted as a single-gene autosomal dominant trait.
  3. *Restrictive cardiomyopathy* (RCM), the rarest of the four cardiomyopathies, is caused by ventricles that restrict filling during diastole. The disease can be primary or caused by endocardial or myocardial disease, such as sarcoidosis or amyloidosis.
  4. *Arrhythmogenic right ventricular* (ARV) *cardiomyopathy* (dysplasia) results from replacement of myocardial tissue with fibrous and fatty tissue, usually as a familial condition, and, despite the name, can affect both the right and left ventricles.

Interprofessional Collaborative Care
Recognize Cues: Assessment
- Assess for signs and symptoms of cardiomyopathy.
  1. Signs of reduced cardiac output, manifested by dyspnea on exertion, decreased exercise capacity, fatigue, and palpitations
  2. Dizziness or syncope
  3. Irregular pulse and abnormal or irregular heart rhythms, especially atrial fibrillation and ventricular dysrhythmias
  4. Some patients die without any symptoms; this is one type of sudden cardiac death.
  5. Left or biventricular heart failure
  6. Enlarged heart on CXR and echocardiography

Take Actions: Interventions
- Care of the patient with cardiomyopathy is similar to that for patients with heart failure (see *Heart Failure*) and dysrhythmias.

Nonsurgical Management
- Care includes:
  1. Administering diuretics, vasodilating agents, and cardiac glycosides to increase cardiac output
  2. Administering antidysrhythmics and agents to slow HR
  3. Providing an implantable defibrillator or defibrillator-pacemaker to control dysrhythmias

Surgical Management
- The type of surgery performed depends on the type of cardiomyopathy.
  1. Ventricular septal myectomy is the excision of a portion of the hypertrophied ventricular septum to create a widened outflow tract. This is the most common surgical treatment for obstructive HCM.
  2. Percutaneous alcohol septal ablation is another option for HCM; it is used to improve forward flow of ventricular blood into the aorta.
  3. Heart transplantation is the treatment of choice for patients with severe DCM; a donor heart from a person of comparable body weight and ABO compatibility is transplanted into a recipient within 6 hours of procurement.
- For the patient who receives a heart transplant, provide postoperative care similar to patients who undergo open heart surgery and organ transplantation.

See Chapter 29 in the main text for more information on cardiomyopathy.

CARDITIS, RHEUMATIC (RHEUMATIC ENDOCARDITIS)

- *Rheumatic carditis (rheumatic endocarditis)* develops after an infection with group A beta-hemolytic streptococci in some individuals.
- Inflammation is evident in all layers of the heart and results in impaired contractile function of the myocardium, thickening of the pericardium, and inflamed endocardium, leading to inflammation of valve leaflets and valvular damage.

Interprofessional Collaborative Care

- Common signs and symptoms include:
  1. Evidence of an existing streptococcal infection: moderate-to-high fever, abrupt onset of sore throat, reddened throat with exudate, enlarged and tender lymph nodes
  2. Tachycardia, cardiomegaly, new-onset murmur, pericardial friction rub, precordial pain, ECG changes, and indications of heart failure
- Management includes antibiotic therapy to manage streptococcal infection and follow-up care to manage heart valve or heart damage (see *Valvular Heart Disease* and *Cardiomyopathy*).

See Chapter 29 in the main text for more information on carditis (rheumatic).

CARPAL TUNNEL SYNDROME

- Carpal tunnel syndrome (CTS) is a condition in which the median nerve in the wrist becomes compressed, causing pain and numbness.
- Risk factors include common repetitive stress injury (RSI), synovitis, excessive hand exercise, edema or hemorrhage into the carpal tunnel, thrombosis of the median artery, Colles fracture of the wrist, and hand burns. CTS is also a common complication of certain metabolic and connective tissue diseases.

Interprofessional Collaborative Care
Recognize Cues: Assessment

- Common signs and symptoms include:
  1. Positive results for the Phalen maneuver, producing paresthesia in the palmar side of the thumb, index, and middle finger and radial half of the ring finger within 60 seconds; the patient is asked to relax the wrist into flexion or place the back of the hands together and flex both wrists simultaneously
  2. Weak pinch, clumsiness, and difficulty with fine movements, which progress to muscle weakness, progressing further to muscle wasting in the affected hand
  3. Wrist swelling and autonomic changes, such as skin discoloration, nail brittleness, and increased or decreased palmar sweating

Take Actions: Interventions
Nonsurgical Management
- Drug therapy with NSAIDs
- Wrist immobilization with a splint or brace to place the wrist in a neutral position or slight extension during the day, during the night, or both

Surgical Management
- Surgery is performed to relieve the pressure on the median nerve by cutting or laser.
  Postoperative Care
- Check the dressing for drainage and tightness and the hand and fingers for neurovascular status.
- Explain to the patient that hand movements may be restricted for 4 to 6 weeks and that discomfort can last that long or longer.

See Chapter 44 in the main text for more information on carpal tunnel syndrome.

✴ CATARACT: SENSORY PERCEPTION CONCEPT EXEMPLAR

Overview
- A cataract is a lens opacity that distorts the image projected onto the retina, reducing visual sensory perception.
- Cataracts can occur at any age; they may be caused by trauma or exposure to toxic agents, result from comorbidities such as diabetes, or occur with aging.

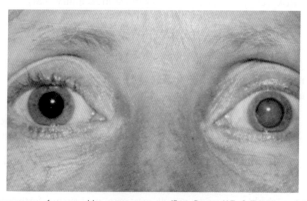

Appearance of an eye with a mature cataract. (From Patton, K.T., & Thibodeau, G.A. [2016]. *Anatomy and physiology* [9th ed.]. St. Louis: Elsevier.)

Interprofessional Collaborative Care
Recognize Cues: Assessment
- Assess the patient for:
  1. Family history for cataracts and exposure to lens-damaging drugs or toxins
  2. Visual acuity (You might say: "Tell me what you can see well and what you have difficulty seeing.")
  3. Decreased color perception or difficulty driving at night

Analyze Cues and Prioritize Hypotheses: Analysis
- The priority collaborative problem for patients with cataracts is:
  1. Impaired visual *sensory perception* due to cataracts

Generate Solutions and Take Actions: Planning and Implementation
- The priority problem for the patient with cataracts is impaired visual *sensory perception*, which is a safety risk. Patients often live with reduced vision for years before the cataract is removed.

Improving Vision
- Surgery is the only cure for cataracts. However, patients often live with reduced vision for years before the cataract is removed. Driving privileges may be restricted or withheld during this period of reduced vision.
  1. The most common surgical procedure is removal of the lens by phacoemulsification and replacement with a clear plastic lens for specific vision correction.
  2. Stress that care after surgery requires the instillation of different types of eye drops several times each day for 2 to 4 weeks.
  3. Instruct the patient on the importance of following the prescribed regimen for eye drops after surgery.
  4. Instruct the patient to notify the surgeon if there is significant swelling or bruising around the eye; pain occurring with nausea or vomiting; increasing redness of the eye; a change in visual acuity, tears, or photophobia; or yellow or green drainage.

! NURSING SAFETY PRIORITY
Action Alert

Instruct the patient who has had cataract surgery to immediately report any reduction of vision in the eye that just had the cataract removed.

Care Coordination and Transition Management
- Help the patient and family plan the eye drop schedule and daily home eye examination.
- Review these indications of complications after cataract surgery with the patient and family:
  1. Sharp, sudden pain in the eye
  2. Bleeding or increased discharge
  3. Thick green or yellow drainage
  4. Lid swelling
  5. Reappearance of a bloodshot sclera after the initial appearance has cleared
  6. Decreased vision
  7. Flashes of light or floating shapes

- Teach the patient to avoid activities that might increase intraocular pressure (IOP). Also teach regarding activity restrictions such as vacuuming because of the forward flexion involved and rapid, jerky movements.

Evaluate Outcomes: Evaluation
- Evaluate the care of the patient with cataracts on the basis of improving visual *sensory perception*. The expected outcomes include that the patient will have improved visual *sensory perception* following surgery and recognize signs and symptoms of complications.

 See Chapter 39 in the main text for more information on cataracts.

CELIAC DISEASE

- Celiac disease is a multisystem autoimmune disease that has cycles of remission and exacerbation characterized by inflammation of small intestinal mucosa, leading to malabsorption syndrome.
- Like other autoimmune inflammatory conditions, it is thought to be caused by a combination of genetic, immunologic, and environmental factors.
- Symptoms include anorexia; diarrhea and/or constipation; steatorrhea (fatty stools); abdominal pain, distention, and weight loss.

Interprofessional Collaborative Care
- Dietary management with a gluten-free diet promotes disease remission.

 See Chapter 49 in the main text for more information on celiac disease.

CHLAMYDIA INFECTION

- *Chlamydia trachomatis* is an intracellular bacterium and the causative agent of cervicitis (in women), urethritis, and proctitis.
- The incubation period ranges from 1 to 3 weeks, but the pathogen may be present in the genital tract for months without producing symptoms. Many infected persons are asymptomatic.
- *C. trachomatis is reportable to local health departments in all states.* In the United States, it is the most frequently reported bacterial sexually transmitted *infection* (CDC, 2022a).
- Men may report penile discharge, urinary frequency, and dysuria.

- Women may have no symptoms or report a mucopurulent vaginal discharge, urinary frequency, and abdominal discomfort or pain. Cervical bleeding may present as spotting between menses and after intercourse. Complications include salpingitis, pelvic inflammatory disease (PID), ectopic pregnancy, infertility, and complications with a newborn that is delivered.

Interprofessional Collaborative Care
Recognize Cues: Assessment

C

- Ask the patient about:
  1. Presence of symptoms, including vaginal or urethral discharge, **dysuria** (painful urination), pelvic *pain,* and any irregular bleeding (for women)
  2. A history of sexually transmitted infections (STIs)
  3. Whether current or past sexual partners have had symptoms or a history of STIs
  4. Whether the patient has had a new partner, or multiple sexual partners
  5. Whether the patient or a current or recent partner has had unprotected intercourse

Take Actions: Interventions
- The primary treatment is antibiotic therapy with doxycycline; other agents can be used.
- Test and treat sexual partners.
- Educate patients about:
  1. The mode of disease transmission and incubation period
  2. Manifestation, including the possibility of asymptomatic infections
  3. Essential elements of treatment with antibiotic
  4. The need for abstinence from sexual intercourse until the patient and partner have completed treatment
  5. No test of cure is required, but all women should be rescreened 3 months after treatment because of the high risk for PID
  6. The need for the patient and partner to return for evaluation if symptoms recur or new symptoms develop

See Chapter 65 in the main text for more information on chlamydia infection.

✴ CHOLECYSTITIS: INFLAMMATION CONCEPT EXEMPLAR

Overview
- Cholecystitis is an *inflammation* of the gallbladder that can occur as an acute or chronic process and results in and alters *nutrition*.
- Acute calculous cholecystitis usually develops in association with cholelithiasis (gallstones).
  1. Gallstones are composed of substances normally found in bile, such as cholesterol, bilirubin, bile salts, calcium, and various proteins.
  2. Gallstones are classified as either cholesterol stones or pigment stones.
- Acalculous cholecystitis occurs in the absence of gallstones and is associated with biliary stasis caused by any condition that affects the regular filling or emptying of the gallbladder, such as decreased blood flow to the gallbladder, or anatomic problems, such as kinking of the gallbladder neck or cystic duct that can result in pancreatic enzyme reflux into the gallbladder.
- Chronic cholecystitis results when repeated episodes of cystic duct obstruction result in chronic *inflammation*, and the gallbladder becomes fibrotic and contracted, resulting in decreased motility and deficient absorption.
- Complications of cholecystitis include pancreatitis and cholangitis (*inflammation* of the bile ducts).
- Jaundice (yellow discoloration of body tissues) and icterus (yellow discoloration of the sclera) can occur in acute disease but are most commonly seen in the chronic form of cholecystitis. Jaundice results from increased bilirubin in the body that collects in the skin and sclera. Itching and a burning sensation result.

Interprofessional Collaborative Care
Recognize Cues: Assessment
- Record patient information:
  1. Height and weight, body mass index, and waist circumference
  2. Fatty food intolerances and related GI symptoms, including flatulence, dyspepsia (indigestion), eructation (belching), anorexia, nausea, vomiting, and abdominal *pain* in relation to fatty food intake
  3. Family history of gallbladder disease
  4. In women, assess for current or history of estrogen replacement therapy
- Assess for signs and symptoms:
  1. Abdominal *pain* of varying intensity in the right upper abdominal quadrant, including radiation to the right upper shoulder; ask the patient to describe the intensity, duration, precipitating factors, and relief measures

NURSING SAFETY PRIORITY

Critical Rescue

The severe pain of biliary colic is produced by obstruction of the cystic duct of the gallbladder or movement of one or more gallstones. When a stone is moving through or is lodged within the duct, tissue spasm occurs in an effort to get the stone through the small duct. Biliary colic may be so severe that it occurs with tachycardia, pallor/ash gray appearance, diaphoresis, and prostration (extreme exhaustion). Assess the patient for possible shock caused by biliary colic. *Notify the health care provider or Rapid Response Team if these symptoms occur.* Stay with the patient and keep the head of the bed flat if shock occurs.

2. Other GI symptoms, including nausea, vomiting, dyspepsia, flatulence, eructation, and feelings of abdominal heaviness, guarding, rigidity, rebound tenderness (Blumberg's sign)
3. Late signs and symptoms of chronic cholecystitis:
   - Jaundice, clay-colored stools, and dark urine
   - Steatorrhea (fatty stools)
   - Elevated temperature with tachycardia and dehydration from fever and vomiting
   - Results of serum liver enzyme and bilirubin tests (may be elevated); amylase (may be elevated if pancreas is involved)
   - Increased WBC count

KEY FEATURES

Cholecystitis

- Episodic or vague upper abdominal **pain** or discomfort that can radiate to the right shoulder
- Pain triggered by a high-fat or high-volume meal
- Anorexia
- Nausea and/or vomiting
- Dyspepsia
- Eructation
- Flatulence
- Feeling of abdominal fullness
- Rebound tenderness (Blumberg's sign)
- Inspiratory arrest (Murphy's sign)
- Fever
- Jaundice, clay-colored stools, dark urine

Analyze Cues and Prioritize Hypotheses: Analysis

- The priority collaborative problems for patients with cholecystitis include:
  1. Acute or persistent *pain* due to gallbladder *inflammation* and/or gallstones
  2. Weight loss due to decreased intake because of *pain*, nausea, and anorexia

Generate Solutions and Take Actions: Planning and Implementation

Managing Acute Pain

Nonsurgical Management

- Nonsurgical management for acute pain is required for most patients.
- Withhold food and oral fluids during nausea and vomiting episodes to avoid airway compromise
- Drug therapy includes:
  1. Opioid analgesics to relieve *pain* and reduce spasm; all opioids may cause some sphincter of Oddi spasm, worsening pain
  2. Ketorolac may be used for mild to moderate *pain*
  3. Antiemetics to provide relief from nausea and vomiting
  4. Oral bile acid dissolution or gallstone stabilizing agents such as ursodiol and chenodiol may be given as long-term therapy to dissolve or stabilize gallstones
- *Extracorporeal shock wave lithotripsy (ESWL)* may be used to break up small stones or for those who are not good surgical candidates.
- Insertion of a percutaneous transhepatic biliary catheter (drain) using CT or ultrasound guidance to open the blocked duct(s) so that bile can flow (cholecystostomy) may be used.

Surgical Management

- Cholecystectomy is the surgical removal of the gallbladder and may be done laparoscopically (minimally invasive surgical approach) or, less often, in a traditional open abdominal approach.
- Preoperative care is similar to other patients having surgery.
- Provide postoperative care for patients with laparoscopic cholecystectomy, including:
  1. Offering the patient food and water when fully awake, and monitoring for the nausea and/or vomiting that can occur with anesthesia
  2. Teaching the patient the importance of early ambulation to absorb the carbon dioxide that is retained in the abdomen after a laparoscopic procedure
  3. Informing the patient that shoulder pain is both expected and common. The pain decreases as the gases expanding the abdomen are dissipated.

4. Instructing the patient to rest for the first 24 hours and then begin to resume usual activities. Most patients are able to resume usual activities within a week.

> ### ! NURSING SAFETY PRIORITY
> #### *Action Alert*
>
> After a laparoscopic cholecystectomy, assess the patient's oxygen saturation level frequently until the effects of the anesthesia have passed. Remind the patient to perform deep-breathing exercises every hour.

- Use of the open surgical approach (abdominal laparotomy) has greatly declined during the past several decades. Patients who have this type of surgery usually have severe biliary obstruction, and the ducts are explored to ensure patency.
- Provide postoperative care for traditional surgery patients:
  1. Postoperative incisional pain after a traditional cholecystectomy is controlled with opioids, IV acetaminophen, and/or IV antiinflammatory drugs.
  2. Advance the diet from clear liquids to solid foods, as tolerated by the patient.
  3. Maintain the patient's surgical drain.
     - This tube is placed in the gallbladder bed to prevent fluid accumulation. The drainage is usually serosanguineous (serous fluid mixed with blood) and is stained with bile in the first 24 hours after surgery. Antibiotic therapy is given to prevent infection.
  4. Assist the patient with early ambulation.

Promoting Nutrition
- Provide small-volume, low-fat, high-fiber meals.
- Weigh patient to assess for concerning weight loss.
- Monitor nutritional parameters, such as blood urea nitrogen (BUN) and serum prealbumin, albumin, and total protein to assess ongoing *nutrition* status.

Care Coordination and Transition Management
- Education needs to be started as soon as a patient has an initial experience with cholecystitis and has been provided with appropriate pain relief.
- Assess the patient's and family's knowledge of the disease, and provide teaching as needed.
- The desired outcomes for discharge planning and education are to avoid further episodes of cholecystitis.

- Key teaching points include reminding the patient to avoid fatty, fried, and "fast" foods, and to report any signs of postoperative complications to the primary health care provider immediately.

Evaluate Outcomes: Evaluation
- Evaluate the care of the patient with cholecystitis based on the identified priority patient problems. The expected outcomes include that the patient will:
  1. Report control of abdominal pain, as indicated by self-report and pain scale measurement
  2. Have adequate *nutrition* available to meet metabolic needs

 See Chapter 51 in the main text for more information on cholecystitis.

CHRONIC OBSTRUCTIVE PULMONARY DISEASE: GAS EXCHANGE CONCEPT EXEMPLAR

Overview
- **Chronic obstructive pulmonary disease (COPD)** is a collection of lower airway disorders that interfere with airflow and *gas exchange*. These disorders include:
  1. Emphysema
     - A destructive problem of lung elasticity that reduces recoil, leading to hyperinflation of the lung and air trapping
  2. Chronic Bronchitis
     - Chronic bronchitis is an inflammation of the bronchi and bronchioles *(bronchiolitis)* caused by exposure to irritants, especially cigarette smoke. The irritant triggers inflammation, vasodilation, mucosal edema, congestion, and bronchospasm. Bronchitis affects only the airways, not the alveoli.
- Cigarette smoking is the greatest risk factor for COPD; other contributing factors include chronic exposure to inhaled particles, fuels, and a history of asthma.
- Complications of COPD include hypoxemia, hypercarbia, respiratory infections, heart failure, dysrhythmias, and respiratory failure.
- Respiratory infection can cause an acute exacerbation (worsening) in COPD symptoms.

Interprofessional Collaborative Care
Recognize Cues: Assessment
- Obtain and record patient information and history:
  1. Age, occupational history, and family history
  2. Smoking history, including the length of time the patient has smoked and the number of packs smoked daily
  3. Occupational or environmental exposure to lung irritants
  4. History of asthma

5. Current breathing problems:
   - Does the patient have difficulty breathing while talking? Can the patient speak in complete sentences, or is it necessary to take a breath between every one or two words?
   - Ask about the presence, duration, or worsening of wheezing, coughing, and shortness of breath, and what activities trigger these problems.
   - If the cough is productive, what is the sputum color and amount, and has the amount increased or decreased?
   - What is the relationship between activity tolerance and dyspnea? How is the patient's activity level and shortness of breath now compared with a month earlier and a year earlier? Is the patient having any difficulty with eating, sleeping, or performing activities of daily living (ADLs)?
6. How are the patient's weight and general appearance? The patient with severe COPD is thin with loss of muscle mass in the extremities, has enlarged neck muscles and a barrel-shaped chest, and is slow moving and slightly stooped.
- Assess for signs and symptoms
  1. Respiratory changes
     - Subjective report of dyspnea using a standard approach such as a Visual Analog Dyspnea Scale
     - Rapid, shallow respirations, paradoxical respirations, or use of accessory muscles
     - Limited diaphragmatic movement (excursion)
     - Abnormal lung sounds
     - Increased anterior-posterior chest diameter
     - Cough with or without sputum production

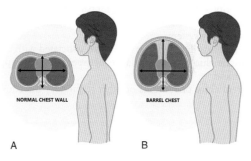

(A) Normal adult. The thorax has an oval shape with an anteroposterior-to-transverse diameter of 1:1.5 or 5:7. **(B)** Barrel chest. Note equal anteroposterior-to-transverse diameter and that ribs are horizontal instead of the normal downward slope. This is associated with chronic obstructive pulmonary disease and severe asthma as a result of hyperinflation of the lungs. (Used with permission from shutterstock.com, Pepermpron.)

2. Cardiovascular changes
   - Tachycardia and dysrhythmias
   - Swelling of feet and ankles
   - Cyanosis, or blue-tinged, dusky appearance
   - Clubbing of the fingers
3. Psychosocial issues
   - Social isolation due to decreased mobility and energy
   - Anxiety and fear related to dyspnea that may reduce the patient's ability to participate in a full life
   - Patient's and family's concerns about COPD progression to a life-limiting disorder
4. Diagnostic and laboratory tests
   - Serial arterial blood gas (ABG) values for hypoxemia and hypercarbia
   - Oxygen saturation by pulse oximetry
   - Sputum cultures
   - Hematocrit and hemoglobin to evaluate polycythemia, a compensation for chronic hypoxia
   - Serum electrolyte levels that support respiratory effort because low phosphate, potassium, calcium, or magnesium levels can reduce (breathing) muscle strength
   - Serum Alpha-1-antitrypsin (AAT) levels in patients with a family history of COPD
   - Chest x-ray
   - Pulmonary function test (PFT)
   - Peak expiratory flow rates
   - Carbon monoxide diffusion test

Analyze Cues and Prioritize Hypotheses: Analysis

- The priority collaborative problems for patients with COPD include:
  1. Decreased gas exchange due to physiological changes in the respiratory system
  2. Weight loss due to decreased intake associated with dyspnea
  3. Fatigue due to an imbalance between oxygen supply and demand
  4. Potential for pneumonia or other respiratory infections

Generate Solutions and Take Actions: Planning and Implementation
Improving Gas Exchange and Reducing Carbon Dioxide Retention
Nonsurgical Management

- Most patients with COPD use nonsurgical management to improve or maintain gas exchange.
- Priority nursing management for patients with COPD focuses on ensuring consistent use of prescribed drug therapy and on airway maintenance, monitoring, breathing techniques, positioning, effective coughing, oxygen therapy, exercise conditioning, suctioning, and hydration.
  1. Drug Therapy
     - Drugs used to manage COPD are the same drugs as for asthma and include beta-adrenergic agents, cholinergic antagonists, xanthines, corticosteroids, and cromones.
     - The focus is on long-term control therapy with longer-acting drugs, such as arformoterol, indacaterol, tiotropium, aclidinium bromide, olodaterol, and the combination drugs, such as fluticasone/vilanterol and a newer triple combination of fluticasone/umeclidinium/vilanterol.
  2. Monitoring
     - Monitoring for changes in respiratory status is key to providing prompt interventions to reduce complications.
     - Assess the hospitalized patient with COPD at least every 2 hours, even when the purpose of hospitalization is not COPD management.
     - Apply prescribed oxygen, assess the patient's response to therapy, and prevent complications.
  3. Breathing Techniques
     - Teach the patient diaphragmatic or abdominal and pursed-lip breathing, as this is helpful for managing dyspneic episodes.
  4. Positioning
     - Having the patient remain in an upright position with the head of the bed elevated can help alleviate dyspnea by increasing chest expansion and keeping the diaphragm in the proper position to contract.
  5. Effective Coughing
     - For effective coughing, teach the patient to sit in a chair or on the side of a bed with feet placed firmly on the floor.
     - Instruct the patient to turn the shoulders inward and to bend the head slightly downward, hugging a pillow against the stomach.

PATIENT AND FAMILY EDUCATION

Breathing Exercises

Diaphragmatic or Abdominal Breathing

- If you can do so comfortably, lie on your back with your knees bent. If you cannot lie comfortably, perform this exercise while sitting in a chair.
- Place your hands or a book on your abdomen to create resistance.
- Begin breathing from your abdomen while keeping your chest still. You can tell if you are breathing correctly if your hands or the book rises and falls accordingly.

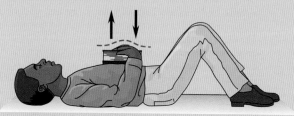

Abdominal breathing.

Pursed-Lip Breathing

- Close your mouth and breathe in through your nose.
- Purse your lips as you would to whistle. Breathe out slowly through your mouth, without puffing your cheeks. Spend at least twice the amount of time it took you to breathe in.
- Use your abdominal muscles to squeeze out every bit of air you can.
- Remember to use pursed-lip breathing during any physical activity. Always inhale before beginning the activity and exhale while performing it. Never hold your breath.

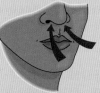
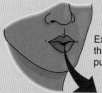

Inhale through the nose

Exhale through pursed lips

Pursed lip breathing. (From Sorrentino, S.A., & Remmert, L.N. [2023]. *Mosby's® Essentials for nursing assistants* [7th ed.]. St. Louis: Elsevier.)

- The patient then takes a few breaths, attempting to exhale more fully.
- After the third to fifth breath (in through the nose, out through pursed lips), instruct the patient to take a deeper breath and bend forward slowly while coughing two or three times ("mini" coughs) from the same breath.
- On return to a sitting position, the patient takes a comfortably deep breath. The entire coughing procedure is repeated at least twice.

6. Oxygen Therapy
   - All hypoxic patients, even those with COPD and hypercarbia, should receive oxygen therapy at rates appropriate to reduce hypoxia and bring Spo_2 levels up between 88% and 92%.

7. Exercise Conditioning
   - Pulmonary rehabilitation involves education and exercise training to prevent muscle deconditioning. Each patient's exercise program is personalized to fit current limitations and planned outcomes.

Surgical Management

- Lung transplantation and lung volume reduction surgery (LVRS) can improve *gas exchange* in the patient with COPD. Transplantation is a relatively rare procedure because of cost and the scarce availability of donor lungs. The more common surgical procedure for patients with emphysema is LVRS.

  1. Lung reduction surgery can improve gas exchange through removal of the hyperinflated lung tissue areas that are useless for gas exchange.

Preventing Weight Loss

- Weight loss occurs in patients with COPD as a result of food intolerance, nausea, early satiety, poor appetite, and meal-related dyspnea.
- The increased work of breathing raises calorie and protein needs.
- Malnourished patients lose muscle mass and strength, lung elasticity, and alveolar-capillary surface area, which contributes to poor gas exchange.
- Collaborate with the registered dietitian nutritionist (RDN) to provide sufficient protein and calories to support the work of breathing.

- Monitor patient weight and other indicators of nutrition, such as skin condition and serum prealbumin levels.
- Manage eating to avoid dyspnea and shortness of breath.
    1. Urge the patient to rest before meals.
    2. Teach the patient to plan the biggest meal of the day for the time when the patient will be most hungry and is well rested. Four to six small meals each day may be preferred to three larger ones.
    3. Suggest the use of a bronchodilator 30 minutes before the meal.
- Encourage the patient to select food that is appealing, easy to chew, and not gas forming.

Decreasing Fatigue and Increasing Endurance
- Decreased endurance is related to fatigue, dyspnea, and an imbalance between oxygen supply and demand.
- Teach energy conservation techniques to plan and pace activities for maximal tolerance and minimal discomfort.
    1. Work with the patient to develop a personal daily schedule for activities and rest periods.
    2. Teach about the use of adaptive tools for housework, such as long-handled dustpans, sponges, and dusters, to reduce bending and reaching.
    3. Suggest how to organize workspaces so that items used most often are within easy reach.
    4. Teach the patient not to talk when engaged in other activities that require energy, such as walking.
- Assist with ADLs of eating, bathing, and grooming based on assessment of the patient's needs and fatigue level.
- Assess the patient's response to activity by noting skin color changes, pulse rate and regularity, BP, and work of breathing.
- Suggest the use of supplemental oxygen during periods of high-energy use, such as bathing or walking.

Preventing Respiratory Infection
- Patients with COPD who have excessive secretions or who have artificial airways are at increased risk for respiratory tract infections.
- Teach patients to avoid large crowds and anyone who is ill.
- Stress the importance of receiving a pneumonia vaccination and a yearly influenza vaccination.

Care Coordination and Transition Management
- Most patients with COPD are managed in the ambulatory care setting and cared for at home.
- Determine what equipment and assistance will be needed in the home setting.
- Teach the patient and family about:
  1. The disease and its course
  2. Drug therapy
  3. Manifestations of infection, especially pneumonia
  4. Avoidance of respiratory irritants, including smoking cessation
  5. Nutrition therapy regimen
  6. Stress and anxiety management
  7. Breathing and coughing techniques
  8. Energy conservation measures while maintaining self-care activities

Evaluate Outcomes: Evaluation
- Evaluate the care of the patient with COPD based on the identified priority patient problems. The expected outcomes of care are that the patient will:
  1. Attain and maintain *gas exchange* at a level within the patient's chronic baseline values
  2. Cough and clear secretions effectively
  3. Maintain a respiratory rate and rhythm appropriate to the patient's activity level
  4. Achieve an effective breathing pattern that decreases the work of breathing
  5. Achieve and maintain a body weight within 10% of the patient's ideal weight
  6. Report increased endurance and decreased fatigue
  7. Avoid serious respiratory infections

See Chapter 24 in the main text for more information on chronic obstructive pulmonary disease.

✳ CIRRHOSIS: CELLULAR REGULATION CONCEPT EXEMPLAR

Overview

- **Cirrhosis** is extensive, irreversible scarring of the liver, usually caused by a chronic reaction to hepatic *inflammation* and necrosis. This scarring process directly impairs *cellular regulation*. The disease typically develops slowly and has a progressive, prolonged, destructive course, resulting in end-stage liver disease.
- Cirrhosis is characterized by widespread fibrotic (scarred) bands of connective tissue that change the liver's normal makeup and its associated cellular regulation.
- Complications of cirrhosis include:
  1. *Portal hypertension:* A persistent increase in pressure within the portal vein develops as a result of increased resistance or obstruction to flow. Blood flow backs into the spleen, causing splenomegaly. Veins in the esophagus, stomach, intestines, abdomen, and rectum become dilated. Dilated vessels develop weakened walls, leading to plasma leak and hemorrhage.
  2. *Ascites:* Free fluid accumulates within the peritoneal cavity. Increased hydrostatic pressure from portal hypertension results in venous congestion of the hepatic capillaries, causing plasma to leak directly from the liver surface and portal vein. Other contributing factors include reduced circulating plasma protein and increased hepatic lymphatic formation. Massive ascites can cause abdominal compartment syndrome.
  3. *Gastroesophageal varices:* Thin-walled, distended esophageal veins result from increased portal hypertension. Varices occur most often in the lower esophagus, stomach, and rectum. Fragile varices can rupture, resulting in gastrointestinal bleeding.
  4. *Splenomegaly* (enlarged spleen) results from the pressure of portal hypertension. The enlarged spleen destroys platelets (thrombocytopenia), adding to the increased risk for bleeding.
  5. *Reduced bile production,* preventing the absorption of fat-soluble vitamins and decreased synthesis of clotting factors depending on vitamin K, leading to coagulopathy manifested by bruising and bleeding
  6. *Jaundice* caused by ineffective excretion of bile from hepatic (hepatocellular disease) or bile duct tracts from scarring (intrahepatic obstruction). Patients with jaundice often report pruritus (itching).

7. *Hepatic encephalopathy* (also called *portal-systemic encephalopathy* [PSE]): This is a complex neurologic syndrome. It is associated with elevated serum ammonia levels. Early symptoms include sleep disturbance, mood disturbance, mental status changes, and speech problems. Later, altered level of consciousness, impaired thinking processes, and neuromuscular disturbances (e.g., "liver flap") are common symptoms.

8. *Hepatorenal syndrome:* Progressive, oliguric kidney failure is associated with hepatic failure, resulting in functional impairment of kidneys with normal anatomic and morphologic features. It is manifested by a sudden decrease in urinary output and elevated serum urea nitrogen and creatinine levels, with abnormally decreased urine sodium excretion and increased urine osmolality.

9. *Spontaneous bacterial peritonitis* from translocation of bowel bacteria to ascitic fluid

Interprofessional Collaborative Care
Recognize Cues: Assessment
- Document patient information and history:
  1. Age, gender, and race
  2. Employment history, including working conditions exposing the patient to toxins
  3. History of individual and family liver disease
  4. Medical conditions, including viral hepatitis (especially B, C, and D), systemic viral infections, biliary tract disorders, autoimmune disorders, heart failure, respiratory disorders, and liver injury. Blood transfusions and bloodborne infections from tattoos may be associated with hepatitis.
  5. Sexual history
  6. History of or present alcohol or substance use
- Because cirrhosis has a slow onset, many of the *early* signs and symptoms are vague and nonspecific. Assess for:
  1. Fatigue
  2. Weight changes (loss or gain)
  3. GI symptoms, such as anorexia and vomiting
  4. Abdominal distention, pain, or tenderness
- The development of late signs of *advanced cirrhosis* (also called *end-stage liver failure*) usually causes the patient to seek medical treatment. GI bleeding, jaundice, ascites, and spontaneous bruising indicate poor liver function and complications of cirrhosis.

Analyze Cues and Prioritize Hypotheses: Analysis
- Priority collaborative problems for patients with cirrhosis include:
  1. Fluid overload due to third spacing of abdominal and peripheral fluid (ascites)
  2. Potential for hemorrhage due to portal hypertension and subsequent GI varices
  3. Acute confusion and other cognitive changes due to increased serum ammonia levels and/or alcohol withdrawal
  4. Pruritus due to increased serum bilirubin and jaundice

KEY FEATURES

Late-Stage Cirrhosis

- **Jaundice** and **icterus** (yellow coloration of the eye sclerae)
- Dry skin
- Pruritus (itchy skin)
- Rashes
- Purpuric lesions, such as **petechiae** (round, pinpoint, red-purple hemorrhagic lesions) or **ecchymoses** (large purple, blue, or yellow bruises)
- Warm and bright red palms of the hands (palmar erythema)
- Vascular lesions with a red center and radiating branches, known as spider angiomas (also called telangiectases, spider nevi, or vascular spiders), on the nose, cheeks, upper thorax, and shoulders
- Ascites
- Peripheral dependent edema of the extremities and sacrum
- Vitamin deficiency (especially fat-soluble vitamins A, D, E, and K)

Generate Solutions and Take Actions: Planning and Implementation
Managing Fluid Volume
- Monitor respiratory status to avoid complications from pulmonary edema.
  1. Monitor Spo$_2$ with vital signs.
  2. Elevate the head of the bed to minimize shortness of breath and position for comfort.
- Provide nutrition therapy
  1. Provide a low-sodium diet initially, restricting sodium to 1 to 2 g/day.
  2. Suggest alternatives to salt, such as lemon, vinegar, parsley, oregano, and pepper.
  3. Collaborate with the registered dietitian nutritionist (RDN) to explain the purpose of diet and meal planning; suggest the elimination of table salt, salty foods, canned and frozen vegetables, and salted butter and margarine.

4. Supplement vitamin intake with thiamine, folate, and multivitamin preparations.
- Provide drug therapy
  1. Administer diuretics as prescribed to reduce intravascular fluid and to prevent cardiac and respiratory impairment.
  2. Monitor intake and output carefully with daily weight.
  3. Monitor serum electrolytes.
- Paracentesis may be indicated if dietary restrictions and drug administration fail to control ascites.
  1. Explain the procedure and verify that informed consent has been obtained.
  2. Obtain vital signs and weight, and check allergies.
  3. Assist the patient to an upright position at the side of the bed.
  4. Monitor vital signs every 15 minutes during the procedure; rapid, drastic removal of ascitic fluid leads to decreased abdominal pressure, which may contribute to vasodilation and shock.
  5. Measure and record drainage; send samples to laboratory if ordered.
  6. Position the patient in a semi-Fowler's position in bed, and maintain bed rest until vital signs are stable.
  7. Assess the patient's lung sounds.

Preventing or Managing Hemorrhage

- All patients with cirrhosis should be screened for esophageal varices by endoscopy to detect them early *before they bleed*. If patients have varices, they are placed on preventive therapy. If acute bleeding occurs, early interventions are used to manage it. *Because massive esophageal bleeding can cause rapid blood loss, emergency interventions are needed.*
  1. The role of early drug therapy is to *prevent* bleeding and infection in patients who have varices. A nonselective *beta-blocking agent* such as propranolol is usually prescribed to prevent bleeding.
  2. Infection is one of the most common indicators that patients will have an acute variceal bleed (AVB). Cirrhotic patients with GI bleeding should receive *antibiotics* when admitted to the hospital.
  3. Support the patient during endoscopic therapy to reduce bleeding from varices.
     - Endoscopic variceal ligation (banding) decreases the blood supply to the varices.
     - Endoscopic sclerotherapy allows varices to be injected with a sclerosing agent to decrease bleeding.

4. Initiate rescue therapy with esophagogastric balloon tamponade to compress bleeding vessels.
   - Very effective way to control bleeding. However, the procedure can cause potentially life-threatening complications, such as aspiration, asphyxia, and esophageal perforation. Similar to a nasogastric tube, the tube is placed through the nose and into the stomach. An attached balloon is inflated to apply pressure to the bleeding variceal area.
5. *Transjugular intrahepatic portal-systemic shunting (TIPS)* is a nonsurgical procedure whereby the physician implants a shunt between the portal vein and the hepatic vein to reduce portal venous pressure and control bleeding.
6. Administer blood products (red blood cells [RBCs] and fresh-frozen plasma) and IV fluids to sustain circulation and perfusion during episodes of bleeding.
7. Monitor vital signs every hour and check coagulation studies, including prothrombin time (PT), partial thromboplastin time (PTT), platelet count, and international normalized ratio (INR).

Preventing or Managing Confusion
- Collaborative interventions are planned around the management of slowing or stopping the accumulation of ammonia in the body to improve mental status and orientation. Assess the patient's neurologic status and monitor during treatment.

Managing Pruritus
- Patients frequently report pruritus and dry skin as a result of jaundice from increased levels of serum bilirubin as cirrhosis progresses.
- Comfort measures include avoiding being too warm, moisturizing the skin, and avoiding irritants to the skin.
- Some patients find that cool compresses and/or corticosteroid creams provide temporary relief.

Care Coordination and Transition Management
- If the patient with late-stage cirrhosis survives life-threatening complications, the patient is usually discharged to home or to a long-term care facility after treatment measures have managed the acute medical problems. A home care referral may be needed if the patient is discharged to home.
- Health teaching is individualized for the patient, depending on the cause of the disease.
- Identify whether the patient needs a family member or friend to help with drugs or needs a home health care nurse or aide.

- Teach the patient and family to:
  1. Follow the prescribed diet.
  2. Restrict sodium intake if ascites occur.
  3. Obtain and record daily weights and report an increase of 5 lb or more over any 3-day period.
  4. Restrict protein intake if the patient is susceptible to encephalopathy.
  5. Take diuretics as prescribed, report symptoms of hypokalemia, and consume foods high in potassium.
  6. Take H_2 receptor antagonist agent or proton pump inhibitor as prescribed.
  7. Avoid all nonprescription drugs.
  8. Avoid alcohol (refer to Alcoholics Anonymous if patient is addicted to alcohol).
  9. Address end-of-life concerns with patients who experience progressive cirrhotic disease; include preferences and values about transplantation in this discussion.

Evaluate Outcomes: Evaluation

- Evaluate the care of the patient with cirrhosis based on the identified priority patient problems. The expected outcomes include that the patient will:
  1. Have a decrease in or have no ascites
  2. Have electrolytes within normal limits
  3. Not have hemorrhage or will be managed immediately if bleeding occurs
  4. Not develop encephalopathy or will be managed immediately if it occurs
  5. Successfully abstain from alcohol or drugs (if disease is caused by one or more of these substances) and have adequate nutrition

 See Chapter 50 in the main text for more information on cirrhosis.

COLITIS, ULCERATIVE: INFLAMMATION CONCEPT EXEMPLAR

Overview

- Ulcerative colitis (UC) creates widespread *inflammation* of the rectum and rectosigmoid colon but can extend to the entire colon when the disease is extensive.
- UC is a disease that is associated with periodic remissions and exacerbations (flare-ups) and is often confused with Crohn's disease.

Differential Features of Ulcerative Colitis and Crohn's Disease

Feature	Ulcerative Colitis	Crohn's Disease
Location	Begins in the rectum and proceeds in a continuous manner toward the cecum	Most often in the terminal ileum, with patchy involvement through all layers of the bowel
Etiology	Unknown	Unknown
Peak age of incidence	15 to 35 yr and 55 to 65 yr	15 to 40 yr
Number of stools	10 to 20 liquid, bloody stools per day	5 to 6 soft, loose stools per day, nonbloody
Complications	Hemorrhage Nutritional deficiencies	Fistulas (common) Nutritional deficiencies
Patient need for surgery	25% to 35%	65% to 75%

- UC is characterized by hyperemic intestinal mucosa (increased blood flow) with resultant edema. In more severe inflammation, the lining can bleed and small ulcers occur.
- Abscesses can form in ulcerative areas and result in tissue necrosis, perforation, and peritonitis.
- Edema and mucosal thickening can lead to a narrowed colon and bowel obstruction.
- Complications of the disease include fistula formation, toxic megacolon, hemorrhage, increased risk for colon cancer, and malabsorption.
- Extraintestinal clinical manifestations include polyarthritis, oral and skin lesions, iritis, and hepatic and biliary disease.
- The patient's stool typically contains blood and mucus. Patients report tenesmus (an unpleasant and urgent sensation to defecate) and lower abdominal colicky pain relieved with defecation. Malaise, anorexia, anemia, dehydration, fever, and weight loss are common.

Interprofessional Collaborative Care
Recognize Cues: Assessment
- Document patient information and history:
  1. Family history of inflammatory bowel disease
  2. Previous and current therapy for illnesses, including surgeries
  3. Diet history, including usual patterns and intolerances of food
  4. History of weight changes
  5. Presence of abdominal pain, cramping, urgency, and diarrhea

6. Bowel elimination patterns; color, consistency, and character of stools; and the presence or absence of blood
7. Relationship between the occurrence of diarrhea and the timing of meals, pain, emotional distress, and activity
8. Extraintestinal symptoms such as arthritis, mouth sores, vision problems, and skin disorders

- Assess signs and symptoms:
  1. Abdominal cramping, pain, and distention
  2. Bloody diarrhea, tenesmus
  3. Fever, tachycardia
  4. Patient's understanding of the disease process
  5. Psychosocial impact of the disease; the inability to control symptoms, especially diarrhea, can be disruptive and stress producing
  6. Abnormal laboratory values: hematocrit, hemoglobin, WBC count, erythrocyte sedimentation rate, C-reactive protein, and electrolytes
  7. Results from most recent colonoscopy or magnetic resonance enterography

Analyze Cues and Prioritize Hypotheses: Analysis

- The priority collaborative problems for patients with UC include:
  1. Diarrhea due to *inflammation* of the bowel mucosa
  2. Acute or persistent *pain* due to *inflammation* and ulceration of the bowel mucosa and skin irritation
  3. Potential for lower GI bleeding and resulting anemia due to UC

Generate Solutions and Take Actions: Planning and Implementation
Managing Diarrhea

- Many measures are used to relieve symptoms and reduce intestinal motility, decrease *inflammation,* and promote intestinal healing. Nonsurgical and/or surgical management may be needed.

Nonsurgical Management

- Record patient responses to interventions, noting changes in the color, volume, frequency, and consistency of stools.
- Monitor the skin in the perianal area for irritation and ulceration resulting from loose, frequent stools.
- Monitor immune function and results of stool or other cultures.
- Drug therapy
  1. Aminosalicylates are used to reduce inflammation.
  2. Glucocorticoids are used during exacerbations of the illness.
  3. Immunomodulators to alter (modulate) the immune response are most effective when given with corticosteroids. Examples include infliximab and adalimumab.

- Nutritional therapy may include:
  1. NPO status with total parenteral nutrition (TPN) for the patient with severe symptoms
  2. Elemental formulas, which are absorbed in the small intestine, minimizing bowel stimulation
  3. Avoiding caffeine, alcohol, or foods that cause symptoms
- Ensure that the patient has easy access to the bedside commode or bathroom.
- Complementary and integrative therapies may include flaxseed, selenium, vitamin C, biofeedback, yoga, acupuncture, and Ayurveda (combination of diet, herbs, and breathing exercises).

Surgical Management

- The need for surgery is based on the patient's response to medical interventions.
- Surgical procedures include:
  1. A temporary or permanent *ileostomy*
     - An ileostomy is a procedure in which a loop of the ileum is placed through an opening in the abdominal wall (stoma) for drainage of fecal material.
  2. Restorative proctocolectomy with ileo pouch–anal anastomosis (RPC-IPAA) has become the gold standard for patients with UC. This is a two-stage procedure.
     - First, the surgeon removes the colon and most of the rectum, leaving the anus and anal sphincter remain intact. The surgeon creates an internal pouch (reservoir) using a portion of the small intestine. The pouch, sometimes called a *J-pouch*, *S-pouch*, or *pelvic pouch*, is then connected to the anus. A temporary ileostomy through the abdominal skin is created to allow healing of the internal pouch.
     - In the *second* surgical stage, the loop ileostomy is closed, and elimination returns through the anus.

✚ NURSING SAFETY PRIORITY
Critical Rescue

The ileostomy stoma is usually placed in the right lower quadrant of the abdomen below the belt line. It should not be prolapsed or retract into the abdominal wall. Assess the stoma frequently. It should be pinkish to cherry red to ensure an adequate blood supply. *If the stoma looks pale/ash gray, bluish, or dark, report these findings to the health care provider immediately.*

---

  3. Total proctocolectomy with a permanent ileostomy. The procedure involves the removal of the colon, rectum, and anus with surgical closure of the anus. The surgeon brings the end

of the ileum out through the abdominal wall and forms a stoma, or permanent ostomy.

Managing Pain
- Assess the patient for changes in pain intensity that may indicate disease or surgical complications, such as peritonitis.
- Assess for pain, including its character, pattern of occurrence (e.g., before or after meals, during the night, before or after bowel movements), and duration.
- Take measures to relieve irritated skin caused by contact with diarrheal stool or ileostomy drainage.

Preventing or Monitoring for Lower GI Bleeding
- Monitor the patient for bright red or black and tarry stools and symptoms of GI bleeding.
- Notify the health care provider immediately of GI bleeding because blood transfusion or surgical interventions may be necessary.

✚ NURSING SAFETY PRIORITY
Critical Rescue

Recognize that it is important to monitor stools for blood loss for the patient with UC. The blood may be bright red (frank bleeding) or black and tarry (melena). Monitor hematocrit, hemoglobin, and electrolyte values, and assess vital signs. Prolonged slow bleeding can lead to anemia. Observe for fever, tachycardia, and signs of fluid volume depletion. Changes in mental status may occur, especially among older adults, and may be the first indication of dehydration or anemia.

If symptoms of GI bleeding begin, respond by notifying the Rapid Response Team or primary health care provider immediately. Blood products are often prescribed for patients with severe anemia. Prepare for the blood transfusion by inserting a large-bore IV catheter if it is not already in place.

Care Coordination and Transition Management
- Health teaching includes the following:
    1. Provide information on the nature of the disease, including acute episodes, remissions, and symptom management.
    2. Self-management strategies to reduce or control pain, promote adequate nutrition, manage clinical manifestations, and monitor for complications
    3. Provide additional information for the patient with an ostomy regarding:
        - Ostomy or pouch care
        - Skin care, including anal and peristomal skin

- Special issues related to drugs (e.g., to avoid taking enteric-coated drugs and capsule drugs); the patient should inform health care providers and the pharmacist of the ostomy
- Symptoms indicating a need to contact the provider, such as increased or no drainage, stomal swelling, or discoloration of the stoma
- Activity limitations, including avoidance of heavy lifting
- The importance of adequate fluid intake, especially during periods of high ostomy output
- Refer the patient to home health care ostomy or outpatient clinics.
- Refer the patient to support groups for ostomy recipients and to organizations that provide education and support for individuals with inflammatory bowel disease.

Evaluate Outcomes: Evaluation

- Evaluate the care of the patient with ulcerative colitis based on the identified priority patient problems. Expected outcomes may include that the patient will:
  1. Experience no diarrhea or a decrease in diarrheal episodes
  2. Verbalize decreased pain
  3. Have absence of lower GI bleeding
  4. Self-manage the ileostomy or ileo-anal pouch (temporary or permanent)

See Chapter 49 in the main text for more information on colitis (ulcerative).

COMPARTMENT SYNDROME

- Compartment syndrome is a serious, limb-threatening condition in which increased pressure within one or more compartments (that contain muscle, blood vessels, and nerves) reduces circulation to the lower leg or forearm.
- It is usually a complication of musculoskeletal trauma in the lower leg or forearm, but it can be seen with severe burns, extensive insect bites, acute arterial occlusion (thrombosis or embolism), or massive infiltration of IV fluids.
- The pressure to the compartment can be from an external or internal source, but fracture is present in most cases of acute compartment syndrome (ACS). Tight, bulky dressings and casts are examples of *external* pressure causes. Blood or fluid accumulation in the compartment is a common source of *internal* pressure.
- If the condition is not treated, cyanosis, tingling, numbness, paresis, and necrosis can occur.

Interprofessional Collaborative Care

- Patients with acute compartment syndrome may need a surgical procedure known as a **fasciotomy**. In this procedure, the surgeon cuts through the fascia to relieve pressure and tension on vital blood vessels and nerves. The wound remains open and requires care to begin to heal from the inside out. The surgeon usually closes the wound with a skin graft in several days.
- Complications of compartment syndrome can include infection, persistent motor weakness in the affected extremity, contracture, and myoglobinuric renal failure.
- In extreme cases, amputation becomes necessary.

See Chapter 44 in the main text for more information on compartment syndrome.

CORNEAL ABRASION, ULCERATION, AND INFECTION

- A *corneal abrasion* is a scrape or scratch injury of the cornea that disrupts the integrity of this structure; it is most commonly caused by the presence of a small foreign body, trauma, or contact lens use.
- The abrasion provides a portal of entry for organisms, leading to *corneal infection*.
- *Corneal ulceration* is a deeper disruption of the corneal epithelium, often occurring with bacterial, fungal, or viral infection. *This problem is an emergency and can lead to permanently impaired vision.*

Interprofessional Collaborative Care
Recognize Cues: Assessment

- Wear gloves when examining the eye.
- Anticipate the cornea to look hazy or cloudy with a patchy area of ulceration.
- When fluorescein stain is used by the health care provider, the patchy area appears green.

Take Actions: Interventions

- Antiinfective therapy is started before the organism is identified because of the high risk for vision loss.
- A broad-spectrum antibiotic is prescribed first and may be changed when culture results are known.
- Steroids may be used with antibiotics to reduce the eye inflammation.
- Drugs can be given topically as eye drops, or injected subconjunctivally or intravenously.

> ## ❗ NURSING SAFETY PRIORITY
> ### *Action Alert*
>
> Stress the importance of applying the drug as often as prescribed, even at night, and to complete the entire course of antibiotic therapy. Treating the infection can save the vision in the infected eye. Remind the patient to make and keep all follow-up appointments.

See Chapter 39 in the main text for more information on corneal abrasion, ulceration, and infection.

CORNEAL OPACITIES AND KERATOCONUS

- The cornea can permanently lose its shape, become scarred or cloudy, or become thinner, reducing useful visual sensory perception.
- *Keratoconus* is the degeneration of the corneal tissue, resulting in an abnormal corneal shape; it can occur with trauma or may occur as part of an inherited disorder.
- *Keratoplasty* is the surgical removal of diseased corneal tissue and replacement with tissue from a human donor cornea (corneal transplant). For a misshaped cornea that is still clear, surgical management involves a corneal implant that adjusts the shape of the cornea.

Interprofessional Collaborative Care

- *Preoperative care* may be short, with little time for teaching because transplantation is performed when the donor cornea becomes available.
  1. Examine the patient's eyes for signs and symptoms of infection, and report any redness/hyperpigmentation, drainage, or edema to the eye care provider.
  2. Instill prescribed antibiotic eye drops, and obtain IV access before surgery.
- *Postoperative care* involves comprehensive patient teaching. Local antibiotics are injected or instilled. Usually the eye is covered with a pressure patch and a protective shield until the patient returns to the surgeon.
  1. Teach the patient to lie on the nonoperative side to reduce intraocular pressure.
  2. Maintain the eye protective shield and dressing care as prescribed by the surgeon.
  3. Educate the patient or caregiver about the instillation of eye drops, typically antibiotics.

4. Teach the patient and caregiver to examine the eye daily for the presence of infection, graft rejection, and reduced visual acuity.
   • Report immediately to the surgeon the presence of purulent discharge, a continuous leak of clear fluid from around the graft site (not tears), or excessive bleeding.
5. Instruct the patient to avoid activities that promote rapid or jerky head motions or increase intraocular pressure for several weeks after surgery.

See Chapter 39 in the main text for more information on corneal opacities and keratoconus.

CORONARY ARTERY DISEASE

See *Acute Coronary Syndrome.*

CROHN'S DISEASE

• Crohn's disease is a chronic inflammatory disease of the small intestine (most often), colon, or both segments of the GI tract.
  1. "Skip lesions" with thickened intestinal walls, alternating with healthy tissue, can result in deep fissures and ulcerations, predisposing the patient to development of bowel fistulas.
  2. Narrowing of the bowel lumen (strictures) contributes to GI symptoms and complications.
  3. Complications of Crohn's disease include malabsorption, fistulas, hemorrhage, abscess formation, and intestinal obstruction. Severe malnutrition and debilitation over time can occur with reduced intestinal absorption of nutrients.

Interprofessional Collaborative Care
Recognize Cues: Assessment
• Assess for:
  1. Abdominal pain, distention, or masses
  2. Frequency and consistency of stools; presence of blood or fat (steatorrhea) in the stool
  3. Weight loss (indicates serious nutritional deficiencies)
  4. Diet history or nutritional intake
  5. Family history of the disease
  6. Distention, masses, or visible peristalsis
  7. Ulcerations or fissures of the perianal area
  8. Bowel sounds may be diminished or absent in the presence of severe inflammation; high-pitched over narrowed bowel loops

9. Results of diagnostic imaging tests that show narrowing, ulcerations, strictures, and fistulas consistent with Crohn's disease
10. Results of laboratory studies, especially CBC and electrolytes
- Low hemoglobin and hematocrit (anemia) may indicate GI bleeding, malnutrition, or both.
- Elevated WBC levels may indicate exacerbation or complications (fistula formation, perforation, or peritonitis).

! NURSING SAFETY PRIORITY
Action Alert

> For the patient with Crohn's disease, be especially alert for manifestations of peritonitis, hemorrhage, small-bowel obstruction, or nutritional and fluid imbalances. Early detection of a change in the patient's status helps reduce these potentially life-threatening complications.

Take Actions: Interventions
- The care of the patient with Crohn's disease is similar to care for the patient with UC (*see Colitis, Ulcerative*).

! NURSING SAFETY PRIORITY
Action Alert

> Adequate **nutrition** and **fluid and electrolyte balance** are priorities in the care of the patient with a fistula. GI secretions are high in volume and rich in electrolytes and enzymes. The patient is at high risk for malnutrition, dehydration, and hypokalemia (decreased serum potassium). Assess for these complications, and collaborate with the health care team to manage them. Carefully monitor urinary output and daily weights. A decrease in either measurement indicates possible dehydration, which should be treated immediately by providing additional fluids.

- Fistulas are common with acute exacerbations of Crohn's disease. They can be between the bowel and bladder (enterovesical), between two segments of bowel (enteroenteric), between the skin and bowel (enterocutaneous), or between the bowel and vagina (enterovaginal).
- Malnutrition can result in poor fistula and wound healing, loss of lean muscle mass, decreased immune system response, and increased morbidity and mortality.

1. Consult with the registered dietitian nutritionist to individualize diet and monitor tolerance to nutritional intake.
2. Assist the patient to select high-calorie, high-protein, high-vitamin, low-fiber meals.
3. Offer oral supplements.
4. Record food intake and accurate calorie count.

- Electrolyte therapy includes:
  1. Fluid and electrolyte replacement by oral liquids and nutrients, as well as IV fluids
  2. Cautious use of antidiarrheal agents to decrease fluid loss
  3. Monitoring of intake, output, and daily weights

- Impaired skin integrity results from fistula formation. The degree of associated problems is related to the location of the fistula, the patient's general health status, and the character and amount of fistula drainage.
  1. In collaboration with the wound enterostomal therapist, apply a pouch or drain to the fistula to prevent skin irritation and to measure the drainage. Negative pressure wound therapy may promote healing when the fistula is large.
  2. Provide skin barriers to prevent skin irritation and excoriation.
  3. Protect the adjacent skin, and keep it clean and dry.
  4. Observe for subtle signs of infection or sepsis such as fever, abdominal pain, or change in mental status.

- Some patients with Crohn's disease require surgery, such as a bowel resection and anastomosis with or without a colon resection, to improve the quality of life.
- Stricturoplasty may be performed for bowel strictures.

 See Chapter 49 in the main text for more information on Crohn's disease.

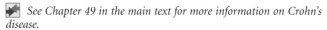 COVID-19: INFECTION CONCEPT EXEMPLAR

Overview
- In December 2019 and continuing into 2022, the world experienced a coronavirus pandemic, COVID-19 (CO = coronavirus; VI = virus; D = disease; 19 = 2019). The virus that causes COVID-19 is referred to as severe acute respiratory syndrome coronavirus 2 (SARS-CoV-2).
- Because COVID-19 is spread via person-to-person contact and is highly transmissible, the primary mode of health promotion is vaccination and prevention methods within the community.

COVID-19 Vaccine Information

- Do not mix products for the primary vaccination series.
- If you have COVID-19, wait to receive any vaccine until isolation is complete.
- If you develop COVID-19 before your next dose of vaccine (primary or booster), you may delay the next vaccine dose by 3 months. If significant risk factors exist, you may opt to get the vaccine as soon as your isolation period ends.
- COVID-19 vaccines are effective at decreasing the risk of getting seriously ill, being hospitalized, or dying.
- Boosters are recommended for most because the protection that is offered with the COVID-19 vaccine decreases over time.
- While COVID-19 vaccines were developed quickly, the science that was used has been in existence for decades.

Adapted from Centers for Disease Control and Prevention. (2022). *Understanding how COVID-19 vaccines work*. https://www.cdc.gov/coronavirus/2019-ncov/vaccines/different-vaccines/how-they-work.h tml; and Centers for Disease Control and Prevention (CDC). (2022). *Why to get a COVID-19 vaccine*. https://www.cdc.gov/coronavirus/2019-ncov/vaccines/vaccine-benefits.html.

Interprofessional Collaborative Care

Recognize Cues: Assessment

- Assess the patient for:
  1. Signs of viral illness (fever, cough, chills, or gastrointestinal upset)
  2. Recent loss of taste or smell
  3. Other household members who are ill
  4. Exposure to COVID-19 and current vaccination status
  5. Risk of progression to severe COVID-19 (aged 65 years or older; cancer; chronic kidney, lung, liver, or heart disease; cystic fibrosis; diabetes mellitus; disabilities such as cerebral palsy; HIV; dementia; mental health disorders; obesity; smoking history; tuberculosis; and/or use of immunosuppressive medications)
  6. Key features of COVID-19
- To confirm COVID-19 diagnosis, the nucleic acid amplification test (NAAT), most commonly using a reverse transcription polymerase chain reaction (RT-PCR) assay is preferred.
- There are also rapid point-of-care tests that can be completed in minutes and include antigen tests and some NAATs. Home tests are also widely available.

KEY FEATURES

COVID-19

Most Common Symptoms
- Fever or chills
- Cough
- Shortness of breath or difficulty breathing
- Fatigue
- Muscle or body aches
- Headache
- New loss of taste (ageusia) or smell (anosmia)
- Sore throat
- Nausea or vomiting
- Diarrhea
- Abdominal pain

Unique Features in Some Patients
- Conjunctivitis
- Prothrombotic state (venous and arterial thromboembolic disease)
- Neurologic findings (encephalopathy with agitated delirium)
- Dermatologic findings, especially reddish nodules on distal digits (in young adults)

Indications for Emergency Interventions
- Trouble breathing
- Persistent pain or pressure in the chest
- New confusion
- Inability to wake or stay awake
- Bluish lips or face

Data from Centers for Disease Control and Prevention (CDC). (2022). *Symptoms of COVID-19*. https://www.cdc.gov/coronavirus/2019-ncov/symptoms-testing/symptoms.html Cuker, A., & Peyvandi, F. (2022). COVID-19: Hypercoagulability. *UpToDate*. https://www.uptodate.com/contents/covid-19-hypercoagulability; and McIntosh, K. (2023). COVID-19 clinical features. *UpToDate*. Retrieved March 5, 2023, from https://www.uptodate.com/contents/ covid-19-clinical-features.

Analyze Cues and Prioritize Hypotheses: Analysis
- The priority interprofessional collaborative problems for patients with COVID-19 include:
    1. Potential to transmit infection due to the highly communicable nature of COVID-19.
    2. Potential for reduced oxygenation due to COVID-19 infection.
    3. Potential for progression to severe/critical COVID-19 infection.

Generate Solutions and Take Actions: Planning and Implementation
Preventing Infection Transmission
- The majority of patients who do not experience dyspnea are managed at home with supportive care.

1. For patients with fever, muscle pain, and headache, antipyretics and analgesics are suggested. Acetaminophen is preferred, but NSAIDs can be used.
2. Nursing priorities include teaching about symptom management, warning signs of disease progression, and preventing the spread of COVID-19 to others.

Infection Control at Home With COVID-19

Patients with confirmed or suspected COVID-19 or those who are awaiting test results for COVID-19 should:
- Stay home and avoid exposing others.
- Separate themselves within the home from people and animals; if this is not possible, remain 6 feet apart.
- Wear a well-fitting face mask. Also, those around the patient should wear a face mask.
- Use a separate bathroom from other members of the household when possible.
- Limit caregivers, and when possible, ensure that caregivers are vaccinated.
- Don't share dishes, eating utensils, and bedding. Ensure that these items are washed thoroughly.
- Clean and disinfect surfaces and spaces that are frequently touched.

- For patients who are hospitalized with COVID-19, it is important to take additional measures to prevent the spread of the infection.
  1. Patients having aerosolized-generating interventions should be placed in an airborne infection isolation room (AIIR).
  2. When caring for a patient with COVID-19, it is critical that health care providers wear a particulate respirator (N95 respirator mask or higher is preferred over face mask), eye protection (goggles or face shield), isolation gown, and nonsterile gloves.

! NURSING SAFETY PRIORITY

Action Alert

When performing procedures that induce coughing or promote aerosolization of particles (e.g., intubation, extubation, suctioning, using a positive-pressure face mask, obtaining a sputum culture, or giving aerosolized treatments) for the patient with COVID-19, protect yourself and other health care workers. Wear a gown, gloves, N95 mask, and protective eyewear during the procedures. Keep the door to the patient's room closed. Avoid touching your face. Wash your hands after removing personal protective equipment (PPE) and when you leave the patient's room. Wear gloves when disinfecting contaminated surfaces or equipment.

Promoting Gas Exchange
- While it is important to allow the body to rest, it is also important to encourage mobility.
  1. Encourage patients to reposition frequently and to self-prone (lie on the stomach).
  2. Teach to cough and deep breathe frequently.
  3. Patients who require oxygen therapy are usually hospitalized to monitor closely for disease progression.

C

Decreasing Risk of COVID-19 Progression
- Mild dyspnea is common with COVID-19; however, an increase in dyspnea, or dyspnea that occurs at rest is a sign of disease progression.
- For patients with symptoms or risk factors for disease progression, specific therapy for COVID-19 can reduce the risk of hospitalization and mortality (Cohen & Gebo, 2023).
  1. Outpatient treatment continues to evolve; current drug therapy includes nirmatrelvir-ritonavir, an oral combination of protease inhibitors. Remdesivir, an antiviral drug, is an available outpatient treatment.
- Because there is such a wide variability in duration, acute COVID-19 ranges up to 4 weeks from the onset of symptoms.
- Post-COVID condition is defined by a broad range of symptoms that occur during or after acute COVID-19 and last for 2 months or more (Mikkelsen & Abramoff, 2023).
  1. Symptoms of post-COVID condition include fatigue, dyspnea, cough, altered taste and smell, problems with attention and memory (referred to as "brain fog"), anxiety, depression, and some degree of functional disability.
  2. These symptoms can vary widely and for some patients can last over a year.

Care Coordination and Transition Management
- Teach the patient to isolate at home when possible and to take the COVID-19 specific therapy (as prescribed).
- Teach warning signs that can indicate disease progression.
- Teach that vaccination (primary or booster) is recommended 3 months after recovery.

Evaluate Outcomes: Evaluation

- Evaluate the care of the patient with COVID-19 based on the identified priority patient problems. The expected outcomes are that the patient will:
  1. Avoid transmission of COVID-19 to others.
  2. Maintain adequate gas exchange with oxygen saturation of 95% or greater.
  3. Recover from COVID-19 without progression to severe/critical COVID-19 or development of post-COVID condition.
  4. Return to a pre-COVID-19 health status.

 See Chapter 25 in the main text for more information on COVID-19.

COVID-19, SEVERE

- This section is specific to severe COVID-19, which is characterized by hypoxemia (oxygen saturation of 94% or less on room air) and the need for oxygen or ventilatory support (Kim & Ghandi, 2022).

Interprofessional Collaborative Care
Recognize Cues: Assessment

- Severe COVID-19 illness typically presents with dyspnea followed by hypoxemia.
  1. Assess for presenting symptoms, which can include: symptoms of severe viral pneumonia, including a respiratory rate greater than 30 breaths per minute, lung infiltrates greater than 50% of the lung field on imaging, and an oxygen saturation of 94% or less on room air (NIH, 2022).
- Severe COVID-19 illness can progress to critical COVID-19 illness, in which multiple organs are affected.
- Critical COVID-19 illness is defined by the presence of respiratory failure, septic shock, and/or multiorgan failure (NIH, 2022).
- In critically ill patients, acute respiratory failure is usually present, which is most often the result of acute respiratory distress syndrome (ARDS).

Take Actions: Interventions

- Management includes supportive care, improving gas exchange, preventing further lung injury, and treating any underlying medical conditions and any complications from COVID-19. This includes ventilator management, rescue strategies, and drug therapies.
- Similar to ARDS, pronation has been found to improve oxygenation in COVID-19 patients.
  1. Review agency policy for prone positioning procedures.
  2. Multiple team members will need to assist to place a patient in the prone position.

Supine Position

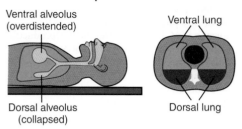

Ventral alveolus
(overdistended)

Ventral lung

Dorsal alveolus
(collapsed)

Dorsal lung

Prone Position

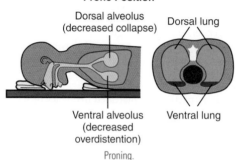

Dorsal alveolus
(decreased collapse)

Dorsal lung

Ventral alveolus
(decreased
overdistention)

Ventral lung

Proning.

- Thromboprophylaxis is essential in the management of COVID-19 because the virus induces a hypercoagulable state, increasing the risk for blood clots.
  1. All patients who are hospitalized for COVID-19 should receive venous thromboembolism (VTE) prophylaxis (unless contraindicated).
- Because there is a high risk of prolonged critical illness and death, advance care planning, determining surrogate medical decision makers, and goals of care should take place on admission.

See Chapter 26 in the main text for more information on Severe/Critical COVID-19.

CUSHING SYNDROME (HYPERCORTISOLISM): FLUID AND ELECTROLYTE BALANCE CONCEPT EXEMPLAR

Overview
- **Hypercortisolism** is a clinical state arising from excessive tissue exposure to cortisol and/or other glucocorticoids (Uwaifo & Hura, 2023).

- Over time, hypercortisolism can lead to **Cushing syndrome,** a set of symptoms caused by the excess of cortisol in the body.
- In certain cases, a pituitary gland tumor secreting adrenocortico-tropic hormone (ACTH) stimulates the overproduction of corti-sol in the body (American Association of Neurological Surgeons, 2023). This condition is called **Cushing disease,** which is a specific type of Cushing syndrome.
- The most common cause of Cushing disease that is unrelated to drug therapy is a pituitary adenoma.

Interprofessional Collaborative Care
Recognize Cues: Assessment
- Obtain patient information about:
  1. History of all health problems and drug therapies
  2. Age, gender, and usual weight
  3. Changes in weight, diet, or eating behaviors
  4. Change in activity or sleep patterns, fatigue, and muscle weakness
  5. Bone pain or a history of fractures
  6. Infections, particularly increased frequency or severity
  7. Easy bruising
  8. Cessation of menses
  9. GI ulcers
- Assess for and document key features of hypercortisolism

KEY FEATURES

Hypercortisolism (Cushing Disease/Syndrome)

General Appearance
Moon face
Buffalo hump
Truncal obesity
Weight gain

Cardiovascular Symptoms
Hypertension
Frequent dependent edema
Bruising
Petechiae

Immune System Symptoms
Increased risk for infection
Reduced immunity
Decreased inflammatory responses
Signs and symptoms of infection and inflammation (possibly masked)

Skin Symptoms
Thinning skin
Increased facial and body hair
Striae and increased pigmentation

Musculoskeletal Symptoms
Muscle atrophy (most apparent in extremities)
Osteoporosis with:
- Pathologic fractures
- Decreased height and vertebral collapse
- Aseptic necrosis of the femur head
- Slow or poor healing of bone fractures

- Diagnostic assessment includes:
    1. Blood, salivary, and urine cortisol levels
    2. Dexamethasone suppression testing
    3. Serum electrolyte values (increased sodium, decreased calcium, decreased potassium)
    4. X-rays, CT scans, or MRI to identify tumors of the adrenal or pituitary glands, lung, GI tract, or pancreas

Analyze Cues and Prioritize Hypotheses: Analysis

- The priority problems for patients with Cushing disease or Cushing syndrome are:
    1. Fluid overload due to hormone-induced water and sodium retention
    2. Potential for injury due to skin thinning, poor wound healing, and bone density loss
    3. Potential for infection due to hormone-induced reduced immunity

Generate Solutions and Take Actions: Planning and Implementation
Restoring Fluid Volume Balance
- Prevent fluid overload leading to pulmonary edema and HF:
    1. Monitor for indicators of increased fluid overload (bounding pulse, increasing neck vein distention, lung crackles, increasing peripheral edema, reduced urine output) at least every 2 hours.
    2. Administer drug therapies as prescribed that interfere with adrenocorticotropic hormone (ACTH) production or adrenal hormone synthesis. Ketoconazole and levoketoconazole are commonly used oral medications used to inhibit one or more steps in cortisol synthesis (Nieman, 2022a). For patients with hypercortisolism resulting from increased ACTH production, cyproheptadine may be used because it interferes with ACTH production.
    3. Nutritional therapy for the patient with hypercortisolism may involve restrictions of both fluid and sodium intake to control fluid volume.
    4. Monitor intake and output and weight to assess therapy effectiveness. Fluid retention may not be visible. Rapid weight gain is the best indicator of fluid retention and overload. Each 1 lb (about 500 g) of weight gained (after the first half pound) equates to 500 mL of retained water.
    5. *Surgical management* of adrenocortical hypersecretion depends on the cause of the problem. When adrenal hyperfunction is due to increased pituitary secretion of ACTH, removal of a pituitary adenoma using minimally invasive techniques

may be attempted. Sometimes a total *hypophysectomy* (surgical removal of the pituitary gland) is needed. If hypercortisolism is caused by an adrenal tumor, an *adrenalectomy* (removal of the adrenal gland) may be needed.

Preventing Injury
- Priority nursing interventions for prevention of injury focus on skin assessment and protection, coordinating care to ensure gentle handling, and patient teaching regarding drug therapy for the prevention of GI ulcers.
- Prevent skin injury by:
  1. Assessing the patient's skin for reddened areas, excoriation, breakdown, and edema
  2. Using pressure-relieving intervention during bed rest, including repositioning or assisting with turns every 2 hours
  3. Teaching the patient activities to avoid trauma
     - Use a soft toothbrush.
     - Use an electric shaver.
     - Keep the skin clean, and dry it thoroughly after washing.
     - Use a moisturizing lotion.
     - Use tape sparingly and take care when removing it.
- Prevent pathologic fractures by:
  1. Using a lift sheet to move the patient instead of grasping the patient
  2. Reminding the patient to call for help when ambulating
  3. Reviewing the use of ambulatory aids (walkers or canes), if needed
  4. Keeping rooms free of extraneous objects that may cause a fall
  5. Teaching AP to use a gait belt when ambulating the patient
  6. Teaching the patient about safety issues and dietary support for bone health
- Prevent GI bleeding by:
  1. Implementing prescribed drug therapy
  2. Encouraging the patient to reduce or eliminate habits that contribute to gastric irritation, such as:
     - Consuming alcohol or caffeine
     - Smoking
     - Using NSAIDs

Preventing Infection
- Continually assess the patient for the presence of infection.
  1. Monitor the daily CBC with differential WBC count and absolute neutrophil count (ANC) to detect and report abnormal values.
  2. Inspect the mouth during every shift for mucosal integrity.

3. Assess the lungs every 8 hours for crackles, wheezes, or reduced breath sounds.
4. Assess all urine for odor and cloudiness.
5. Ask the patient about any urgency, burning, or pain present on urination.
6. Take vital signs at least every 4 hours to assess for fever.
- Urge the patient to cough and deep breathe or to perform sustained maximal inhalations every 1 to 2 hours while awake.

C

Care Coordination and Transition Management

- Teach the patient who must take corticosteroid replacement drugs after surgery to:
  1. Take the drug in divided doses, with the first dose in the morning and the second dose between 4:00 and 6:00 p.m. and to take the drug with food.
  2. Weigh daily, record it, and compare with previous weights.
     - Call the health care provider if more than 3 lb are gained in a week or more than 1 to 2 lb is gained within 24 hours.
  3. Increase the dosage as directed for increased physical stress or severe emotional stress, including surgery, dental work, influenza, fever, pregnancy, and family problems.
  4. *Never skip a dose of the drug.* If the patient has persistent vomiting or severe diarrhea and cannot take the drug by mouth for 24 to 36 hours, call the primary health care provider. If the patient cannot reach the primary health care provider, go to the nearest ‾emergency department because an injection may be needed in place of the usual oral drug.
  5. Always wear a medical alert bracelet or necklace.
  6. Make regular visits for health care follow-up.
  7. Urge attention to handwashing and personal hygiene to reduce exposure to transmissible disease.
- The patient with hypercortisolism usually has muscle weakness and fatigue for some weeks after surgery and remains at risk for falls and other injury.
- Immediately after returning home, the patient may need a support person to stay and provide more attention than could be given by a visiting nurse or home care aide.

Evaluate Outcomes: Evaluation

- Evaluate the care of the patient with hypercortisolism based on the identified priority patient problems. The expected outcomes of interventions are that the patient will:
  1. Maintain fluid and electrolyte balance as indicated by blood pressure at or near the normal range, stable body weight, and normal serum sodium and potassium levels

2. Remain free from injury as indicated by having intact skin, minimal bruising, absence of bone fractures, and no occult blood in vomitus, stools, or GI secretions
3. Remain free from infection as indicated by absence of fever, purulent drainage, cough, and pain or burning on urination
4. Participate in infection prevention strategies of social distancing and obtaining appropriate immunizations
5. Avoid episodes of acute adrenal insufficiency

See Chapter 54 in the main text for more information on Cushing disease (hypercortisolism).

CYSTIC FIBROSIS

- **Cystic fibrosis (CF)** is an autosomal recessive genetic disease that affects many organs, with most impairment occurring to pancreatic and/or lung function. Although CF is present from birth and usually is first seen in early childhood, almost half of patients with CF in the United States are adults (Cystic Fibrosis Foundation [CFF], 2021).
- The underlying problem of CF is blocked chloride transport in cell membranes, causing the formation of thick and sticky mucus.
- This mucus plugs up glands in the lungs, pancreas, liver, salivary glands, and testes, causing atrophy and organ dysfunction.
- Nonpulmonary problems include pancreatic insufficiency with malnutrition and intestinal obstruction, poor growth, male sterility, diabetes, and cirrhosis of the liver.
- The primary cause of death in the patient with CF is respiratory failure.

Interprofessional Collaborative Care
Recognize Cues: Assessment
- The major diagnostic test is sweat chloride analysis, and additional genetic testing can be performed to determine which specific mutation a person may have.
- Assess for these nonpulmonary manifestations: abdominal distention, gastroesophageal reflux, rectal prolapse, foul-smelling stools, steatorrhea (excessive fat in stools), small stature, and underweight for height.
- Assess for these common pulmonary manifestations: frequent or chronic respiratory infections, chest congestion, limited exercise tolerance, cough, sputum production, use of accessory muscles, and decreased pulmonary function (especially forced

vital capacity and forced exhalation volume over 1 second [FEV$_1$]).

Take Actions: Interventions

- The patient with CF needs daily therapy to slow disease progress and enhance **gas exchange**. There is no cure for CF.
- Nutrition management focuses on weight maintenance, vitamin supplementation, diabetes management, and pancreatic enzyme replacement (enzymes must be taken with food).
- Pulmonary management is focused on preventive maintenance and management of pulmonary exacerbation.
  1. Preventive or maintenance therapy involves the use of a regimen of chest physiotherapy, positive expiratory pressure, active cycle breathing technique, and an individualized regular exercise program. Drug therapy includes bronchodilators, antiinflammatory agents, mucolytics, and antibiotics.
  2. Exacerbation therapy is needed when the patient with CF has a change in manifestations from baseline. Management focuses on mucous clearance, oxygenation, and, if infection is present, antibiotic therapy. These drugs target the CFR channel so that the transporter can move chloride across the cell membrane, reducing sodium.
  3. *Gene therapy* for CF is available for use in patients with specific gene mutations.
- The surgical management of the patient with CF involves lung transplantation.
  1. Antirejection drug regimens must be started immediately after surgery. The drugs generally are used long-term to prevent rejection after organ transplantation. Antirejection drugs are immunosuppressive and increase the risk for serious infection.

See Chapter 24 in the main text for more information on cystic fibrosis.

CYSTITIS (URINARY TRACT INFECTION)

- Cystitis is an inflammatory condition of the bladder. Commonly, it refers to inflammation from an infection of the bladder. However, cystitis can be caused by inflammation without infection. For example, drugs, chemicals, or local radiation therapy cause bladder inflammation without an infecting organism.
  1. Cystitis with infection is a "urinary tract infection" (UTI).
     - A UTI is further categorized as *uncomplicated* or *complicated*.

Urinary Tract Infection Types

Type	Description
Acute Uncomplicated Cystitis	Acute UTI—bladder involvement only No signs/symptoms of upper UTI No anatomic or functional abnormality of the urinary tract or condition that increases the risk for infection or possibility of treatment failing to resolve the infection
Acute Complicated Cystitis	Involves more than the bladder Symptoms of upper UTI: fever, flank pain, chills/rigors, malaise, costovertebral angle tenderness, and pelvic and/or perineal pain in men.

👤 PATIENT-CENTERED CARE: GENDER HEALTH
Urinary Tract Infections

Females are 30 times more likely to have a UTI than men (U.S. Department of Health and Human Services [USDHHS], 2021). The female urethra is shorter than the male urethra, and this makes it easier for bacteria to get into the bladder. In addition, the female urethra is closer to the anus, which is a source of *E. coli*, a main source of UTIs (USDHHS, 2021).

- Noninfectious inflammation causes include chemical exposure, radiation therapy, and immunologic responses in chronic inflammatory disease.
  1. *Interstitial cystitis* is a chronic inflammation of the lower urinary tract (bladder, urethra, and adjacent pelvic muscles).
  2. Cystitis may sometimes occur as a complication of other disorders, such as gynecologic cancers, PIDs, endometriosis, Crohn's disease, diverticulitis, lupus, or tuberculosis.

Interprofessional Collaborative Care
Recognize Cues: Assessment
- Assess for:
  1. Increased frequency or urgency in voiding
  2. Urgency and pain or discomfort on urination
  3. Change in urine color, clarity, or odor; presence of pus (WBCs) or blood (RBCs)
  4. Presence of nitrogen or leukocyte esterase with urinalysis
  5. Positive urine culture
  6. Elevated plasma WBCs
  7. Abdominal or back pain

8. Bladder distention
9. Feelings of incomplete bladder emptying
10. Difficulty in initiating urination

Take Actions: Interventions

- Drug therapy includes:
  1. Antibiotics: In uncomplicated UTIs (also called acute bacterial cystitis), oral antibiotic treatment is recommended. A longer course of oral or parenteral antibiotics may be needed for complicated UTIs and for urosepsis.
  2. Analgesics or antipyretics may be used to promote comfort.
  3. Antispasmodics may be used to decrease bladder spasm and promote complete bladder emptying in certain chronic conditions or with recurrent UTI.

- Diet therapy includes:
  1. Some urologists recommend sufficient fluid intake to result in at least 1.5 L of urine output or 7 to 12 voidings daily.
  2. Cranberry juice or tablets taken daily may reduce the frequency of recurrent UTIs but should be avoided with interstitial cystitis.

- Other therapy includes providing warm sitz baths to relieve perineal discomfort.

- Surgical interventions for the management of noninfectious cystitis include urologic procedures for structural abnormalities or endourologic procedures to manipulate or pulverize kidney stones if these conditions are associated with cystitis.

Care Coordination and Transition Management

- Teach the patient to:
  1. Self-administer drugs and complete all of the prescribed antibiotic or antimicrobial agent.
  2. Expect changes in the color of urine with some treatments.
  3. Use appropriate techniques to prevent discomfort with sexual activities and to prevent postcoital infections.
  4. Consume a liberal amount of fluids to maintain urine color as clear or light yellow.
  5. Clean the perineum after urination.
  6. Empty the bladder as soon as the urge is felt.
  7. Avoid known irritants, such as caffeine, carbonated beverages, tomato products, chemicals in bath water (e.g., bubble baths), vaginal washes, and scented toilet tissue.
  8. Seek prompt medical care if symptoms recur.

See Chapter 58 in the main text for more information on cystitis.

CYSTOCELE

- A cystocele is a protrusion of the bladder through the vaginal wall, resulting from weakened pelvic structures.
    1. Causes include obesity, advanced age, childbearing, or genetic predisposition.

Interprofessional Collaborative Care

- Assess for:
    1. Difficulty in emptying the bladder
    2. Urinary frequency and urgency or other symptoms of UTI
    3. Stress urinary incontinence
    4. Bulging of the anterior vaginal wall, especially when the woman is asked to bear down during a pelvic examination
- Diagnostic tests may include cystography, measurement of residual urine, IV urography (IVU), voiding cystourethrography (VCUG), cystometrography, and uroflowmetry.
- Management of patients with mild symptoms is conservative and may include:
    1. Use of a pessary for bladder support
    2. Kegel exercises to strengthen perineal muscles
- Surgical intervention for severe symptoms is usually a vaginal sling or an anterior colporrhaphy (anterior repair) to tighten the pelvic muscles for better bladder support.

 See Chapter 63 in the main text for more information on cystocele.

DEHYDRATION: FLUID AND ELECTROLYTE CONCEPT ✳ EXEMPLAR

Overview

- In **dehydration**, fluid intake or retention is less than what is needed to meet the body's fluid needs, resulting in a deficit of fluid volume, especially plasma volume. It is a condition rather than a disease and can be caused by many factors.
  1. It may be an *actual* decrease in total body water caused by either too little intake of fluid or too great a loss of fluid; or it can occur as a *relative* deficit, without an actual loss of total body water, such as when water shifts from the plasma into the interstitial space.

 PATIENT-CENTERED CARE: OLDER ADULT HEALTH

Dehydration

Older adults are at high risk for dehydration because they have less total body water than younger adults, resulting from age-related muscle mass loss. Many older adults have decreased thirst sensation and may have difficulty with walking or other motor skills needed for obtaining fluids. They also may take diuretics, antihypertensives, and laxatives that increase fluid excretion. Assess the ***fluid and electrolyte balance*** status of older adults in any setting, and especially among those in long-term care (Morton, 2022).

  2. *Isotonic dehydration* is the most common type of fluid volume deficit, in which fluid is lost from the extracellular fluid (ECF) space, including both the plasma and the interstitial spaces. See common causes of dehydration.

Common Causes of Fluid Imbalances: Dehydration

- Hemorrhage
- Vomiting
- Diarrhea
- Profuse salivation
- Fistulas
- Ileostomy
- Profuse diaphoresis
- Burns
- Severe wounds
- Long-term NPO status
- Diuretic therapy
- GI suction
- Hyperventilation
- Diabetes insipidus
- Difficulty swallowing
- Impaired thirst
- Unconsciousness
- Fever
- Impaired motor function

Interprofessional Collaborative Care
Recognize Cues: Assessment
- Obtain and record patient information:
  1. Nutritional history
  2. Fluid history
     - Intake and output volumes
     - Weight: Because 1 L of water weighs 2.2 lb (1 kg), changes in daily weights are the best indicators of fluid losses or gains. A weight change of 1 lb corresponds to a fluid volume change of about 500 mL.
  3. Drug therapy (especially diuretics and laxatives)
  4. Medical history
- Physical assessment/signs and symptoms
  1. Vital signs, including orthostatic heart rate (HR) and blood pressure (BP) if patient is able to sit or stand
  2. Cardiovascular changes
     - Tachycardia at rest
     - Weak peripheral pulses
     - Low systolic or mean arterial BP
     - Decreased pulse pressure
     - Flat neck and hand veins in dependent position
  3. Respiratory changes
     - Increased respiratory rate
  4. Skin changes
     - Dry mucous membranes
     - Tongue has a paste-like coating or fissures
     - Dry, flaky skin
     - Poor skin turgor (skin "tents" when pinched)

PATIENT-CENTERED CARE: OLDER ADULT HEALTH
Skin Turgor

Assess skin turgor in an older adult by pinching the skin over the sternum rather than the back of the hand. With aging the skin loses elasticity and tents on hands and arms even when the person is well hydrated.

  5. Neurologic changes
     - Changes in cognition (especially confusion)
     - Fever
  6. Kidney function
     - Urine output below 500 mL/day for a patient without kidney disease is cause for concern (Ellison & Farrar, 2018)
     - The urine may be concentrated, with a specific gravity greater than 1.030 and have a dark amber color and a strong odor

- Diagnostic assessment: No single laboratory test result confirms or rules out dehydration. Instead, it is determined by laboratory findings along with signs and symptoms. Common laboratory findings for dehydration include:
  1. Elevated levels of hemoglobin and hematocrit
  2. Increased serum osmolality, glucose, protein, blood urea nitrogen, and various electrolytes

Analyze Cues and Prioritize Hypotheses: Analysis
- The priority problems for the patient who has dehydration are:
  1. Altered fluid and electrolyte balance due to excess fluid loss or inadequate fluid intake
  2. Potential for injury due to poor *perfusion* associated with decreased fluid volume

Generate Solutions and Take Actions: Planning and Implementation
- Goals of care for the patient with dehydration are to prevent further fluid loss, increase fluid volumes to normal, and prevent injury.

Restoring Fluid and Electrolyte Balance
- Mild to moderate dehydration is corrected with oral fluid replacement if the patient is alert enough to swallow and can tolerate oral fluids.
  1. Encourage fluid intake and measure the amount ingested.
  2. When dehydration is severe or the patient cannot tolerate oral fluids, IV fluid replacement is needed. Calculation of how much fluid is needed for replacement is based on the patient's weight loss and symptoms. The rate of fluid replacement depends on the degree of dehydration and the patient's cardiac, pulmonary, and kidney status.
  3. The two most important areas to monitor during rehydration are pulse rate and quality and urine output.
  4. Drug therapy may correct some causes of the dehydration.
     - Antidiarrheal drugs are prescribed when diarrhea causes dehydration.
     - Antimicrobial therapy may be used in patients with bacterial diarrhea.
     - Antiemetics may be used when vomiting causes dehydration.
     - Antipyretics to reduce fever are helpful when fever makes dehydration worse.

Preventing Injury
- Assess muscle strength, gait stability, and level of alertness.
  1. Implement fall precautions for safety.
  2. Instruct the patient to get up slowly from a lying or sitting position and to immediately sit down if feeling light-headed.
  3. Stress the importance of asking for assistance to ambulate.

Care Coordination and Transition Management
- Because dehydration is a symptom or complication of another health problem or drug therapy, even severe dehydration is resolved before patients return home or to residential care.
- Education is an important management strategy to prevent recurrence among adults who remain at some risk for recurrence, such as patients who have diabetes insipidus or diabetes mellitus.

Evaluate Outcomes: Evaluation
- Most patients return to an acceptable fluid balance with proper management.

 See Chapter 13 in the main text for more information on dehydration.

DEMENTIA

See *Alzheimer's Disease.*

DIABETES INSIPIDUS (ARGININE VASOPRESSIN DEFICIENCY / ARGININE VASOPRESSIN RESISTANCE)

- Diabetes insipidus is a disorder of the posterior pituitary gland in which water loss is caused by a deficiency in vasopressin (antidiuretic hormone [ADH]) or an inability of the kidneys to respond to vasopressin (ADH). In early 2023, new terminology for diabetes insipidus was adopted globally. Arginine vasopressin deficiency (AVP-D) refers to central diabetes insipidus, and arginine vasopressin resistance (AVP-R) refers to nephrogenic diabetes insipidus.

Interprofessional Collaborative Care
Recognize Cues: Assessment
- Most patients with moderate to severe AVP-D or AVP-R report polyuria, nocturia, and polydipsia (Bichet, 2023b).

Take Actions: Interventions
- Management focuses on controlling symptoms using drug therapy with desmopressin (Bichet, 2023a; Burchum & Rosenthal, 2022). As a synthetic drug, it serves to replace natural vasopressin (ADH) and decrease urination. It is available orally, as a sublingual "melt," or intranasally in a metered spray. The frequency of dosing varies with patient responses.

- Drug therapy induces water retention. Teach patients to weigh themselves daily to identify weight gain.
- If weight gain of more than 2.2 lb (1 kg) and other signs of water toxicity occur (e.g., persistent headache, acute confusion, nausea, vomiting), instruct the patient to go immediately to the emergency department or call 911.
- Instruct the patient to wear a medical alert bracelet identifying the disorder and drug.
- Treatment of AVP-R is selected based on cause. Urine output can be lowered with a low-salt, low-to-normal protein diet and diuretics (Bichet, 2023c). In adults, restricting sodium intake to less than 2.3 g/day and reducing protein intake to <1.0 mg/kg daily diminishes urine output (Bichet, 2023c). A thiazide diuretic induces mild volume depletion; even a weight loss of 1 to 1.5 kg can reduce urine output significantly (Bichet, 2023c). Other treatments are dependent on the patient's individualized needs.

D

⬮ NURSING SAFETY PRIORITY

Drug Alert

> The parenteral form of desmopressin is 10 times stronger than the oral form, and the dosage must be reduced.

- For the hospitalized patient, nursing management focuses on early detection of dehydration and maintaining adequate hydration.
  1. Actions include accurately measuring fluid intake and output, checking urine specific gravity, and recording the patient's weight daily.
  2. Encourage the patient to drink fluids in an amount equal to urine output. If fluids are given IV, ensure the patency of the access catheter and accurately monitor the amount infused hourly.
  3. Some patients may require lifelong drug therapy. Check the patient's ability to assess symptoms and adjust dosages as prescribed for changes in condition. Teach that polyuria and polydipsia indicate the need for another dose.

🏹 *See Chapter 54 in the main text for more information on diabetes insipidus (arginine vasopressin deficiency / arginine vasopressin resistance).*

DIABETES MELLITUS: GLUCOSE REGULATION CONCEPT ✳ EXEMPLAR

Overview

- **Diabetes mellitus** (DM) is a common chronic, complex disorder of impaired nutrient metabolism (especially of glucose) that can affect the function of every body system.
  1. *Glucose regulation* is the process of maintaining optimal blood glucose levels, also known as *glycemic control*.
  2. DM is classified by the underlying problem causing a lack of insulin and the severity of the insulin deficiency.

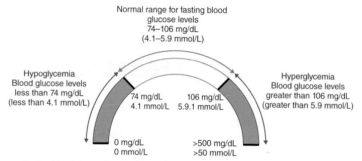

Fasting blood glucose levels. When **glucose regulation** is adequate, fasting levels remain in the normal range. With insufficient insulin usage, hyperglycemia results. Excess insulin or insufficient glucose results in hypoglycemia.

Acute Complications of DM

- Three glucose-related emergencies can occur in patients with DM:
  1. Diabetic ketoacidosis (DKA) caused by absence of insulin and generation of ketoacids
  2. Hyperglycemic-hyperosmolar state (HHS) caused by insulin deficiency and profound dehydration
  3. Hypoglycemia from too much insulin or too little glucose

  All three problems require emergency treatment and can be fatal if treatment is delayed or incorrect.

Classification of Diabetes Mellitus

Type 1 Diabetes (T1DM)
- Beta-cell destruction leading to absolute insulin deficiency
- Autoimmune
- Idiopathic

Type 2 Diabetes (T2DM)
- Ranges from insulin resistance with relative insulin deficiency to secretory deficit with insulin resistance

Latent Autoimmune Diabetes of Adulthood (LADA)
- Slow, progressive form of autoimmune disease
- Sometimes referred to as Type 1.5
- Varying degrees of insulin resistance
- Diagnosed >30 years of age

Maturity-Onset Diabetes of the Young (MODY)
- Inherited mutation in one of at least six known genes that results in loss of insulin function and hyperglycemia
- Usually diagnosed in younger adults but can be found at any time in adulthood
- Resembles type 1 DM with insulin requirements and potential for DKA
- Is not an autoimmune problem

Gestational Diabetes Mellitus (GDM)
- Glucose intolerance with onset or first recognition during pregnancy. (All pregnant women should be screened.)

D

Chronic Complications of DM

- DM can lead to organ complications and early death because of changes in large blood vessels (*macrovascular*) and small blood vessels (*microvascular*) in tissues and organs. These blood vessel changes lead to complications from poor tissue **perfusion** and cell ischemia.
  1. Macrovascular complications
     - Cardiovascular disease
     - Reduced immunity
  2. Microvascular complications
     - Eye and vision complications
     - Diabetic peripheral neuropathy
     - Diabetic autonomic neuropathy
     - Diabetic nephropathy
     - Sexual dysfunction
     - Cognitive dysfunction

PATIENT-CENTERED CARE: HEALTH EQUITY

Screening for DM

Racial and ethnically diverse populations have a higher prevalence and greater burden of T2DM. The rate of DM is 14.5% among American Indians and Alaska Natives, 12.1% among non-Hispanic Blacks, 11.8% among those with Hispanic origin, 9.5% among non-Hispanic Asians, and 7.4% among non-Hispanic Whites. (CDC, 2022c). Be alert to the risk for DM whenever you are interviewing or assessing adults. The ADA has identified indications for asymptomatic screening. Be familiar with these screening indications and advocate for early screening to promote early intervention for all adults.

Interprofessional Collaborative Care

Recognize Cues: Assessment

- Ask about and record patient history:
  1. Age and weight
  2. Birth weight of children or diagnosis of GDM or glucose intolerance during pregnancy
  3. History of recent illness, infection, or extreme stress
  4. Omission of insulin or oral diabetic drugs if the patient is known to have DM
  5. Change in eating habits
  6. Change in exercise schedule or activity level
  7. Presence and duration of polyuria, polydipsia, polyphagia, and loss of energy
  8. Presence of cardiovascular disease such as hyperlipidemia, hypertension, heart failure, or stroke
- Laboratory assessment
  1. Diabetes can be diagnosed by assessing the blood glucose levels listed in the Laboratory Profile.

Analyze Cues and Prioritize Hypotheses: Analysis

- The priority collaborative problems for patients with diabetes DM include:
  1. Potential for injury due to hyperglycemia
  2. Potential for surgical complications due to the health complexities with DM
  3. Potential for injury due to peripheral neuropathy
  4. Potential for kidney disease due to reduced kidney *perfusion*
  5. Potential for acute complications associated with glucose-related emergencies

Laboratory Profile

Blood Glucose Values

Test	Normal Range	Prediabetes	Diabetes
Glycosylated hemoglobin (A1C)	4%–5.7% (20–39 mmol/mol)	5.7%–6.4% (39–47 mmol/mol)	≥6.5% (48 mmol/mol)
Fasting blood glucose	74–100 mg/dL (4.1–5.6 mmol/L)	100–125 mg/dL (5.6–6.9 mmol/L)	≥126 mg/dL (7.0 mmol/mol)
Glucose tolerance (2-hour postprandial glucose [PPG])	<140 mg/dL (<7.8 mmol/L)	140–199 mg/dL (7.8–11.0 mmol/L)	≥200 mg/dL (11.1 mmol/mol)

Data from American Diabetes Association Standards of Medical Care Abridged for Primary Care Providers (2022); and Pagana, K. D., Pagana, T. J., & Pagana, T. N. (2022). *Mosby's manual of diagnostic and laboratory tests* (7th ed.). St. Louis: Elsevier.

D

Generate Solutions and Take Actions: Planning and Implementation

Preventing Injury From Hyperglycemia

- Patients are expected to manage DM and prevent disease progression by maintaining blood glucose levels within their target range. Management of DM involves **nutrition** interventions, blood glucose monitoring, a planned exercise program, and, often, drugs to lower blood glucose levels.

Nonsurgical Management

- Management of DM involves the following:
  1. **Nutrition** interventions
  2. Glucose monitoring
  3. Regular physical activity
  4. Stress management and reduction
  5. Drugs to lower blood glucose levels
- Nurses, the interprofessional team members, and the patient plan, coordinate, and deliver care.

Drug Therapy

- Drug therapy is indicated when a patient with type 2 DM does not achieve blood glucose control with diet changes, regular exercise, and stress management.
- Patients with type 1 DM require insulin therapy for blood glucose control and may use other antidiabetic drugs as well.
- See Drug Therapy for Diabetes Mellitus box.

Common Examples of Drug Therapy

Diabetes Mellitus

Drug Category	Nursing Implications

For all drugs used in the treatment of DM, teach patient the signs and symptoms of hypoglycemia (hunger, headache, tremors, sweating, confusion) because many antidiabetic drugs lower blood glucose levels even when hyperglycemia is not present.

Biguanides

Lower blood glucose by inhibiting liver glucose production, decreasing intestinal absorption of glucose, and increasing insulin sensitivity

- Metformin
  - Instruct patients not to drink alcohol while taking this drug *to reduce the risk for lactic acidosis.*
  - Remind patients that this drug must be stopped before certain imaging tests using contrast agents *because of the increased risk for kidney damage and lactic acidosis.*
  - Warn patients that GI problems are common side effects of this drug class. The medication should be taken with food *to lessen GI side effects.*

Incretin Mimetics (GLP-1 Agonists)

Act like natural "gut" hormones that work with insulin to lower blood glucose levels by reducing pancreatic glucagon secretion, reducing liver glucose production, and delaying gastric emptying

- Dulaglutide
- Exenatide
- Exenatide extended release
- Liraglutide
- Lixisenatide
- Semaglutide

  - Instruct patient how to inject themselves *because most drugs in this class are only available as subcutaneous formulations.*
  - Instruct patients to read dosing schedule carefully for exenatide, dulaglutide and injected semaglutide *because they are injected **weekly** rather than daily.*
  - Teach patients to report persistent abdominal pain and nausea to the health care provider *because these drugs increase the risk for pancreatitis and are contraindicated in gastroparesis.*

Sodium-Glucose Cotransport 2 (SGLT-2) Inhibitors

Lower blood glucose levels by preventing kidney reabsorption of glucose and sodium that was filtered from the blood into the urine. This filtered glucose is excreted in the urine rather than moved back into the blood

- Canagliflozin
- Dapagliflozin
- Empagliflozin
- Ertugliflozin

  - Teach the patient the signs and symptoms of dehydration (increased thirst, light-headedness, dry mouth and mucous membranes, orthostatic hypotension) *because these drugs increase urine output and increase dehydration risk.*
  - Teach the signs and symptoms of hyponatremia (muscle weakness, abdominal cramping, rapid heart rate, orthostatic hypotension) *because these drugs increase sodium loss.*

Common Examples of Drug Therapy—cont'd

Diabetes Mellitus

Drug Category	Nursing Implications
	• Teach patients the signs and symptoms of urinary tract infection (frequency, pain and burning on urination, foul urine odor) *because the increased glucose in the urinary tract predisposes to infection.*
	• Instruct to be alert for genital itching and vaginal discharge in females *because these drugs increase the risk for genital yeast infection.*
	• Teach patients to report any swelling, tenderness, or redness/hyperpigmentation of the genitals or perineal skin *because these drugs increase the risk for Fournier gangrene with perineal fasciitis.*

D

DPP-4 Inhibitors (*Gliptins*)

DPP-4 inhibitors are oral agents that prevent the enzyme DPP-4 from breaking down the natural gut hormones (GLP-1 and GIP); this allows these natural substances to work with insulin to lower glucagon secretion from the pancreas, which reduces liver glucose production. These oral drugs also reduce blood glucose levels by delaying gastric emptying and slowing the rate of nutrient absorption into the blood

• Alogliptin	• Instruct patients to be alert for rash or other sign of allergic reaction *because this class of drugs is associated with a moderate incidence of drug allergy.*
• Linagliptin	
• Saxagliptin	
• Sitagliptin	• Teach patients to report persistent abdominal pain and nausea to the health care provider *because these drugs increase the risk for pancreatitis.*
	• Instruct patients to notify the primary health care provider if shortness of breath, dyspnea on exertion, or cough, especially when lying down, is experienced *because this class of drugs is associated with heart failure.*

Insulin Stimulators (Secretagogues)

Lower blood glucose levels by triggering the release of preformed insulin from beta cells

Sulfonylureas	• Instruct patients to take these drugs with or just before meals *to prevent hypoglycemia.*
• Glipizide	
• Glyburide	• Instruct patients taking a sulfonylurea to check with their health care provider or a pharmacist before taking any over-the-counter drug or supplement *because these drugs interact with many other drugs.*
• Glimepiride	
Meglitinide ***(Glinides)***	
• Repaglinide	
• Nateglinide	

Continued

Common Examples of Drug Therapy—cont'd

Diabetes Mellitus

Drug Category	Nursing Implications

Insulin Sensitizers

Lower blood glucose by decreasing liver glucose production and improving the sensitivity of insulin receptors

Thiazolidinediones (TZDs or Glitazones)
- Pioglitazone
- Rosiglitazone

- Teach patients with any cardiovascular disease to weigh themselves daily and report a weight gain of more than 2 lb (1 kg) in one day or 4 lb (2 kg) in a week to the prescriber *because these drugs increase the risk for heart failure.*
- Instruct patients to report vision changes immediately *because these drugs increase the risk for macular edema.*
- Warn patients that weight gain and peripheral edema are *common side effects of these drugs.*

Alpha-Glucosidase Inhibitors

Act in the intestine to delay the absorption of carbohydrates, preventing after-meal hyperglycemia

- Acarbose
- Miglitol

- Teach patients to take these drugs only with a meal *because the action is in the intestinal tract.*
- Warn patients that abdominal discomfort and bloating, flatulence, nausea, diarrhea, and indigestion are common side effects of this drug class.

Amylin Analogs

These drugs are similar to amylin, a naturally occurring hormone produced by beta cells in the pancreas that is co-secreted with insulin and lowers blood glucose levels by decreasing endogenous glucagon, delaying gastric emptying, and triggering satiety

- Pramlintide

- Instruct patient how to inject themselves *because these drugs are only available as subcutaneous formulations.*
- Warn patients that nausea and vomiting are *common side effects of this drug class.*
- Do not mix in the same syringe with insulin *because their pH is not compatible.*

- *Insulin Therapy*: Insulin therapy is required for type 1 DM and often is used for type 2 DM. Many types of insulin and regimens are available to achieve normal blood glucose levels. Because insulin is a small protein that is quickly inactivated in the GI tract, it is usually injected.
    1. *Types of insulin* vary with the source and manufacturing techniques. Insulin analogs are synthetic human insulins in which

the structure of the insulin molecule is altered to change the rate of absorption and duration of action within the body (e.g., Lispro insulin).

2. Rapid-, short-, intermediate-, and long-acting forms of insulin can be injected separately, and some can be mixed in the same syringe. Insulin is available in concentrations of 100 units/mL (U-100), 200 units/mL (U-200), 300 units/mL (U-300), and 500 units/mL (U-500). U-500 insulin concentration is less common and reserved for when very large doses of insulin are required.

3. Teach the patient that the insulin types, the injection technique, and the site of injection all affect the absorption, onset, degree, and duration of insulin activity.

D

Timed Activity of Selected Pharmaceutical Insulin

Preparation	Onset (min)	Peak (hr)	Duration (hr)
Rapid-Acting Insulin Analogs			
Insulin aspart	10–20	1–3	3–5
Insulin glulisine	10–15	1–1.5	3–5
Insulin lispro (Humalog)	15–30	0.5–2.5	3–6
Short-Acting Insulin			
Regular insulin	30–60	1–5	6–10
Intermediate Acting Insulin			
NPH insulin	60–120	6–14	16–24
Long-Acting Insulin Analogs			
Insulin glargine U-100	70	None[a]	18–24
Insulin detemir	60–120	None[a]	12–24
Ultra Long–Acting Insulin			
Insulin degludec	30–90	None	24+

[a]Levels are steady with no discernible peak.
Data from Burchum, J., & Rosenthal, L. (2022). *Lehne's Pharmacology for nursing care* (11th ed.). St. Louis: Elsevier.

4. Injection site area affects the speed of insulin absorption. Absorption is fastest in the abdomen and, except for a 2-inch radius around the navel, is the preferred injection site.
5. Rotating injection sites allow each injection site to heal completely before the site is used again.
6. Rotation *within* one anatomic site is preferred to rotation from one area to another to prevent day-to-day variability in absorption.

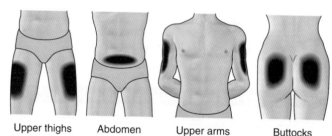

Upper thighs   Abdomen   Upper arms   Buttocks

Common insulin injection areas and sites. (From Peate, I. [2020]. *Alexander's Nursing practice: Hospital and home* [5th ed.]. London: Elsevier, Ltd.)

🗡 NURSING SAFETY PRIORITY
Drug Alert

Do not mix any other insulin type with insulin glargine, insulin detemir, or any of the premixed insulin formulations such as Humalog Mix 75/25.
- *Proper dose preparation* is critical for insulin effectiveness and safety. Teach patients that the person giving the insulin needs to inspect the vial before each use for changes (e.g., clumping, frosting, precipitation, or change in clarity or color) that may indicate loss in potency.
- Methods of insulin administration vary. These include syringes, insulin pens, smart pens, continuous subcutaneous insulin infusion, and dry powder inhalers.
- Preparations containing NPH insulin are uniformly cloudy after gently rolling the vial between the hands. Other insulins should be clear.

👪 PATIENT AND FAMILY EDUCATION

Subcutaneous Insulin Administration

With Vial and Syringe

- Wash your hands.
- Inspect the bottle for the type of insulin and the expiration date.
- Gently roll the bottle of intermediate-acting insulin in the palms of your hands to mix the insulin.
- Clean the rubber stopper with an alcohol swab.
- Remove the needle cover and pull back the plunger to draw air into the syringe. The amount of air should be equal to the insulin dose. Push the needle through the rubber stopper and inject the air into the insulin bottle.
- Turn the bottle upside down and draw the insulin dose into the syringe.
- Remove air bubbles in the syringe by tapping on the syringe or injecting air back into the bottle. Redraw the correct amount.
- Make certain the tip of the plunger is on the line for your dose of insulin. Magnifiers are available to assist in measuring accurate doses of insulin.
- Remove the needle from the bottle. Recap the needle if the insulin is not to be given immediately.
- Select a site within your injection area that has not been used in the past month.
- Clean your skin with an alcohol swab. Lightly grasp an area of skin and insert the needle at a 90-degree angle.
- Push the plunger all the way down. This will push the insulin into your body. Release the pinched skin.
- Pull the needle straight out quickly. Do not rub the place where you gave the shot.
- Dispose of the syringe and needle without recapping in a puncture-proof container.

❗ NURSING SAFETY PRIORITY

Action Alert

The Institute for Safe Medication Practices (ISMP) identifies insulin as a *High-Alert* drug. (High-Alert drugs are those that have an increased risk of causing patient harm if given in error.) The ISMP cautions that digital displays on some insulin pens can be misread. If the pen is held upside down, as a left-handed person might do, a dose of 52 units actually appears to be a dose of 25 units, and a dose of 12 units looks like a dose of 21 units.

Blood Glucose Monitoring

- The patient needs to know how to perform all aspects of blood glucose monitoring (BGM).
  1. Meter systems now require a very small blood sample, which allows for alternate testing sites (e.g., arm, thigh, hand).
  2. *Accuracy of the blood glucose monitor* is ensured when the manufacturer's directions are followed. If the meter requires calibration, teach patients to properly calibrate the machine.
  3. Teach the patient how to clean the equipment to prevent infection. The chance of becoming infected from blood glucose monitoring processes is reduced by handwashing before monitoring and by not reusing lancets.
  4. *Continuous blood glucose monitoring* (CGM) systems monitor glucose levels in interstitial fluid to provide real-time glucose information to the user. The system consists of three parts: a disposable sensor that measures glucose levels, a transmitter that is attached to the sensor, and a receiver that displays and stores glucose information.
- After an initiation or warm-up period, the sensor gives glucose values every 1 to 5 minutes. Sensors may be used for 3 to 7 days, depending on the manufacturer.
- CGM provides information about the current blood glucose level, provides short-term feedback about results of treatment, and provides warnings when glucose readings become dangerously high or low.

Nutrition Therapy

- Effective self-management of DM requires that **nutrition**, including the meal plan, education, and counseling programs, be individualized for each patient.
- Suggestions include:
  1. *Carbohydrate* intake avoids nutrient-deficient sources ("empty calories") and focuses on sources from vegetables, fruits, whole grains, legumes, and dairy products.
  2. Adults with diabetes should eat at least 25 g of fiber daily.
  3. *Dietary fat and cholesterol* intake for adults with DM focuses on the quality of fat rather than on the quantity of fat.
  4. *Alcohol* consumption affects blood glucose levels, especially with high alcohol use or when DM is poorly controlled. Teach patients that two alcoholic beverages for males and one for females can be ingested with, and in addition to, the usual meal plan.

PATIENT-CENTERED CARE: OLDER ADULT HEALTH

Nutritional Patterns

Factors that increase the risk for poor **nutrition** in older adults with DM include dental issues, financial stress, changes in appetite, and changes in the ability to obtain and prepare food. Older adults may have reduced awareness of either hypoglycemia or hyperglycemia, and dehydration, increasing the risk for hyperglycemic-hyperosmolar state (HHS) (Touhy & Jett, 2023). They may eat out or live in situations in which they have little control over meal preparation. Visits by home health nurses can help older patients follow a diabetic meal plan.

Changing the eating habits of 60 to 70 years is difficult and requires a realistic approach. The nurse, registered dietition nutritionist (RDN), and patient assess the patient's usual eating patterns. Teach the older patient taking antidiabetic drugs the importance of eating meals and snacks at the same time every day and eating the same amount of food from day to day.

Physical Activity

- Collaborate with the patient and rehabilitation specialist to develop an exercise program that includes at least 150 min/week of moderate-to-intensive aerobic physical activity divided into 5 days (ADA, 2022).

! NURSING SAFETY PRIORITY

Action Alert

Teach patients with T1DM to perform vigorous exercise only when blood glucose levels are 100 to 250 mg/dL (5.6 to 13.8 mmol/L) and no ketones are present in the urine.

- Teach the patient the following regarding exercise:
  1. Exercise helps control blood glucose levels, blood lipid levels, and helps reduce the complications of diabetes.
  2. Examine your feet daily and after exercising.
  3. Stay hydrated and do not exercise in the extreme heat or cold.
  4. Do not exercise within 1 hour of insulin injection or near time of peak insulin action.

Blood Glucose Control in Hospitalized Patients

- Current guidelines recommend treatment protocols that maintain blood glucose levels between 140 and 180 mg/dL (7.8 and 10.0 mmol/L) for critically ill patients.
- For most non–critically ill patients, premeal glucose targets are lower than 140 mg/dL (7.8 mmol/L), with random blood glucose values less than 180 mg/dL (10.0 mmol/L).
- To prevent hypoglycemia, insulin regimens are reviewed if blood glucose levels fall below 100 mg/dL (5.6 mmol/L) and are modified when blood glucose levels are less than 70 mg/dL (3.9 mmol/L) (ADA, 2022).

Surgical Management

- The most common surgical intervention for DM is pancreas transplantation. When successful, this procedure eliminates the need for insulin injections, blood glucose monitoring, and many dietary restrictions.
  1. Drug therapy is needed for life to prevent graft rejection.
  2. Complications include venous thrombosis, rejection, and infection.
  3. Most pancreatic transplants involve cadaver donors using a whole pancreas still attached to the exit of the pancreatic duct. The recipient's pancreas is left in place, and the donated pancreas is placed in the pelvis.
  4. Complications of DM increase the risk for surgical problems. Patients with DM are at higher risk for hypertension, ischemic heart disease, cerebrovascular disease, myocardial infarction (MI), and cardiomyopathy.

Preventing Surgical Complications

- Complications of DM increase the risk for surgical problems. Patients with DM are at higher risk for hypertension, ischemic heart disease, cerebrovascular disease, myocardial infarction (MI), and cardiomyopathy.
  1. Before surgery, blood glucose levels are optimized to reduce the risk for complications.
  2. Sulfonylureas are discontinued 1 day before surgery.
  3. Metformin is stopped at least 24 hours before surgery.
  4. Patients taking long-acting insulin may need to be switched to intermediate-acting insulin forms 1 to 2 days before surgery.
  5. IV infusion of insulin, glucose, and potassium is standard therapy for perioperative management of DM, and infusion rates are based on hourly capillary glucose testing.

6. Guidelines recommend insulin dosing to maintain blood glucose between 140 and 180 mg/dL (7.8 and 10.0 mmol/L) for critically ill patients (ADA, 2022).
7. Continue glucose and insulin infusions as ordered until the patient is stable and can tolerate oral feedings.
8. Short-term insulin therapy may be needed after surgery for the patient who usually uses oral agents.
9. For those receiving insulin therapy, dosage adjustments may be required until the stress of surgery subsides.

Preventing Injury From Peripheral Neuropathy

- Patients with DM need intensive teaching about foot care because foot injury is a common complication. Once a failure of ***tissue integrity*** has occurred and an ulcer has developed, there is an increased risk for wound progression that may eventually lead to amputation.

D

Assessment of the Diabetic Foot

Assess the patient's risk for diabetic foot problems:
- History of previous ulcer
- History of previous amputation

Assess the foot for abnormal skin and nail conditions:
- Dry, cracked, fissured skin
- Ulcers
- Toenails: thickened, long nails; ingrown nails
- Tinea pedis; onychomycosis (mycotic nails)

Assess the foot for status of circulation:
- Symptoms of claudication
- Presence or absence of dorsalis pedis or posterior tibial pulse
- Prolonged capillary filling time (greater than 25 seconds)
- Presence or absence of hair growth on the top of the foot

Assess the foot for evidence of deformity:
- Calluses, corns
- Prominent metatarsal heads (metatarsal head is easily felt under the skin)
- Toe contractures: clawed toes, hammertoes
- Hallux valgus or bunions
- Charcot foot ("rocker bottom")

Assess the foot for loss of strength:
- Limited ankle joint range of motion
- Limited motion of great toe

Assess the foot for loss of protective sensation:
- Numbness, burning, tingling
- Semmes-Weinstein monofilament testing at 10 points on each foot

Data from American Diabetes Association (ADA). (2022). Standards of medical care in diabetes—2022. *Diabetes Care 45*(Suppl. 1). https://diabetesjournals.org/care/issue/45/Supplement_1.

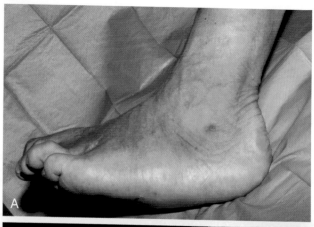

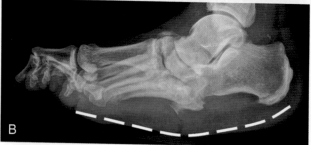

(A) Clinical presentation and **(B)** lateral radiograph of the rocker-bottom deformity of end-stage Charcot foot. (From Iaquinto, J.M., & Leslie, M.E. [2023]. *Foot and ankle biomechanics*. St. Louis: Elsevier Inc.)

- Foot care education includes:
  1. Recommending that the patient have shoes fitted by an experienced shoe fitter such as a certified podiatrist. Instruct the patient to change shoes at midday and in the evening and to wear socks with shoes.
  2. Teach patients about preventive care and the need for examination of the feet and legs at each visit to a diabetes health care provider or primary health care provider. A mirror placed on the floor can help the patient visually examine the plantar surface of the foot.
  3. Wound care for diabetic ulcers includes a moist wound environment, débridement of necrotic tissue, and offloading or elimination of pressure.

🏥 PATIENT AND FAMILY EDUCATION
Foot Care Instructions

- Inspect your feet daily, especially the area between the toes.
- Wash your feet daily with lukewarm water and soap. Dry thoroughly.
- Apply a moisturizer to your feet (but not between your toes) after bathing.
- Change into clean cotton socks every day.
- Do not wear the same pair of shoes 2 days in a row and wear only shoes made of breathable materials, such as leather or cloth.
- Check your shoes for foreign objects (nails, pebbles) before putting them on. Check inside the shoes for cracks or tears in the lining.
- Buy shoes that have plenty of room for your toes. Buy shoes later in the day, when feet are normally larger. Break in new shoes gradually.
- Wear socks to keep your feet warm.
- Trim your nails straight across with a nail clipper and smooth them with an emery board.
- See your diabetes health care provider immediately if you have blisters, sores, or infections. Protect the area with a dry, sterile dressing. Do not use tape to secure dressing to the skin.
- Do not treat blisters, sores, or infections with home remedies.
- Do not smoke or use nicotine products.
- Do not step into the bathtub without checking the temperature of the water with your wrist or a thermometer.
- Do not use very hot or cold water. Never use hot-water bottles, heating pads, or portable heaters to warm your feet.
- Do not treat corns, blisters, bunions, calluses, or ingrown toenails yourself.
- Do not go barefooted.
- Do not wear sandals with open toes or straps between the toes.
- Do not cross your legs or wear tight stockings that constrict blood flow.

Data from American Diabetes Association (ADA). (2022). Standards of medical care in diabetes—2022. Diabetes Care 45(Suppl. 1). https://diabetesjournals.org/care/issue/45/Supplement_1.

Reducing the Risk for Kidney Disease

- Diabetic kidney disease is more likely to develop in patients with poor blood glucose control. Progression to end-stage kidney disease can be delayed or prevented by normalizing blood pressure using drugs from either the angiotensin-converting enzyme inhibitor (ACEI) class or the angiotensin receptor blocker (ARB) class.
  1. Hypertension greatly accelerates the progression of diabetic kidney disease.
  2. An annual test to quantify urine albumin is performed for patients who have had T1DM for over 5 years and in all those with T2DM starting at diagnosis (ADA, 2022).

3. Use of angiotensin-converting enzyme inhibitors (ACEIs) or angiotensin receptor blockers (ARBs) is recommended for all patients with persistent albuminuria or advanced stages of nephropathy (ADA, 2022).
4. ACE inhibitors reduce the level of albuminuria and the rate of progression of kidney disease, although they do not appear to prevent albuminuria. Monitor serum potassium levels for development of hyperkalemia (ADA, 2022).
5. Dialysis for patients with DM and kidney failure is the same as for patients without diabetes.

Preventing Complications of Glucose Related Emergencies
Preventing Hypoglycemia

- Hypoglycemia is a low blood glucose level that induces specific symptoms and resolves when blood glucose concentration is raised.
- The most common causes of hypoglycemia are:
  1. Too much insulin compared with food intake and physical activity
  2. Insulin injected at the wrong time relative to food intake and physical activity
  3. The wrong type of insulin injected at the wrong time
  4. Decreased food intake resulting from missed or delayed meals
  5. Delayed gastric emptying from gastroparesis
  6. Decreased liver glucose production after alcohol ingestion
  7. Decreased insulin clearance due to progressive kidney failure
- Monitor blood glucose levels before giving antidiabetic drugs, before meals, before bedtime, and when the patient is symptomatic.
- All patients who take insulin, those taking sulfonylureas, and those taking metformin in combination with sulfonylureas are at risk for hypoglycemia.
- In the hospital setting, mealtime insulin *must* be coordinated with timely monitoring and food delivery to avoid episodes of hypoglycemia. Blood glucose should be checked no more than 1 hour before a meal and rapid-acting insulin given just before the meal to avoid hypoglycemia.
- In hospitalized patients most protocols for management of hypoglycemia follow the 15-15 rule for hypoglycemia management (Watts et al., 2020).
  1. With this rule 15 grams of carbohydrate are given if the blood glucose level is less than 70 mg/dL (3.9 mmol/L) (or 30 grams if less than 50 mg/dL [2.8 mmol/L]) or if the patient is experiencing symptoms of hypoglycemia.
  2. If the patient can swallow, give a liquid form of carbohydrate, although any fast-acting carbohydrate source can be used (avoid high-potassium options such as orange juice).

3. If the blood glucose recheck within 15 minutes is still low, the same treatment is given again.
4. If at any time the patient is unable to swallow, an IV dose of 50% dextrose or subcutaneous glucagon is indicated.
- Glucagon is the main balancing hormone to insulin and is used as first-line therapy for severe hypoglycemia.
- Take care to prevent aspiration in patients receiving glucagon because it often causes vomiting.
- Give concentrated dextrose carefully to avoid extravasation because it is hyperosmolar and can damage tissue.
- The effects of glucagon and dextrose are temporary. Evaluate response by monitoring blood glucose levels for several hours because symptoms may persist.
- A target blood glucose level is 70 to 110 mg/dL (3.9 to 6.2 mmol/L).

D

✚ NURSING SAFETY PRIORITY

Critical Rescue

Assess patients to recognize the presence and severity of hypoglycemia. For the patient with *severe* hypoglycemia respond by:
1. Giving prescribed dose of glucagon
2. Repeating the dose in 10 minutes if the patient remains unconscious
3. Notifying the diabetes health care provider immediately, and following instructions

Preventing Diabetic Ketoacidosis

- **Diabetic ketoacidosis (DKA)** is a complication of diabetes characterized by uncontrolled hyperglycemia, metabolic acidosis, and increased production of ketones.
  1. This condition results from the combination of insulin deficiency and an increase in hormone release that leads to increased liver and kidney glucose production. These changes increase ketoacid production with metabolic acidosis.
  2. The most common precipitating factor for DKA is infection or illness.
  3. Classic symptoms of DKA include:
     - Polyuria
     - Polydipsia
     - Polyphagia
     - A rotting citrus fruit odor to the breath
     - Vomiting
     - Abdominal pain
     - Dehydration

- Weakness
- Confusion
- Shock and coma
- Mental status, which can vary from total alertness to profound coma

4. If ketoacidosis occurs, interventions include the following:
   - Give insulin bolus as prescribed, usually followed by a continuous IV infusion.
   - Check the patient's BP, pulse, and respirations every 15 minutes until stable.
   - Replace both fluid volume and ongoing losses, monitoring for heart failure symptoms and pulmonary edema if large volume of IV fluid is administered.
   - Record urine output, temperature, and mental status every hour.
   - Assess the patient's level of consciousness and blood glucose levels at least every hour until stable (more frequently may be ordered); once stable, assess every 4 hours.
   - Monitor the patient for dehydration and hypokalemia (symptoms are muscle weakness, abdominal distention or paralytic ileus, hypotension, and weak pulse). Hypokalemia is a common cause of death in the treatment of DKA. Before administering potassium, ensure that the patient's urine output is at least 30 mL/hr.

5. Instruct the patient about how to prevent future episodes of DKA by contacting the primary health care provider when the blood glucose is greater than 250 mg/dL, when ketonuria is present for longer than 24 hours, when unable to take food or fluids, and when illness persists for longer than 1 to 2 days.

Preventing Hyperglycemic-Hyperosmolar State

- HHS is a hyperosmolar (increased blood osmolarity) state caused by hyperglycemia. Both HHS and DKA are caused by hyperglycemia and dehydration. HHS differs from DKA in that ketone levels are absent or low and blood glucose levels are much higher. Blood glucose levels may exceed 600 mg/dL (33.3 mmol/L), and blood osmolarity may exceed 320 mOsm/L.

1. Administer IV fluids and insulin as indicated, and monitor and assess the patient's response to therapy.
2. Assess for signs of cerebral edema, and immediately report to the health care provider a change in the level of consciousness; a change in pupil size, shape, or reaction to light; or seizure activity.

Differences Between Diabetic Ketoacidosis and Hyperglycemic-Hyperosmolar State

	Diabetic Ketoacidosis (DKA)	Hyperglycemic-Hyperosmolar State (HHS)
Onset	Sudden	Gradual
Precipitating factors	Infection	Infection
	Other stressors	Other stressors
	Inadequate insulin dose	Poor fluid intake
Symptoms	Ketosis: Kussmaul respiration, "rotting fruit" breath, nausea, abdominal pain	Altered central nervous system function with neurologic symptoms
	Dehydration or electrolyte loss: polyuria, polydipsia, weight loss, dry skin, sunken eyes, soft eyeballs, lethargy, coma	Dehydration or electrolyte loss: same as for DKA

Laboratory Findings

Serum glucose	>300 mg/dL (16.7 mmol/L)	>600 mg/dL (33.3 mmol/L)
Osmolarity/Osmolality	Variable	>320 mOsm/L (mOsm/kg)
Serum ketones	Positive at 1:2 dilutions	Negative
Serum pH	<7.35	>7.4
Serum HCO_3^-	<15 mEq/L (mmol/L)	>20 mEq/L (mmol/L)
Serum Na^+	Low, normal, or high	Normal or low
BUN	>30 mg/dL (10 mmol/L); elevated because of dehydration	Elevated
Creatinine	>1.5 mg/dL (60 mmol/L); elevated because of dehydration	Elevated
Urine ketones	Positive	Negative

BUN, Blood urea nitrogen; HCO_3^-, bicarbonate; Na^+, sodium.

Care Coordination and Transition Management
- Discharge planning includes:
  1. Ensuring that the patient understands the significance, symptoms, causes, and treatment of hypoglycemia and hyperglycemia
  2. Assisting the patient to identify the items needed for the administration of insulin and for glucose monitoring

3. Teaching the patient how to monitor blood sugar level
4. Teaching the patient how to administer drugs and prevent hypoglycemia
5. In collaboration with the dietitian, teaching the patient the skills associated with food choices and meal planning
6. Referring the patient to a diabetes educator for the necessary instruction
7. Helping the patient adapt to DM, including teaching stress management techniques and identifying coping mechanisms
8. Referring the patient to the American Diabetes Association and its resources
9. Providing information about community resources, such as diabetic education programs

---

Outcome Criteria for Diabetes Teaching

Before self-management begins at home, the patient with diabetes or the significant other should be able to:

- Tell why insulin or a noninsulin antidiabetic drug is being prescribed
- Name which insulin or noninsulin antidiabetic drug is being prescribed, and name the dosage and frequency of administration
- Discuss the relationship between mealtime and the action of insulin or the other antidiabetic agent
- Discuss plans to follow diabetic diet instructions
- Prepare and inject insulin accurately
- Test blood for glucose or state plans for having blood glucose levels monitored
- Test urine for ketones and state when this test should be done
- Describe how to store insulin
- List symptoms that indicate a hypoglycemic reaction
- Tell which carbohydrate sources are used to treat hypoglycemic reactions
- Tell which symptoms indicate hyperglycemia
- Tell which dietary changes are needed during illness
- State when to call the diabetes health care provider or the nurse (frequent episodes of hypoglycemia, symptoms of hyperglycemia)
- Describe the procedures for proper foot care

Evaluate Outcomes: Evaluation

- Evaluate the care of the patient with DM based on the identified priority patient problems. Outcome success for diabetes education is the ability of the patient to maintain blood glucose levels within their established target range. See Outcome Criteria for Diabetes Teaching.

See Chapter 56 in the main text for more information on diabetes mellitus.

DIVERTICULAR DISEASE

- Diverticular disease includes diverticulosis and diverticulitis.
    1. *Diverticula* are pouchlike herniations of the mucosa through the muscular wall of any portion of the gut, but most commonly the colon.
    2. *Diverticulosis* is the presence of many abnormal pouchlike herniations (diverticula) in the wall of the intestine.
    3. *Diverticulitis* is the inflammation or infection of diverticula.
    4. Complications of diverticula and diverticulitis are abscess formation and perforation followed by peritonitis.

Interprofessional Collaborative Care
Recognize Cues: Assessment
- Patients with diverticulosis are usually asymptomatic; a minor history of left lower quadrant pain or constipation may be reported.
- Diverticula are identified by colonoscopy; a screening abdominal ultrasound may reveal thickened bowel wall.
- Assess for signs and symptoms of diverticulitis:
    1. Abdominal *pain* that may begin as intermittent and may progress to continuous; pain may be localized to the left lower quadrant and increase with coughing, straining, or lifting
    2. Fever
    3. Nausea and vomiting
    4. Abdominal distention
    5. Blood in the stool (microscopic to larger amounts)
    6. Elevated WBCs; reduced hematocrit and hemoglobin if bleeding occurs
    7. Hypotension and dehydration occur if bleeding occurs (see *Shock*)
    8. Signs of septic shock occur if peritonitis has occurred
    9. Intake and output, including NG tube (amount, color, and quality) if used for gastric decompression or to manage vomiting

Take Actions: Interventions
- Drug therapy is used to treat infection and inflammation from diverticulitis.
    1. Administer broad-spectrum antibiotics, such as metronidazole plus trimethoprim/sulfamethoxazole, or ciprofloxacin.
    2. Implement management for mild or moderate pain; if pain is severe, use opioids.
    3. Laxatives and enemas are not given because they increase intestinal motility.
- An NG tube is inserted if nausea, vomiting, or abdominal distention is severe.

- Diet therapy:
    1. Provide IV fluids for hydration during the acute phase of the disease or when the patient is NPO.
    2. Consult with a dietitian to promote healthy food choices.

Surgical Management
- Patients with diverticulitis need emergent surgery if any of the following occurs:
    1. Rupture of the diverticulum with subsequent peritonitis
    2. Abdominal or pelvic abscess
    3. Bowel obstruction
    4. Fistula
    5. Persistent fever or **pain**
    6. Uncontrolled bleeding
- Surgical management includes a colon resection with or without a colostomy, and is the most common surgical procedure for patients with diverticular disease.
- Postoperative care includes:
    1. Maintaining a drainage system at the abdominal incision site
    2. If a colostomy was created, monitoring colostomy stoma for color and integrity, anticipating that a gray or black color or separation between the mucous membranes and skin is indicative of poor healing and requires immediate communication with the surgeon
    3. Providing the patient with an opportunity to express feelings about the colostomy
    4. Consulting with the wound or ostomy specialist
    5. Providing written postoperative instructions on:
        - Wound care
        - Avoidance of activities that increase intra-abdominal pressure
        - Pain management, including prescriptions
- Teach the patient and family to:
    1. Follow dietary considerations for diverticulosis, which include consultation with the dietitian. Keep a food diary to note food associations with symptoms and to implement the following:
        - Eat a diet high in cellulose and hemicellulose, which are found in wheat bran, whole-grain breads, cereals, fresh fruit, and vegetables.
        - A bulk-forming laxative such as psyllium hydrophilic mucilloid may be used to increase fecal size and consistency.
        - Encourage fluids to prevent bloating, which may accompany a high-fiber diet.
        - Avoid alcohol, which has an irritant effect on the bowel.
    2. Avoid all fiber when symptoms of diverticulitis are present because high-fiber foods are then irritating. As **inflammation** resolves, gradually add fiber back into the diet.

3. Monitor for signs and symptoms of diverticulitis (e.g., fever, abdominal pain, bloody stools).

See Chapter 49 in the main text for more information on diverticular disease.

DUMPING SYNDROME

- Dumping syndrome is a term that refers to a group of vasomotor symptoms that occur after eating in patients who had a gastrectomy. A gastrectomy is a surgical procedure to reduce the size of the stomach as a treatment for cancer, for perforation from peptic ulcer disease, or as bariatric surgery to reduce complications from morbid obesity.
- This syndrome is believed to occur as a result of the rapid emptying of food contents into the small intestine, which shifts fluid into the gut, causing abdominal distention.
- *Early dumping syndrome* typically occurs within 30 minutes of eating. Symptoms include vertigo, tachycardia, syncope, sweating, pallor/ash gray skin, palpitations, and the desire to lie down. Report these signs and symptoms to the surgeon in the postoperative recovery period, and encourage the patient to lie down.
- *Late dumping syndrome,* which occurs 1 to 3 hours after eating, is caused by a release of an excessive amount of insulin. The insulin release follows a rapid rise in the blood glucose level that results from the rapid entry of high-carbohydrate food into the jejunum. Observe for signs and symptoms, including dizziness, light-headedness, palpitations, diaphoresis, and confusion, and encourage the patient to lie down and reconsider dietary choices.

Interprofessional Collaborative Care
- Dumping syndrome is managed by **nutrition** changes that include decreasing the amount of food taken at one time and eliminating liquids ingested with meals. In collaboration with the registered dietitian nutritionist, teach the patient to eat a high-protein, high-fat, low- to moderate-carbohydrate diet.

See Chapter 47 in the main text for more information on dumping syndrome.

DYSRHYTHMIAS

- Cardiac dysrhythmias are abnormal rhythms of the heart's electrical system that can affect its ability to effectively pump oxygenated blood throughout the body.

- Some dysrhythmias are life-threatening, and others are not. They are the result of disturbances in cardiac electrical impulse formation, conduction, or both.
- Any disorder of the heartbeat is called a dysrhythmia.

⚓ *Refer to the appendix: Electrocardiographic Complexes, Segments, and Intervals to view sample rhythms of each type.*

Normal Sinus Rhythm
- Originates from the sinoatrial (SA) node (dominant pacemaker) and meets these ECG criteria:
  1. Rate: atrial and ventricular rates of 60 to 100 beats/min
  2. Rhythm: atrial and ventricular rhythms are regular
  3. P waves: present, consistent configuration; one P wave before each QRS complex
  4. PR interval: 0.12 to 0.20 second and constant
  5. QRS duration: 0.06 to 0.11 second and constant

Sinus Arrhythmia
- Sinus arrhythmia has all the characteristics of normal sinus rhythm (NSR) except for its irregularity. The PP and RR intervals vary, with the difference between the shortest and the longest intervals being greater than 0.12 second.

Common Dysrhythmias
Premature Complexes
- *Premature complexes* are early complexes that occur when a cardiac cell or group of cells other than the SA node becomes irritable and fires an impulse before the next sinus impulse is generated.
  1. *Bigeminy* occurs when normal complexes and premature complexes occur alternately in a repetitive two-beat pattern, with a pause occurring after each premature complex so that complexes occur in pairs.
  2. *Trigeminy* is a repetitive three-beat pattern, usually occurring as two sequential normal complexes followed by a premature complex and a pause, with the same pattern repeating itself in triplets.
  3. *Quadrigeminy* is a repetitive four-beat pattern, usually occurring as three sequential normal complexes followed by a premature complex and a pause, with the same pattern repeating itself in a four-beat pattern.

Bradydysrhythmias
- *Bradydysrhythmias* are characterized by a HR less than 60 beats/min.
  1. The patient may tolerate a low HR if BP is adequate.
  2. Symptomatic bradydysrhythmias lead to hypotension, myocardial ischemia or infarction, other dysrhythmias, and heart failure.

Tachydysrhythmias

- *Tachydysrhythmias* are HRs greater than 100 beats/min.
  1. Signs and symptoms include palpitations; chest discomfort; pressure or *pain* from myocardial ischemia or infarction; restlessness; anxiety; pale/ash gray, cool skin; and syncope from hypotension.
  2. They may cause heart failure, as indicated by dyspnea, orthopnea, pulmonary crackles, distended neck veins, fatigue, and weakness.
- Dysrhythmias are further classified according to their site of origin.

Sinus Dysrhythmias

- Sinus tachycardia occurs when the SA node discharge exceeds 100 beats/min.
  1. Treatment is based on identifying the underlying cause (e.g., angina, fever, hypovolemia, pain).
- Sinus bradycardia is a decreased rate of SA node discharge of less than 60 beats/min.
  1. If the patient is symptomatic, treatment may include atropine, a pacemaker, and avoidance of parasympathetic stimulations such as prolonged suctioning.

D

! NURSING SAFETY PRIORITY

Action Alert

For patients with sinus tachycardia, assess for fatigue, weakness, shortness of breath, orthopnea, decreased oxygen saturation, increased pulse rate, and decreased blood pressure. Also assess for restlessness and anxiety from decreased cerebral *perfusion* and for decreased urine output from impaired renal *perfusion*. The patient may also have anginal pain and palpitations. The ECG pattern may show T-wave inversion or ST-segment elevation or depression in response to myocardial ischemia.

Atrial Dysrhythmias

- *Premature atrial complex* (PAC) occurs when atrial tissue becomes irritable. This ectopic focus fires an impulse before the next sinus impulse is due.
  1. No intervention is generally needed except to treat the cause, such as heart failure or valvular disease.
- *Supraventricular tachycardia* (SVT) involves the rapid stimulation of atrial tissue at a rate of 100 to 280 beats/min.
  1. Drug therapy is prescribed for some patients to convert SVT to an NSR. Adenosine is used to terminate the acute episode and is given rapidly (over several seconds) followed by a normal saline bolus.

2. Oxygen therapy, antidysrhythmic drugs, vagal maneuvers, or synchronized cardioversion may be needed.
3. Sustained SVT may need to be treated with radiofrequency catheter ablation.

⬥ NURSING SAFETY PRIORITY
Drug Alert

Side effects of adenosine include significant bradycardia with pauses, nausea, and vomiting. When administering adenosine, be sure to have emergency equipment readily available!

- *Atrial fibrillation* (AF) is characterized by chaotic depolarization of the atria, decreasing cardiac output and ***perfusion***. It is considered uncontrolled when the ventricular rate is 120 to 200 beats/min. See *Atrial Fibrillation*.
  1. Drug treatment is used to prevent embolus formation related to irregular cardiac rhythm and to slow the cardiac rate from an altered conduction pattern or to return the rhythm to normal.

Ventricular Dysrhythmias

- Ventricular dysrhythmias are potentially more life-threatening than atrial dysrhythmias because the left ventricle pumps oxygenated blood throughout the body to perfuse vital organs and other tissues.
  1. *Premature ventricular complexes* (PVCs) (also called premature ventricular contractions) result from irritability of ventricular cells.
     - Premature ventricular contractions are common, and their frequency increases with age.
     - They may be insignificant or may occur with problems such as myocardial infarction, chronic heart failure, chronic obstructive pulmonary disease (COPD), and anemia.
     - PVCs may also be present in patients with hypokalemia or hypomagnesemia.
     - If there is no underlying heart disease, PVCs are not usually treated other than by eliminating or managing any contributing cause (e.g., caffeine, stress).
     - Potassium or magnesium is given for replacement therapy if hypokalemia or hypomagnesemia is the cause.
     - If the number of PVCs in a 24-hour period is excessive, the patient may be placed on beta-adrenergic blocking agents (beta blockers).

2. *Ventricular tachycardia* (VT), sometimes referred to as *V tach,* occurs with repetitive firing of an irritable ventricular ectopic focus, usually at a rate of 140 to 180 beats/min or more. VT may result from increased automaticity or a reentry mechanism. It may be intermittent (nonsustained VT) or sustained, lasting longer than 15 to 30 seconds. The rapid rate and loss of atrial volume results in decreased cardiac output.
   - Patients are at risk for VT during acute coronary syndromes, following surgical manipulation of the heart or pericardium, or with electrolyte imbalances.

D

✚ NURSING SAFETY PRIORITY

Critical Rescue

In some patients, VT causes cardiac arrest. Assess the patient's circulation, airway, breathing, level of consciousness, and oxygenation level. For the *stable* patient with sustained VT, administer oxygen and confirm the rhythm via a 12-lead ECG. Amiodarone, lidocaine, or magnesium sulfate may be ordered.

   - Current Advanced Cardiac Life Support (ACLS) guidelines state that elective cardioversion is highly recommended for stable VT.
   - The primary health care provider may order an oral antidysrhythmic agent to prevent further occurrences.
   - Patients who persist with episodes of stable VT may require radiofrequency catheter ablation.
   - *Unstable* VT without a pulse is treated the same way as ventricular fibrillation.

3. *Ventricular fibrillation* (VF), sometimes called *V fib,* is the result of electrical chaos in the ventricles and is *life-threatening!* Impulses from many irritable foci fire in a totally disorganized manner so that ventricular contraction cannot occur. *There is no cardiac output or pulse and therefore no cerebral, myocardial, or systemic **perfusion**. This rhythm is rapidly fatal if not successfully ended within 3 to 5 minutes.*
   - The priority is to defibrillate the patient immediately according to ACLS protocol.
   - If a defibrillator is not readily available, high-quality cardiopulmonary resuscitation (CPR) must be initiated and continued until the defibrillator arrives. An automated external defibrillator (AED) is frequently used because it is simple for both medical and lay personnel.

NURSING SAFETY PRIORITY

Critical Rescue

Early defibrillation is critical in resolving pulseless VT or VF. It must not be delayed for any reason after the equipment and skilled personnel are present. The earlier defibrillation is performed, the greater the chance of survival! *Do not defibrillate ventricular asystole.* The purpose of defibrillation is disruption of the chaotic rhythm, allowing the SA node signals to restart. In ventricular asystole, no electrical impulses are present to disrupt.

Before defibrillation, loudly and clearly command all personnel to clear contact with the patient and the bed, and check to see that they are clear before the shock is delivered. Deliver the shock and immediately resume CPR for five cycles, or about 2 minutes. Reassess the rhythm every 2 minutes and, if indicated, charge the defibrillator to deliver an additional shock at the same energy level previously used. During the 2-minute intervals, while high-quality CPR is being delivered, the ACLS team administers medications and performs interventions to try to restore an organized cardiac rhythm. *Discussion of ACLS protocol is beyond the scope of this text.*

- Antidysrhythmic drugs may be used after return of an organized rhythm; the most common drug used is amiodarone.
4. Ventricular asystole, sometimes called *ventricular standstill,* is the complete absence of any ventricular rhythm. There are no electrical impulses in the ventricles and therefore *no* ventricular depolarization, no QRS complex, no contraction, no cardiac output, and no perfusion to the rest of the body.
   - CPR must be initiated immediately when asystole occurs.
   - When finding an unresponsive patient, confirm unresponsiveness and call 911 (in a community or long-term care setting) or the emergency response team (in the hospital). Gather the AED or defibrillator *before initiating CPR.* Guidelines for CPR have changed from an ABC (airway-breathing-compressions) approach to the initial priorities of CAB (compressions-airway-breathing).
   - Check for a carotid pulse for 5 to 10 seconds.
   - If a carotid pulse is absent, start chest compressions of 100 to 120 compressions per minute and a compression depth of at least 2 inches with no more than 2.4 inches. Push hard and fast! Avoid leaning into the chest after each compression to allow for full chest wall recoil.
   - Maintain a patent airway.

- Ventilate (**b**reathing) with a mouth-to-mask device. Give rescue breaths at a rate of 10 to 12 breaths/min. If an advanced airway is in place, one breath should be given every 6 to 8 seconds (8 to 10 breaths/min).
- Ventilation-to-compression ratio should be maintained at 30 compressions to 2 breaths if advanced airway is not in place.
- Limit interruptions to compressions to less than 10 seconds.
- When possible, compressors should be changed every 2 minutes to maintain effective compressions.
- A CPR coach should be assigned to cardiac arrest response teams to coordinate, communicate, and maintain effective CPR (Craig-Branagan & Day, 2021)

Interprofessional Collaborative Care

- Assess patients with dysrhythmias for a decrease in cardiac output, resulting in inadequate oxygenation and *perfusion* to vital organs; assess VS, pulses, and level of consciousness unless the monitored rhythm is VF. If VF, initiate the Rapid Response Team and begin CPR.
- Interpret common dysrhythmias, especially bradycardia, tachycardia, AF, VT, VF, PVCs, and asystole, using the steps of ECG analysis. Respond with immediate communication to the primary health care provider when a patient has a new abnormal rhythm.
- Identify and intervene in life-threatening situations by providing CPR, electrical therapy (cardioversion or defibrillation), or drug administration.
- Anticipate blood collection for evaluation of serum electrolytes and possibly serum levels of antidysrhythmic drugs if these types of drugs have been prescribed.
- Anticipate the need for IV access and fluids, and place a peripheral catheter if one is not present and functioning.
- If sinus rhythm or spontaneous circulation returns during treatment, transport the patient to the ICU, and use best practices to hand off the patient (SBAR or agency format).
- Some institutions allow or encourage family members to be present at a resuscitation event; contact the chaplain or social worker to provide family members with support and debriefing if they witness urgent care around a dysrhythmia.

Care Coordination and Transition Management

- If an implantable defibrillator or pacemaker is newly placed for treatment, teach the patient about incisional care and safe practice.

- Teach patients with dysrhythmias the correct drug, dose, route, time, and side effects of prescribed drugs, and teach them to notify their primary care provider if adverse effects occur.
- Teach patients taking anticoagulant therapy to report any signs of bruising or unusual bleeding immediately to their primary health care provider.
- Teach family members where to learn CPR to decrease their anxiety while living with a patient with dysrhythmias or an ICD/pacemaker.

See Chapter 28 in the main text for more information on dysrhythmias.

ENDOCARDITIS, INFECTIVE

- Infective endocarditis (previously called bacterial endocarditis) refers to a microbial *infection* (virus, bacterium, fungus) involving the endocardium.
- Infective endocarditis occurs primarily in patients with a history of injection drug use (IDU), valve replacements, or systemic infection, or in patients with structural cardiac defects.
- The incidence of infective endocarditis is rising in conjunction with the opioid epidemic in the United States.
- Portals of entry for infecting organisms include:
  1. Oral cavity, especially if dental procedures have been performed
  2. Skin rashes, lesions, or abscesses
  3. Infections (cutaneous, genitourinary, gastrointestinal [GI], or systemic)
  4. Surgical or invasive procedures, including IV line placement

Interprofessional Collaborative Care
Recognize Cues: Assessment

- Because the mortality rate remains high, early detection of infective endocarditis is essential. Without treatment, infective endocarditis is fatal.
- Signs and symptoms typically occur within 2 weeks of a bacteremia. See key features of infective endocarditis.

KEY FEATURES
Infective Endocarditis

- Fever associated with chills, night sweats, malaise, and fatigue
- Anorexia and weight loss
- Cardiac murmur (newly developed or change in existing)
- Development of heart failure
- Evidence of systemic embolization
- Petechiae
- Splinter hemorrhages
- Osler nodes (on palms of hands and soles of feet)
- Janeway lesions (flat, reddened maculae on hands and feet)
- Roth spots (hemorrhagic lesions that appear as round or oval spots on the retina)
- Positive blood cultures

- Assess for:
  1. Signs of infection, including fever, chills, malaise, night sweats, and fatigue
  2. Heart murmurs: almost all patients with infective endocarditis develop murmurs.
  3. *Heart failure is the most common complication of infective endocarditis.*
     - Right-sided heart failure, evidenced by:
       - Peripheral edema
       - Weight gain
       - Anorexia
     - Left-sided heart failure, evidenced by:
       - Fatigue
       - Shortness of breath
       - Crackles
  4. Evidence of arterial embolization from fragments of vegetation on valve leaflets, which may travel to other organs and compromise function. Signs of acute embolization include:
     - Splenic emboli: sudden abdominal pain and radiation to the left shoulder
     - Kidney infarction: flank pain that radiates to the groin and is accompanied by hematuria or pyuria
     - Mesenteric emboli: diffuse abdominal pain, often after eating and abdominal distention
     - Brain emboli: signs of stroke, confusion, reduced concentration, and difficulty speaking
     - Pulmonary emboli: pleuritic chest pain, dyspnea, and cough
  5. Petechiae of the neck, shoulders, wrists, ankles, mucous membranes, or conjunctivae
  6. Splinter hemorrhages, black longitudinal lines, or small red streaks in the nail bed
- The most reliable criteria for diagnosing endocarditis include positive blood cultures, a new regurgitant murmur, and evidence of endocardial involvement by echocardiography.

Take Actions: Interventions

- Interventions include:
  1. Administering IV antimicrobial therapy as prescribed
  2. Monitoring the patient's tolerance to activity
  3. Protecting the patient from contact with potentially infective organisms

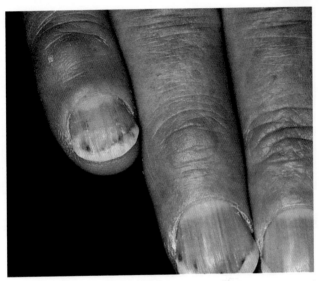

Splinter hemorrhages on the nail bed of the fingers. (From Callen, Jeffrey P., et al. [2017]. *Dermatological signs of systemic disease* [5th ed.]. Philadelphia: Elsevier.)

E

- Surgical intervention includes removal of the infected valve, repair or removal of congenital shunts, repair of injured valves and chordae tendineae, and draining abscesses in the heart or elsewhere.
- Preoperative and postoperative care for the patient having surgery involving the valves is similar to that described for patients undergoing coronary artery bypass grafting or valve replacement.

Care Coordination and Transition Management

- Teach the patient and family:
  1. Information on the cause of the disease and its course, drug regimens, signs and symptoms of infection, and practices to prevent future infections
  2. How to administer IV antibiotics and care for the IV or peripherally inserted central catheter (PICC) site, ensuring that all supplies are available to the patient discharged to home
  3. The importance of good personal and oral hygiene, such as using a soft toothbrush, brushing the teeth twice each day, and rinsing the mouth with water after brushing
  4. To avoid the use of dental irrigation devices and dental floss

> ### ❗ NURSING SAFETY PRIORITY
> #### *Action Alert*
>
> Patients must remind health care providers (including their dentists) of their endocarditis. Guidelines for antibiotic prophylaxis have been revised and are recommended only if the patient with a prosthetic valve, a history of infective endocarditis, or an unrepaired cyanotic congenital heart disease undergoes an invasive dental or oral procedure (Wilson et al., 2021; Habib et al., 2015).
>
> Instruct patients to note any indications of recurring endocarditis, such as fever. Remind them to monitor and record their temperature daily for up to 6 weeks. Teach them to report fever, chills, malaise, weight loss, increased fatigue, sudden weight gain, or dyspnea to their primary care provider.

 See Chapter 29 in the main text for more information on infective endocarditis.

❇ END-OF-LIFE CARE: COMFORT CONCEPT EXEMPLAR

Overview
- Although dying is part of the normal life cycle, it is often feared as a time of pain and suffering.
- **Hospice** is considered to be the model for quality, compassionate care for people facing a life-limiting illness or injury. Hospice uses a team-oriented approach, providing expert medical care, pain management, and emotional and spiritual support expressly tailored to the person's needs and wishes.
- **Palliative care** is a philosophy of care for people with life-threatening disease that assists patients and families in identifying their outcomes for care, assists them with informed decision making, and facilitates quality symptom management.

Components of Advance Care Planning
- **Advance care planning** is a process in which patients and families discuss end-of-life care, clarifying values and goals and then expressing those goals in an advance directive (HPNA, 2018).
- Documentation of self-determination is accomplished by completing an advance directive.
- Advance directives vary from state to state; however, most have a section to name the durable power of attorney for health care (DPOAHC). This is not the same as the power of attorney for

Comparison of Hospice and Palliative Care

Hospice Care	Palliative Care
Patients have a prognosis of 6 months or less to live.	Patients can be in any stage of serious illness.
Care is provided when curative treatment such as chemotherapy has been stopped.	A consultation is provided that is concurrent with curative therapies or therapies that prolong life.
Care is provided in 60- and 90-day periods with an opportunity to continue if eligibility criteria are met. Medicare does cover hospice for 6 months	Care is not limited by specific time periods and may be covered by insurance, Medicare, or Medicaid.
Ongoing care is provided by RNs, social workers, chaplains, and volunteers.	The primary health care provider can refer the patient. The palliative care team includes doctors, nurses, social workers, nutritionists, and chaplains; the team will vary based on the patient's needs.
Hospice care can be provided in any care environment, including the hospital, home, or in a separate hospice center.	Palliative care can be provided in almost any care environment, including the hospital or home.

finances. It may be the same person, depending on whom the patient designates. This person does not make decisions until the health care provider states that the patient lacks the capacity to make personal health care decisions.
- A **living will** (LW) is part of the advance directive and identifies what individual patients would (or would not) want if they were near death. Treatments that are discussed include cardiopulmonary resuscitation (CPR), artificial ventilation, and artificial nutrition or hydration.
- Another part of the advance directive is a do-not-resuscitate (DNR) or do-not-attempt-to-resuscitate (DNAR) order, signed by a physician or other authorized primary health care provider, which instructs that CPR not be attempted in the event of cardiac or respiratory arrest.
  1. DNRs/DNARs are intended for people with life-limiting conditions, for whom resuscitation is not prudent.

2. Some states also have directives referred to as *POLST* (physician orders for life-sustaining treatment), which document additional instructions in case of cardiac or pulmonary arrest.
- By law, all primary health care providers in the United States must initiate CPR for a person who is not breathing or is pulseless unless that person has a DNR order.
- Many patients and families do not understand the limitations of CPR and do not realize that it was never intended to be performed on patients with end-stage disease.

Interprofessional Collaborative Care
Recognize Cues: Assessment
- As death nears, patients often have signs and symptoms of decline in physical function, such as:
  1. Weakness
  2. Sleeping more
  3. Anorexia
  4. Changes in cardiovascular function
  5. Changes in breathing patterns
     - Cheyne-Stokes respirations: apnea alternating with periods of rapid breathing
  6. Change in genitourinary function
  7. Level of consciousness decreases

Analyze Cues and Prioritize Hypotheses: Analysis
- The priority collaborative problem for a patient near the end of life is:
  1. Potential for symptoms of distress that would prevent a peaceful death

Generate Solutions and Take Actions: Planning and Implementation
Interventions are planned to meet the physical, psychological, social, and spiritual needs of patients, using a coordinated interprofessional health team approach to end-of-life care. *Although the perception of hospice is that it provides care for the dying, the major focus of hospice care is on quality of life.*

Managing Symptoms of Distress
- The most common end-of-life symptoms that can cause the patient distress are:
  1. Pain
  2. Weakness
  3. Breathlessness/dyspnea

4. Nausea and vomiting
5. Agitation and delirium
6. Seizures

- Interventions to relieve symptoms of distress include positioning, administration of medications, and a variety of complementary and integrative therapies. When medications are used, they are often scheduled around the clock to maintain **comfort** and prevent recurrence of the symptom.

Managing Pain

- Assess distressing symptom(s) by intensity, frequency, duration, quality, and exacerbating (worsening) and relieving factors.
- Use a consistent method for rating the intensity of symptoms to facilitate ongoing assessments and evaluate treatment response.
- Both nonopioid and opioid analgesics play a role in pain management.
- The use of medical marijuana, or cannabinoid-based medicines (CBMs) is increasing in palliative and end-of-life care.
    1. CBM has been shown to reduce pain, especially pain associated with cancer. However, CBM is only recommended for refractory cancer pain as an adjunct to other prescribed analgesics (Cyr et al., 2018).
- Complementary and integrative health concepts are often integrated into the pain management plan.
    1. Massage
    2. Music therapy
    3. Therapeutic touch
    4. Guided imagery
    5. Aromatherapy with essential oils can be used; lavender is the most researched.

Managing Weakness

- For palliation, collaborate with physical and occupational therapists to reduce energy expenditure and maintain muscle strength and integrity.
- For patients at end of life, consider bed rest to avoid falls and injuries.
- Weakness combined with decreased neurologic function may impair the ability to swallow (dysphagia).
- For palliative care, consult with a speech-language pathologist to improve swallowing ability.
- For end-of-life care, limit oral intake and teach families about the risk for aspiration; with great sensitivity, reinforce that having no appetite or desire for food or fluids is expected.

NURSING SAFETY PRIORITY

Drug Alert

Dysphagia near death presents a problem for oral drug therapy. Although some tablets may be crushed, drugs such as sustained-release capsules should not be taken apart. Reassess the need for each medication. Collaborate with the primary health care provider about discontinuing drugs that are not needed to control pain, dyspnea, agitation, nausea, vomiting, cardiac workload, or seizures. In collaboration with a pharmacist experienced in palliation, identify alternative routes and/or alternative drugs to promote **comfort** and maintain control of symptoms. Choose the least invasive route, such as oral, buccal mucosa (inside cheek), transdermal (via the skin), or rectal. Some oral drugs can be given rectally. Depending on the patient's needs, the subcutaneous or IV routes may be used if access is available. The intramuscular route is almost never used at the end of life because it is considered painful, and drug distribution varies among patients.

Managing Breathlessness or Dyspnea
- Perform a thorough assessment of the patient's dyspnea.
  1. Include onset, severity (e.g., on a 0-to-10 scale), and precipitating factors.
  2. Precipitating factors may include time of day, position, anxiety, pain, cough, or emotional distress.
- *Oxygen therapy* for dyspnea near death has not been established as a standard of care for all patients. However, those who do not respond promptly to morphine or other drugs should be placed on oxygen to assess its effect. Patients often feel more comfortable when the oxygen saturation is greater than 90%.
- Administer drug therapy, including the following:
  1. *Bronchodilators,* such as albuterol or ipratropium bromide via a metered dose inhaler (MDI) or nebulizer, may be given for symptoms of bronchospasm (heard as wheezes).
  2. *Corticosteroids,* such as prednisone, may be given for bronchospasm and inflammatory problems.
  3. *Diuretics,* such as furosemide, may be given to decrease blood volume, reduce vascular congestion, and reduce the workload of the heart.
  4. *Antibiotics* may be indicated for dyspnea related to a respiratory infection.
  5. Opioids such as morphine sulfate are the standard treatment for dyspnea near death. They work by:
     - Altering the perception of air hunger by reducing anxiety and associated oxygen consumption
     - Reducing pulmonary congestion.

6. Loud, wet respirations (referred to as **death rattle**) are disturbing to family and caregivers even when they do not seem to cause dyspnea. This can be managed with *anticholinergics,* such as atropine ophthalmic solution or hyoscyamine, which are given sublingually to dry up secretions.

- Provide nonpharmacologic interventions, including:
  1. Limiting exertion to avoid exertional dyspnea
  2. Insertion of a long-term urinary (Foley) catheter to avoid dyspnea on exertion
  3. Positioning the patient with the head of the bed up, either in a hospital bed or a reclining chair, to increase chest expansion
  4. Applying wet cloths to the patient's face
  5. Encouraging imagery and deep breathing

Managing Nausea and Vomiting

- Assess for bowel obstruction and constipation.
  1. If constipation is identified as the cause of nausea and vomiting, give the patient a biphosphate enema (e.g., Fleet) to remove stool quickly.
- Administer antiemetic agents, such as ondansetron, dexamethasone, or metoclopramide.
- Aromatherapy, using chamomile, camphor, fennel, lavender, peppermint, or rose, may reduce or relieve vomiting. Some patients, however, may have worse nausea with aromatherapy. Ask the patient and family about preferences.

Managing Agitation and Delirium

- Delirium is an acute and fluctuating change in mental status and is accompanied by inattention, disorganized thinking, or an altered level of consciousness. It can be hyperactive, hypoactive, or mixed (both). *Hypoactive (quiet)* delirium is probably not uncomfortable for patients. *Agitated (noisy)* delirium with psychotic and behavioral symptoms (e.g., yelling, hallucinations) can be uncomfortable, especially for family members.
  1. When delirium occurs in the week or two before death, it is referred to as terminal delirium.
  2. Assess for pain or urinary retention, constipation, or another reversible cause.
  3. Ideally antipsychotic drugs are given only to control psychotic symptoms such as hallucinations and delusions. However, if they are needed to facilitate **comfort**, they should be available.

⬥ NURSING SAFETY PRIORITY
Drug Alert

> *Do not give the patient more than one antipsychotic drug at a time because of the risk for adverse drug events (ADEs). A neuroleptic drug such as a low dose of haloperidol orally, IV, subcutaneously, or rectally is commonly used at the end of life. Although haloperidol has the potential to cause extrapyramidal symptoms or adverse cardiovascular events and death in older adults with dementia, the benefits of treating psychosis associated with delirium usually outweigh the risks.*

    4. Music therapy may produce relaxation by quieting the mind and promoting a restful state.

    5. Aromatherapy with chamomile may also help overcome anxiety, tension, stress, and insomnia.

Managing Seizures
- Seizures are uncommon at the end of life, but they may occur in patients with brain tumors, advanced AIDS, or preexisting seizure disorders.
  1. Benzodiazepines, such as diazepam and lorazepam, are the drugs of choice and can be administered as a rectal gel or sublingual solution.

Managing Refractory Symptoms of Distress at End of Life
- Drug therapy for symptoms of distress at end of life is guided by protocols, using medications believed to be safe with the intent of alleviating suffering.
- *There is no evidence that administering medications for symptoms of distress using established protocols hastens deaths.*
- The ethical responsibility of the nurse in caring for patients near death is to follow guidelines for drug use to manage symptoms and to facilitate prompt and effective symptom management until death.

Meeting Psychosocial Needs
- Use a spiritual assessment tool to identify sources of strength and support. One strategy is to use the classic HOPE mnemonic as a guide:

    H: Sources of hope and strength

    O: Organized religion (if any) and role that it plays in one's life

    P: Personal spirituality, rituals, and practices

    E: Effects of religion and spirituality on care and end-of-life decisions

- Regardless of whether individuals have had an affiliation with a religion or a belief in God or other Supreme Being, they can experience what is referred to as *spiritual* or *existential distress*.
  1. Existential distress is brought about by the actual or perceived threat to one's continued existence.
- Acknowledge the patient's spiritual pain, and encourage verbalization.
- Provide opportunity for uninterrupted time with family members, friends, and other individuals who support the patient's health.
- Establish and review patient preferences and values regarding quality of life and treatment options.

PATIENT-CENTERED CARE: CULTURE AND SPIRITUALITY

E

Religion

Spirituality is whatever or whoever gives ultimate meaning and purpose in one's life that invites particular ways of being in the world in relation to others, oneself, and the universe. A person's spirituality may or may not include belief in God. **Religions** are formal belief systems that provide a framework for making sense of life, death, and suffering and responding to universal spiritual questions. Religions often have beliefs, rituals, texts, and other practices that are shared by a community. Spirituality and religion can help some patients cope with the thought of death, contributing to quality of life during the dying process.

Assisting Patients During the Grieving Process

- Nursing interventions are aimed at providing appropriate emotional support to allow patients and their families verbalize their fears and concerns. Support includes keeping the patient and family involved in health care decisions and emphasizing that the goal is to keep the patient as comfortable as possible until death.
- *Intervene with those grieving an impending death by "being with" as opposed to "being there."*
  1. "Being with" implies that you are physically and psychologically with the grieving patient, empathizing to provide emotional support.
  2. Listening and acknowledging the legitimacy of the patient's and/or family's impending loss are often more therapeutic than speaking; this concept is often referred to as **presence.**
  3. *Do not minimize a patient's or family member's reaction to an impending loss/death.*

- *Storytelling through reminiscence and life review can be an important activity for patients who are dying.*
  1. **Life review** is a structured process of reflecting on what one has done through one's life. This is often facilitated by an interviewer.
  2. **Reminiscence** is the process of randomly reflecting on memories of events in one's life.
- Assess coping ability of the patient and family or other caregiver. Prepare the family for the patient's death.

PATIENT AND FAMILY EDUCATION

Physical Signs Indicating That Death Has Occurred

- Breathing stops.
- Heart stops beating.
- Pupils become fixed and dilated.
- Body color becomes pale/ash gray and waxen.
- Body temperature drops.
- Muscles and sphincters relax.
- Urine and stool may be released.
- Eyes may remain open, and there is no blinking.
- The jaw may fall open.

Postmortem Care

- If the death was in the home and expected, emergency assistance (911) should not be called.
- If the person was a patient in a hospice program, the family calls hospice.
- If a death is unexpected or suspicious, the medical examiner is notified. Otherwise, the primary health care provider performs the pronouncement and completes a death certificate.
- Postmortem care includes the following:
  1. Provide all care with respect to communicate that the person was important and valued.
  2. Ask the family or significant others if they wish to help wash the patient or comb the patient's hair; respect and follow their cultural practices for body preparation.
  3. If no autopsy is planned, remove or cut all tubes and lines according to agency policy.
  4. Close the patient's eyes unless the cultural/religious practice is for a family member or other person to close the eyes.
  5. Insert dentures if the patient wore them.
  6. Straighten the patient and lower the bed to a flat position.
  7. Place a pillow under the patient's head.

8. Wash the patient as needed, and comb and arrange the patient's hair unless the family desires to perform bathing and body preparation.

9. Place waterproof pads under the patient's hips and around the perineum to absorb any excrement.

10. Clean the patient's room or unit.

11. Allow the family or significant others to see the patient in private and to perform any religious or cultural customs they wish (e.g., prayer).

12. Assess that all who need to see the patient have done so before transferring to the funeral home or morgue.

13. Notify the hospital chaplain or appropriate religious leader if requested by the family or significant others.

14. Ensure that the nurse or physician has completed and signed the death certificate.

15. Prepare the patient for transfer to either a morgue or funeral home; wrap the patient in a shroud (unless the family has a special shroud to use), and attach identification tags per agency policy.

Evaluate Outcomes: Evaluation

- In end-of-life care, evaluation is not related to improvements in overall condition, rather, it is specific to promoting a peaceful death. The expected outcomes are that the patient with end-of-life care will:

1. Have needs and preferences acknowledged and met
2. Have control/management of symptoms of distress
3. Experience meaningful interactions with family and other loved ones
4. Experience a peaceful death

See Chapter 8 in the main text for more information on end-of-life care.

EPIDIDYMITIS

- *Epididymitis* is an inflammation of the epididymis, often caused by *Neisseria gonorrhoeae* or *Chlamydia trachomatis* in men under 35. In older men, it often occurs in association with obstructive uropathy from benign prostatic hypertrophy (BPH). For men of any age who practice insertive anal intercourse, this condition is often associated with exposure to rectal coliform bacteria.

- Signs and symptoms include localized testicular pain and tenderness and swelling on palpation of the epididymis. Patients may have scrotal edema.

Interprofessional Collaborative Care

- Teach the patient the following:
  1. Take the full course of antibiotics, even if you begin to feel better.
  2. Ibuprofen can be used for pain.
  3. Elevate the scrotum and apply ice intermittently.
  4. Refrain from sexual intercourse until treatment is completed.
  5. Always use a condom when engaging in sexual intercourse.
  6. Report the development of fever, chills, and/or lower urinary tract symptoms to the health care provider right away.

See Chapter 64 in the main text for more information on epididymitis.

ERECTILE DYSFUNCTION

- **Erectile dysfunction (ED),** also known as *impotence,* is the inability to achieve or maintain an erection for sexual intercourse. There are two major types of ED: organic and psychogenic.
  1. *Organic ED* is a gradual deterioration of function. The man may first notice diminishing firmness and a decrease in frequency of erections. Causes include (Rogers, 2023):
     - Vascular, endocrine, or neurologic disease
     - Chronic disease (e.g., diabetes mellitus, renal failure)
     - Penile disease or trauma
     - Surgery or pharmaceutical therapies
     - Obesity
     - Psychological conditions
  2. If the patient has episodes of ED, it usually has a *psychogenic* cause. Men with this type of ED usually still have normal nocturnal (nighttime) and morning erections. Onset is usually sudden and follows a period of high stress.

Interprofessional Collaborative Care

- Diagnostic testing may include evaluating glycated hemoglobin, a lipid panel for cardiac risk factors, thyroid-stimulating hormone to rule out thyroid disease, and serum total testosterone (Khera, 2022).
- Doppler ultrasonography to determine blood flow to the penis. Treatment depends on the underlying cause, and may include (Khera, 2022):
  1. Lifestyle modifications (e.g., smoking cessation, weight loss, management of hypertension)
  2. Management of medications that may cause ED (e.g., antidepressants)

3. Penile self-injection with prostaglandin E1: Vasoconstrictive drugs can be injected directly into the penis to reduce blood outflow and make the penis erect.
4. Phosphodiesterase-5 (PDE5) drug therapy: works by relaxing the smooth muscles in the corpora cavernosa so that blood flow to the penis is increased
5. Psychotherapy
6. Testosterone and PDE5 drug therapy (for men with hypogonadism)
7. Surgery (prosthesis): Penile implants can be surgically placed when other modalities fail. Devices include semirigid, malleable, or hydraulic inflatable and multicomponent or one-piece instruments.
8. Vacuum-assisted erection devices: A vacuum device is a cylinder that fits over the penis, and a vacuum is created with a pump. The vacuum draws blood into the penis to maintain an erection.

E

💊 NURSING SAFETY PRIORITY
Drug Alert

Instruct patients taking PDE5 inhibitors to abstain from alcohol before sexual intercourse because it may impair the ability to have an erection. Common side effects of these drugs include dyspepsia (heartburn), headaches, facial flushing, and stuffy nose. If more than one pill a day is being taken, leg and back cramps, nausea, and vomiting also may occur. *Teach men who take nitrates to avoid PDE5 inhibitors because the vasodilation effects can cause a profound hypotension and reduce blood flow to vital organs* (Burchum & Rosenthal, 2022).

See Chapter 64 in the main text for more information on erectile dysfunction.

ESOPHAGEAL TUMORS

- Esophageal tumors can be benign, but most are malignant (cancerous).
- Esophageal tumors grow rapidly because there is no serosal layer to limit their extension. Because the esophageal mucosa is richly supplied with lymph tissue, there is early spread of tumors to lymph nodes.
- Primary risk factors associated with the development of esophageal cancer include:
  1. Alcohol intake
  2. Diets chronically deficient in fresh fruits and vegetables

3. Diets high in nitrates and nitrosamines (found in pickled and fermented foods)
4. Malnutrition
5. Obesity (especially with increased abdominal pressure)
6. Smoking
7. Untreated gastroesophageal reflux disease

Interprofessional Collaborative Care

Recognize Cues: Assessment

- Cancer of the esophagus is a silent tumor in its early stages, with few observable signs. By the time the tumor causes symptoms, it usually has spread extensively.
  1. One of the most common symptoms of esophageal cancer is dysphagia. This symptom may not be present until the esophageal opening has narrowed.
  2. Weight loss often accompanies progressive dysphagia and can exceed 20 lb over several months.
  3. Assess for signs and symptoms of esophageal tumors.

KEY FEATURES

Esophageal Tumors

- Persistent and progressive dysphagia (most common feature)
- Feeling of food sticking in the throat
- Odynophagia (painful swallowing)
- Halitosis
- Chronic hiccups
- Chronic cough with increasing secretions
- Hoarseness
- Severe, persistent chest or abdominal pain or discomfort
- Anorexia
- Regurgitation
- Nausea and vomiting
- Weight loss (often more than 20 lb)
- Changes in bowel habits (diarrhea, constipation, bleeding)

4. Common diagnostic tests, including:
   - Esophagogastroduodenoscopy (EGD) with biopsy is performed to inspect the esophagus and obtain tissue specimens for cell studies and disease staging.

Take Actions: Interventions

- Treatment of patients with esophageal cancer depends on staging at diagnosis. Multimodal therapy is often necessary to treat esophageal cancer as it is often advanced at diagnosis. Along with treatment of the cancer itself, patients with cancer of the esophagus experience many physical problems, and symptom management becomes essential.

Nonsurgical Management

- Nonsurgical treatment options for cancer of the esophagus that can assist in both disease and **nutrition** management may include:
  1. Nutritional therapy
     - Conduct a screening assessment.
     - Consult a registered dietitian nutritionist (RDN).
     - Perform daily weights.
     - Keep the head of the bed elevated to help keep the esophagus patent.
  2. Swallowing therapy
     - Semisoft foods and thickened liquids are preferred because they are easier to swallow.
     - Enteral feedings may be needed if dysphagia is severe.
     - Collaborate with a speech-language pathologist (SLP) to assist the patient with oral exercises to improve swallowing.
  3. Chemotherapy and radiation therapy
     - *Chemotherapy* may be given preoperatively or in concurrence with other treatments.
     - *Radiation therapy* can also be used alone, but is used most frequently in combination with other treatments.
     - *Chemoradiation* is a treatment for esophageal cancer that involves the use of chemotherapy at the same time as radiation therapy.
  4. Photodynamic therapy
     - Used as palliative treatment for patients with advanced esophageal cancer; it can relieve pain or make swallowing somewhat easier
  5. Esophageal dilation: *dilation* may be performed as necessary throughout the course of the disease to achieve temporary but immediate relief of dysphagia.

✚ NURSING SAFETY PRIORITY

Critical Rescue

When the patient with an esophageal tumor is eating or drinking, recognize that you must monitor for signs and symptoms of aspiration, which can cause airway obstruction, pneumonia, or both, especially in older adults. In coordination with a speech-language pathologist, respond by teaching caregivers how to feed the patient, how to monitor for aspiration, and how to respond quickly if choking occurs.

Surgical Management

- The purposes of surgical resection vary from palliation to cure.
- Esophagectomy is the removal of all or part of the esophagus.
- Preoperative nursing care focuses on teaching and on psychological support regarding the surgical procedure and preoperative and postoperative instructions.
- The patient requires intensive postoperative care and is at risk for multiple serious complications.
  1. Keep the postoperative patient in a semi-Fowler's or high-Fowler's position to support ventilation and prevent reflux.
  2. Monitor for symptoms of fluid overload and dehydration.

❗ NURSING SAFETY PRIORITY

Action Alert

Respiratory care is the highest postoperative priority for patients having an esophagectomy. For those who had traditional surgery, intubation with mechanical ventilation is necessary for at least the first 16 to 24 hours. Pulmonary complications include atelectasis and pneumonia. The risk for postoperative pulmonary complications is increased in the patient who has received preoperative radiation. Once the patient is extubated, support deep breathing, turning, and coughing every 1 to 2 hours. Assess the patient for decreased breath sounds and shortness of breath every 1 to 2 hours. Provide incisional support and adequate analgesia to enhance effective coughing.

---

  3. Monitor for atrial fibrillation that results from irritation of the vagus nerve during surgery.
  4. Monitor for wound healing and anastomotic leak for as long as 10 days after surgery. *Mediastinitis* (inflammation of the mediastinum) resulting from an anastomotic leak can lead to fatal sepsis.

➕ NURSING SAFETY PRIORITY

Critical Rescue

After esophageal surgery, recognize signs of fever, fluid accumulation, signs of inflammation, and symptoms of early shock (e.g., tachycardia, tachypnea). Respond immediately by reporting any of these findings to the surgeon **and** Rapid Response Team!

Care Coordination and Transition Management

- Treatment for esophageal tumors can result in long-lasting fatigue and weakness; help the patient plan for sequencing activities of daily living to reflect reduced energy.
- *Once the patient is discharged to home, ongoing respiratory care remains a priority.* Give the patient and caregiver instructions for ambulation and use of an incentive spirometer. Encourage the patient to be as active as possible and to avoid excessive bed rest because this can lead to complications of immobility.
- *Nutritional support is important.* Encourage the patient to continue to increase oral feedings as prescribed by the surgeon. Remind the patient to eat small, frequent meals containing high-calorie, high-protein foods that are soft and easily swallowed. Teach the value of using supplemental shakes. Emphasize the importance of sitting upright to eat and remaining upright after meals.
- Despite radical surgery, the patient with cancer of the esophagus often still has a terminal illness and a relatively short life expectancy. Emphasis is placed on maximizing quality of life. Help family members explore sources of support and arrange for hospice care when it becomes necessary.

E

See Chapter 46 in the main text for more information on esophageal tumors.

FLAIL CHEST

- Flail chest is the inward movement of the thorax during inspiration, with outward movement during expiration, usually involving only one side of the chest.
- It results from three or more adjacent rib fractures, usually associated with blunt chest trauma; it can also occur as a complication of cardiopulmonary resuscitation.
- *Gas exchange*, the ability to cough, and the ability to clear secretions are impaired.

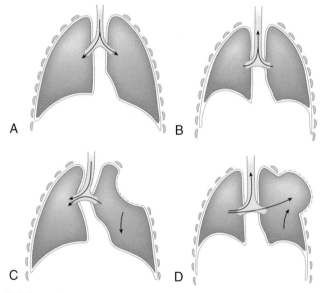

Flail chest. Normal respiration: (A) Inspiration; (B) Expiration. Paradoxical motion: (C) Inspiration-area of the lung underlying unstable chest wall sucks in on inspiration; (D) Expiration-unstable area balloons out. Note movement of mediastinum toward opposite lung during inspiration.

Interprofessional Collaborative Care
Recognize Cues: Assess
- Assess the patient for and document:
    1. Paradoxical chest movement (inward movement of the loose chest area during inspiration and an outward movement of the same area during expiration)

2. Pain
3. Dyspnea
4. Cyanosis
5. Tachycardia
6. Hypotension

Take Actions: Interventions
- Interventions include:
  1. Humidified oxygen
  2. Pain management
  3. Promotion of lung expansion through deep breathing and positioning
  4. Secretion clearance by coughing and tracheal suction
- The patient with a flail chest may be managed with vigilant respiratory care. Mechanical ventilation is needed if respiratory failure or shock occurs. Usually flail chest is stabilized by positive-pressure ventilation. Surgical stabilization is used only in extreme cases of flail chest.

 See Chapter 26 in the main text for more information on flail chest.

FLUID OVERLOAD

- Fluid overload, also called overhydration, is an excess of body fluid.
- It is a clinical sign of a problem in which fluid intake or retention is greater than the body's fluid needs.
- The most common type of fluid overload is hypervolemia because the problems result from excessive fluid in the extracellular fluid (ECF) space.
  1. Most problems caused by fluid overload are related to fluid volume excess in the vascular space or to dilution of specific electrolytes and blood components.
  2. Causes of fluid overload are related to excessive intake or inadequate excretion of fluid and include:
     - Excessive fluid replacement
     - Kidney failure (late phase)
     - Heart failure
     - Long-term corticosteroid therapy
     - Syndrome of inappropriate antidiuretic hormone (SIADH)
     - Psychiatric disorders with polydipsia
     - Water intoxication

Interprofessional Collaborative Care
Recognize Cues: Assessment
- Assess the patient for and document key features of fluid overload.

KEY FEATURES

Fluid Overload

Cardiovascular Changes
- Increased pulse rate
- Bounding pulse quality
- Elevated blood pressure
- Decreased pulse pressure
- Elevated central venous pressure
- Distended neck and hand veins
- Engorged varicose veins
- Weight gain

Respiratory Changes
- Increased respiratory rate
- Shallow respirations
- Shortness of breath
- Moist crackles present on auscultation

Skin and Mucous Membrane Changes
- Pitting edema in dependent areas
- Skin pale/ash gray and cool to touch

Neuromuscular Changes
- Altered level of consciousness
- Headache
- Visual disturbances
- Skeletal muscle weakness
- Paresthesias

Gastrointestinal Changes
- Increased motility
- Enlarged liver

 NURSING SAFETY PRIORITY

Critical Rescue

Assess the patient with fluid overload at least every 2 hours to recognize pulmonary edema, which can occur very quickly and can lead to death. If signs of worsening overload are present (bounding pulse, increasing neck vein distention, lung crackles, increasing peripheral edema, reduced urine output), respond by notifying the primary health care provider.

1. Fluid overload is diagnosed based on assessment findings and the results of laboratory tests. Usually serum electrolyte values are normal, but decreased hemoglobin, hematocrit, and serum protein levels may result from excessive water in the vascular space *(hemodilution)*.

Take Actions: Interventions
- The focus of priority nursing interventions is to ensure patient safety, restore normal fluid balance, provide supportive care until the imbalance is resolved, and prevent future fluid overload.
  1. Assess particularly for symptoms of pulmonary edema and heart failure that may indicate a need for increased surveillance or additional interventions.

2. Drug therapy focuses on removing excess fluid.
   - High-ceiling (loop) diuretics, such as furosemide
   - If there is concern that too much sodium and other electrolytes would be lost using loop diuretics or if the patient has SIADH, conivaptan or tolvaptan may be ordered
3. Monitor patient for response to restricted fluid or sodium intake and drug therapy, especially weight loss and increased urine output.
4. Observe for signs of electrolyte imbalance.
   - Changes in electrocardiographic patterns
   - Changes in sodium and potassium values
5. Collaborate with the dietitian to meet fluid and sodium restriction goals.
   - For more severe fluid overload, the patient may be restricted to 2 to 4 g/day of sodium.
6. Reduce the risk for pressure ulcers in patients with edema by using a pressure-reducing or pressure-relieving overlay on the mattress and over bony prominences (e.g., heel protectors, padding at elastic bands for holding oxygen delivery devices in place).
   - Assess skin pressure areas daily, especially the coccyx, elbows, hips, and heels, for signs of redness/hyperpigmentation or open areas, and document findings.
   - Assist the patient to change positions at least every 2 hours.
7. Fluid retention may not be visible. Rapid weight gain is the best indicator of fluid retention and overload.

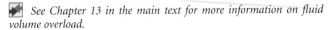 *See Chapter 13 in the main text for more information on fluid volume overload.*

FOOD POISONING

See *Gastritis*.

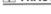 FRACTURE: MOBILITY CONCEPT EXEMPLAR

Overview
- A fracture is a break or disruption in the continuity of a bone and often results in impaired *mobility* and *pain*.
- Fractures are identified by the extent of the break.
  1. *Complete fracture:* The break is across the entire width of the bone in such a way that the bone is divided into two distinct sections.
  2. *Incomplete fracture:* The fracture does not divide the bone into two portions because the break is through only part of the bone.

- Fractures are also described by the extent of associated soft-tissue damage.
  1. A *simple fracture* does not extend through the skin and therefore has no visible wound.
  2. An *open (compound) fracture* has a disrupted skin surface that causes an external wound.

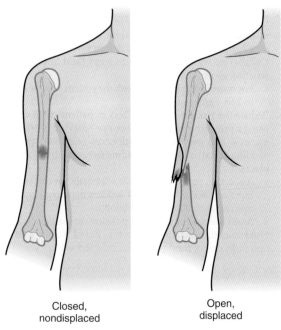

Closed,
nondisplaced

Open,
displaced

Common types of fractures.

- Fractures are also described by their cause.
  1. *Fragility fractures (also known as pathologic or spontaneous fractures)* occur after minimal trauma to a bone that has been weakened by disease.
  2. *Fatigue (stress) fractures* result from excessive strain and stress on the bone.
  3. *Compression fractures* are produced by a loading force applied to the long axis of cancellous bone.
- Bone healing occurs in five stages.
  1. Stage 1 occurs within 24 to 72 hours after the injury, with hematoma formation at the site of the fracture.

2. Stage 2 occurs in 3 days to 2 weeks, when granulation tissue begins to invade the hematoma, stimulating the formation of fibrocartilage.

3. Stage 3 of bone healing usually occurs within 2 to 6 weeks as a result of vascular and cellular proliferation. The fracture site is surrounded by new vascular tissue known as a *callus* that begins the nonbony union.

4. Stage 4 usually takes 3 to 8 weeks as the callus is gradually resorbed and transformed into bone.

5. Stage 5 consists of bone consolidation and remodeling. This stage can continue for up to 1 year.

- Bone healing requires adequate nutrition, especially calcium, phosphorus, vitamin D, and protein.
- Common acute complications of fractures include:
  1. Venous thromboembolism, which includes deep vein thrombosis and its major complication, pulmonary embolism
  2. Wound infections, which are the most common type of infection resulting from orthopedic trauma
  3. Bone infections (osteomyelitis), which is most common with open fractures
- Rare but serious side effects of fractures include the following:
  1. *Acute compartment syndrome* (ACS) is a serious, limb-threatening condition in which increased pressure within one or more compartments (that contain muscle, blood vessels, and nerves) reduces circulation to the lower leg or forearm.
  2. *Fat embolism syndrome* (FES) is a serious complication in which fat globules are released from the yellow bone marrow into the bloodstream within 12 to 48 hours after an injury. These emboli clog small blood vessels that supply vital organs, most commonly the lungs, and impair organ **perfusion**. FES usually results from long bone fractures and pelvic bone or fracture repair, but it is occasionally seen in patients who have a total joint replacement. Signs and symptoms include decreased level of consciousness, anxiety, respiratory distress, tachycardia, tachypnea, fever, hemoptysis, and petechiae, a macular, measleslike rash that may appear over the neck, upper arms, or chest and abdomen.
- Chronic complications of fractures include the following:
  1. Avascular necrosis can occur when the blood supply to the bone is disrupted.
  2. *Delayed union* is a fracture that has not healed within 6 months of injury. Some fractures never achieve union; that is, they never completely heal (nonunion). Others heal incorrectly (malunion).

F

KEY FEATURES

Acute Compartment Syndrome

Physiologic Change	Clinical Findings
Increased compartment pressure	No change
Increased capillary permeability	Edema
Release of histamine	Increased edema
Increased blood flow to area	Pulses present
	Pink tissue
Pressure on nerve endings	Acute pain
Increased tissue pressure	Referred pain to compartment(s)
Decreased tissue perfusion	Increased edema
Decreased oxygen to tissues	Pallor/ash gray skin
Increased production of lactic acid	Unequal pulses
	Flexed posture
Anaerobic metabolism	Cyanosis
Vasodilation	Increased edema
Increased blood flow	Tense muscle swelling
Increased tissue pressure	Tingling
	Numbness
Increased edema	Paresthesia
Muscle ischemia	Severe pain unrelieved by drugs
Tissue necrosis	Paresis/paralysis

3. *Complex regional pain syndrome (CRPS),* formerly called reflex sympathetic dystrophy (RSD), is a poorly understood dysfunction of the central and peripheral nervous systems that leads to severe, persistent ***pain***. Genetic factors may play a role in the development of this devastating complication. CRPS most often results from fractures or other traumatic musculoskeletal injury and commonly occurs in the feet and hands.

Interprofessional Collaborative Care
Recognize Cues: Assessment
- Obtain patient history, including:
  1. Cause of the fracture
  2. Events leading to the fracture and immediate postinjury care

3. Drug history, including substance and alcohol abuse
4. Medical history
5. Occupation and recreational activities
6. Nutritional history
- Assess the patient for and document:
  1. Life-threatening complications of the respiratory, cardiovascular, and neurologic systems (priority assessment)
  2. Fracture site:
     - Change in bone alignment
     - Neurovascular status (pulse, warmth, movement, and sensation) distal to fracture

---

! NURSING SAFETY PRIORITY

Action Alert

Swelling at the fracture site is rapid and can result in marked neurovascular compromise due to decreased arterial *perfusion*. *Gently perform a thorough neurovascular assessment and compare extremities.* Assess skin color and temperature, *sensory perception*, *mobility*, *pain*, and pulses distal to the fracture site. If the fracture involves an extremity and the patient is not in severe pain, check the nails for capillary refill by applying pressure to the nail and observing for the speed of blood return (usually less than 3 seconds). If nails are brittle or thick, assess the skin next to the nail. Checking for capillary refill is not as reliable as other indicators of *perfusion*.

---

3. Soft-tissue damage: color, width, length, depth, drainage, and appearance of surrounding skin
4. Amount of overt bleeding
5. Muscle spasm
- Diagnostic tests for fractures may include:
  1. X-rays
  2. Computed tomography (CT) scanning
  3. Magnetic resonance imaging (MRI)

Analyze Cues and Prioritize Hypotheses: Analysis
- The priority collaborative problems for patients with fractures include:
  1. Acute *pain* due to fractured bone(s), soft-tissue damage, muscle spasm, and edema
  2. Decreased *mobility* due to *pain*, muscle spasm, and soft-tissue damage
  3. Potential for neurovascular compromise related to impaired tissue *perfusion*

Generate Solutions and Take Actions: Planning and Implementation
Manage Acute Pain

- After a head-to-toe assessment (secondary survey) and patient stabilization by the prehospital team, pain is managed with short-term IV opioids such as fentanyl, hydromorphone, or morphine sulfate. Cardiac monitoring for patients older than 50 years is established before drug administration.

- To prevent further tissue damage, reduce *pain*, and increase circulation, the prehospital or emergency team immobilizes the fracture by splinting.

✚ NURSING SAFETY PRIORITY
Critical Rescue

For any patient who experiences trauma in the community, first call 911 and assess for airway, breathing, and circulation (ABCs, or primary survey). Then, provide lifesaving care if needed before being concerned about the fracture.

Nonsurgical Management

- Nonsurgical management includes bone reduction and immobilization with a bandage, splint, boot, cast or, less commonly, traction. For some small, closed incomplete or "hairline" bone fractures in the hand or foot, reduction is not required. Immobilization with an orthotic device or special orthopedic shoe or boot may be the only management needed for healing to occur.

  1. *Closed reduction* is the manipulation of the bone ends for realignment while applying a manual pull, or traction, on the bone.

  2. *Splints and orthopedic boots/shoes* may be used to immobilize certain areas of the body, such as the scapula or clavicle or foot and ankle.

  3. *Casts* are rigid devices that immobilize the affected body part while allowing other body parts to move. A cast allows early mobility, correction of deformity, prevention of deformity, and reduction of pain.
     - The most common cast material is fiberglass.
     - Special considerations for casts include:
       - Arm cast
         - When a patient is in bed, elevate the arm above the heart to reduce swelling; the hand should be higher than the elbow.
         - When the patient is out of bed, support the arm with a sling placed around the neck so that the weight is distributed over a large area of the shoulders and trunk, not just the neck.

- A leg cast may require the patient to use an ambulatory aid.
- A boot may be removed for hygiene but should be in place for all weight bearing.

⚠ NURSING SAFETY PRIORITY
Action Alert

Check to ensure that any type of cast is not too tight, and frequently monitor and document neurovascular status—usually every hour for the first 24 hours after application if the patient is hospitalized. You should be able to insert a finger between the cast and the skin. Teach the patient to apply ice for the first 24 to 36 hours to reduce swelling and inflammation.

- Cast care
  1. Inspect the cast at least once every 8 to 12 hours for drainage, alignment, and fit.
  2. Immediately report to the primary health care provider any sudden increases in the amount of drainage or change in the integrity of the cast.
  3. Assessing for and reporting complications from injury, casting, or immobility:
     - Infection
     - Circulation impairment
     - Peripheral nerve damage
     - Skin breakdown
     - Pneumonia or atelectasis
     - Thromboembolism
- **Traction** is the application of a pulling force to a part of the body to provide bone reduction or as a last resort to decrease muscle spasm (thus reducing *pain).* A patient in traction is often hospitalized, but in some cases home care is possible even for skeletal traction.
  1. Types of traction
     - *Skin traction* involves the use of a Velcro boot (Buck traction), belt, or halter securely placed around a body part to decrease painful muscle spasms. Weight is limited to 5 to 10 lb (2.3 to 4.5 kg) to prevent injury to the skin.
     - *Skeletal traction* uses pins, wires, tongs, or screws that are surgically inserted directly into bone to allow the use of longer traction time and heavier weights, usually 15 to 30 lb (6.8 to 13.6 kg). It aids in bone realignment.
  2. Care for the patient in traction includes:
     - Inspecting the skin at least every 8 hours for signs of irritation or inflammation
     - Removing (when possible) the belt or boot that is used for skin traction every 8 hours to inspect under the device

F

! NURSING SAFETY PRIORITY

Action Alert

When patients are in traction, weights usually are not removed without a primary health care provider's order. They should not be lifted manually or allowed to rest on the floor. Weights should be freely hanging at all times. Teach this important point to assistive personnel on the unit, to other personnel such as those in the radiology department, and to visitors. Inspect the skin at least every 8 hours for signs of irritation or inflammation. When possible, remove the belt or boot that is used for skin traction every 8 hours to inspect under the device. Assess neurovascular status of the affected body part per agency or primary health care provider protocol to detect impaired **perfusion** and **tissue integrity**. The patient's circulation is usually monitored every hour for the first 24 hours after traction is applied and every 4 hours thereafter.

Drug Therapy

- For patients with persistent, severe pain, opioid and nonopioid drugs are alternated or given together to manage pain both centrally in the brain and peripherally at the site of injury.
  1. For severe or multiple fractures, short-term patient-controlled analgesia (PCA) with morphine, fentanyl, or hydromorphone is used.
  2. Oxycodone, oxycodone with acetaminophen, or hydrocodone with acetaminophen are common oral opioid drugs that are very effective for most patients with fracture pain.
  3. NSAIDs are given to decrease associated tissue inflammation; however, they can slow bone healing.

Physical Therapy

- Collaborate with the physical therapist (PT) to assist with pain control and edema reduction by using:
  1. Ice/heat packs
  2. Electrical muscle stimulation
  3. Special treatment, such as dexamethasone iontophoresis
     - Iontophoresis is a method for absorbing dexamethasone, a synthetic steroid, through the skin near the painful area to decrease inflammation and edema. A small device delivers a minute amount of electricity via electrodes placed on the skin.

Surgical Management

- *Open reduction with internal fixation* (ORIF) permits early mobilization. Open reduction allows direct visualization of the fracture site, and internal fixation uses metal pins, screws, rods, plates, or prostheses to immobilize the fracture during healing. An incision is made to gain access to the broken bone and allow implanting one or more devices into bone tissue.

- *External fixation* involves fracture reduction and the percutaneous implantation of pins into the bone. The pins are then held in place by an external metal frame to prevent bone movement but allow patient mobility. A disadvantage of external fixation is the increased risk for pin site infection and osteomyelitis.
- Provide preoperative care, and explain whether a device or cast will be used after surgery to maintain alignment.
- Provide postoperative care and:
  1. Monitor neurovascular status at least every hour for the first 24 hours after surgery and then as often as agency policy, surgeon preference, and patient condition indicate.
  2. Communicate neurovascular compromise or other complications urgently to the provider.
  3. Promote self-management and mobility in collaboration with the physical therapist.
- Additional procedures may be needed when surgical repairs are unsuccessful and the bone does not heal (nonunion).
  1. *Electrical bone stimulation* may be noninvasive or invasive. It involves using electrical current stimulators near or into a fracture site. This procedure, when used for about 6 months, has resulted in bone healing for some patients.
  2. *Bone grafting* is the use of bone chips from the patient's iliac crest or other site, a cadaver donor, or a living donor and packing or wiring the chips between the bone ends to facilitate union.
  3. *Bone banking* from living donors is becoming increasingly popular. If qualified, patients undergoing total hip arthroplasty may donate their femoral heads to the bank for later use as bone grafts for others.
  4. *Low-intensity pulsed ultrasound* involves the application of ultrasound treatments for about 20 minutes each day to the fracture site.

Increase Mobility. Many patients with musculoskeletal trauma, including fractures, are referred by their primary health care provider for rehabilitation therapy with a PT (usually for lower extremity injuries) and/or occupational therapist (OT) (usually for upper extremity injuries). The timing for this referral depends on the nature, severity, and treatment modality of the fracture(s) or other musculoskeletal trauma.

- The use of crutches, knee-scooter, or a walker increases **mobility** and assists in ambulation.

F

- The patient may progress to using a walker or cane after crutches.
- *Crutches* are the most commonly used ambulatory aid for many types of lower extremity musculoskeletal trauma (e.g., fractures, sprains, amputations).
- A *walker* is most often used by the older patient who needs additional support for balance.
- A *cane* is sometimes used if the patient needs only minimal support for an affected leg.

Prevent and Monitor for Neurovascular Compromise

- Perform neurovascular (NV) assessments (also known as "circ checks" or circulation, movement, and sensation [CMS] assessments) frequently before and after fracture treatment.
- Patients who have extremity casts, splints with elastic bandage wraps, and ORIF or external fixation are especially at risk for NV compromise.
- If **perfusion** to the distal extremity is impaired, the patient reports **pain**, impaired **mobility**, and decreased **sensory perception**. If these symptoms are allowed to progress, patients are at risk for ACS.

✚ NURSING SAFETY PRIORITY
Critical Rescue

Monitor for and document early signs and symptoms of ACS. If early indicators are not recognized, ACS may progress and result in the "six Ps" of **p**ain, **p**ressure, **p**aralysis, **p**aresthesia, **p**allor, and **p**ulselessness as a result of decreased arterial perfusion to the affected area. **Pain** is increased even with passive motion and may seem out of proportion to the degree of injury. Analgesics that had controlled pain become less effective or ineffective. *Numbness and tingling (paresthesia) are often among the first signs of the problem.*

If ACS is suspected, notify the primary health care provider immediately and, if possible, implement interventions to relieve the pressure. For example, for the patient with tight, bulky dressings, loosen the bandage or tape. If the patient has a cast, follow agency protocol about who may cut the cast. Do not elevate or ice the extremity because that could compromise blood flow.

- If ACS is verified, the surgeon may perform a fasciotomy, or opening in the fascia, by making an incision through the skin and subcutaneous tissues into the fascia of the affected compartment.

Care Coordination and Transition Management

- Collaborate with the case manager or the discharge planner in the hospital to plan care for the patient with a fracture who is being discharged.

- Assess the patient's ability to safely use a wheelchair or ambulatory aid.
- Arrange for a home health care nurse to check that the home is safe and that the patient and family are able to follow the interdisciplinary plan of care.
- Provide verbal and written instructions on the care of bandages, splints, casts, or external fixators.
- Emphasize the importance of follow-up visits with the health care provider and other therapists.
- Teach the patient and family about:
  1. Care of the extremity after removal of the cast
     - Remove scaly, dead skin carefully by soaking; do not scrub.
     - Move the extremity carefully. Expect discomfort, weakness, and decreased range of motion (ROM).
     - Support the extremity with pillows or an orthotic device until strength and movement return.
     - Exercise as instructed by the physical therapist.
  2. Wound assessment and dressing
  3. Recognition of complications and when and where to seek professional health care if complications occur

Evaluate Outcomes: Evaluation

- Evaluate the care of the patient with one or more fractures based on the identified priority patient problems. The expected outcomes include that the patient:
  1. States that adequate **pain** control (a 2 or 3 on a 0-to-10 pain scale) is achieved to accomplish ADLs
  2. Ambulates independently with or without an assistive device (if not restricted by traction or other device)
  3. Is free of physiologic consequences of decreased **mobility**
  4. Has adequate blood flow to maintain tissue **perfusion** and function
  5. Is free of **fracture complications**

 See Chapter 44 in the main text for more information on fractures.

FRACTURES OF SPECIFIC SITES

- Hip fracture: Hip fracture is the most common injury in older adults and one of the most frequently seen injuries in any health care setting or community. It has a high mortality rate as a result of multiple complications related to surgery, depression, and decreased **mobility**.
  1. *Hip (intracapsular):* This fracture involves the upper third of the femur within the joint capsule. Injury is managed with surgical repair.

2. *Hip (extracapsular):* This fracture involves the upper third of the femur outside of the joint capsule.
3. The treatment of choice is surgical repair by ORIF, when possible, to reduce pain and allow the older patient to be out of bed and ambulatory.

👤 PATIENT-CENTERED CARE: OLDER ADULT HEALTH
Fragility Hip Fractures

Teach older adults about the risk factors for fragility hip fractures, including physiologic aging changes, disease processes, drug therapy, and environmental hazards. Physiologic changes include sensory changes, such as diminished visual acuity and hearing; changes in gait, balance, and muscle strength; and joint stiffness. Disease processes such as osteoporosis, foot disorders, bony metastases, and changes in cardiac function increase the risk for fracture. Drugs, such as diuretics, antihypertensives, antidepressants, sedatives, opioids, and alcohol, are factors that increase the risk for falling in older adults. Use of three or more drugs at the same time drastically increases the risk for falls. Throw rugs, loose carpeting, floor clutter, inadequate lighting, uneven walking surfaces or steps, and pets are environmental hazards that also may cause falls.

❗ NURSING SAFETY PRIORITY
Action Alert

Patients who have a hemiarthroplasty are at risk for hip dislocation or subluxation. Be sure to prevent hip adduction and rotation to keep the operative leg in proper alignment. Regular pillows or abduction devices can be used for patients who are confused or restless. If straps are used to hold the device in place, make sure that they are not too tight and check the skin every 2 hours for signs of pressure. Perform neurovascular assessments to ensure that the device is not interfering with arterial circulation or peripheral nerve conduction.

- Fractures of the chest and pelvis
    1. *Ribs and sternum:* These fractures have the potential to puncture the lungs, heart, or arteries by bone fragments or ends. *Assess airway, breathing, and circulation status **first** for any patient having chest trauma!* Fractures of the lower ribs may damage underlying organs, such as the liver, spleen, or kidneys.
    2. These fractures tend to heal on their own without surgical intervention. Patients are often uncomfortable during the

healing process and require analgesia. They also have a high risk for pneumonia because of shallow breathing caused by *pain* on inspiration. Encourage them to breathe normally if possible, and ensure that their pain is well managed.

3. *Pelvis: Because the pelvis is very vascular and is close to major organs and blood vessels, associated internal damage is the major focus in fracture management.* Pelvic fractures are the second most common cause of death from trauma. The major concern related to pelvic injury is venous oozing or arterial bleeding. Loss of blood volume leads to hypovolemic shock. When a non–weight-bearing part of the pelvis is fractured, management can be as minimal as bed rest on a firm mattress or bed board. A weight-bearing pelvis fracture requires external fixation with multiple pins, ORIF, or both. Progression to weight bearing depends on the stability of the fracture after fixation.

- Compression fractures of spine
  1. These fractures are associated with severe pain, deformity (kyphosis), and possible neurologic compromise. Nonsurgical management includes bed rest, analgesics, nerve blocks, and physical therapy to maintain muscle strength. Compression fractures that remain painful and impair mobility may be surgically treated with vertebroplasty or kyphoplasty, in which bone cement is injected through the skin (percutaneously) directly into the fracture site to provide stability and immediate pain relief.

 See Chapter 44 in the main text for more information on fractures.

FROSTBITE

- Frostbite is a significant cold-related injury that occurs as a result of inadequate insulation against cold weather.
- Contributors to frostbite include wearing wet clothing, fatigue, dehydration, poor nutrition, smoking, alcohol consumption, and impaired peripheral circulation.

Interprofessional Collaborative Care
Recognize Cues: Assessment

- Severity of frostbite is related to the degree of tissue freezing and the resultant damage it produces.
  1. *Frostnip* is a superficial cold injury with initial pain, numbness, and pallor/ash gray appearance of the affected area. It is easily remedied with application of warmth and does not cause impaired *tissue integrity*.
  2. *Grade I frostbite* is the least severe type of frostbite, with hyperemia of the involved area and edema formation.

3. *Grade 2 frostbite* has large, clear to milky fluid-filled blisters that develop with partial-thickness skin necrosis.
4. *Grade 3* is a full-thickness injury that appears as small blisters containing dark fluid and an affected body part that is cool, numb, blue, or red and does not blanch.
5. *Grade 4* is the most severe; the part is numb, cold, and bloodless. The full-thickness necrosis extends into the muscle and bone.

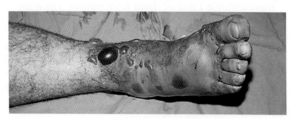

Edema and blister formation 24 hours after frostbite injury, occurring in an area covered by a tightly fitted boot. (From Auerbach, P. S. [2008]. *Wilderness medicine* [5th ed.]. Philadelphia: Mosby; courtesy Cameron Bangs, MD.)

Take Actions: Interventions

- Recognize frostbite by observing for a white, waxy appearance of exposed skin, especially on the nose, cheeks, and ears.
- Seek shelter from the wind and cold.
- Use body heat to warm up superficial frostbite-affected areas by placing warm hands over the affected areas on the face or placing cold hands under the arms in the axillary region.

Hospital Care

- Rapidly rewarm in a water bath at a temperature range of 98.6°F to 102.2°F (37°C to 39°C) is indicated to thaw the frozen part.
- Provide analgesic agents, IV opiates, and IV rehydration.
- Ibuprofen should also be administered every 8 hours as prescribed, as it decreases thromboxane production in the inflammatory cascade and may reduce secondary tissue injury in frostbite (McIntosh et al., 2019).

! NURSING SAFETY PRIORITY

Action Alert

Recognize that dry heat or massage should not be used as part of the warming process for frostbitten areas because these actions can produce further damage to **tissue integrity**. Respond by using other interventions, such as a rapid rewarming water bath of 98.6°F to 102.2°F (37°C to 39°C), to preserve tissue.

1. Handle the injured areas gently, and elevate them above heart level if possible to decrease tissue edema.
2. Use splints to immobilize extremities during the healing process.
3. Assess frequently for the development of compartment syndrome.
4. Immunize the patient for tetanus prophylaxis.
5. Apply only loose, nonadherent, sterile dressings to the damaged areas.
6. Avoid compression of the injured tissues.
7. Topical and systemic antibiotics may be prescribed.
8. Management of severe, deep frostbite requires the same types of surgical intervention as deep or severe burns.

 See Chapter 11 in the main text for more information on frostbite.

F

GASTRITIS

- Gastritis is *inflammation* of the gastric mucosa (stomach lining).
- Gastritis can be erosive (causing ulcers) or nonerosive.
- Prostaglandins provide a protective mucosal barrier. If there is a break in the barrier, mucosal injury occurs, allowing hydrochloric acid to diffuse into the mucosa and injure small vessels, resulting in edema, bleeding, and erosion of the gastric lining.
- Gastritis can be classified as acute or chronic.
  1. *Acute gastritis,* the inflammation of gastric mucosa or submucosa, may result from food poisoning; the onset of infection *(Helicobacter pylori, Escherichia coli);* after exposure to local irritants such as alcohol, aspirin, nonsteroidal antiinflammatory drugs (NSAIDs), or bacterial endotoxins; after ingestion of corrosive substances; or from the lack of stimulation of normal gastric secretions.
     - Gastritis related to food poisoning often occurs within 5 hours of eating contaminated food.
     - Complete regeneration and healing usually occurs within a few days without any residual damage.

▨ PATIENT AND FAMILY EDUCATION

Gastritis Prevention

- Eat a well-balanced diet and exercise regularly.
- Avoid drinking excessive amounts of alcoholic beverages.
- Do not take large doses of aspirin, other NSAIDs (e.g., ibuprofen), or corticosteroids.
- Avoid excessive intake of coffee (even decaffeinated).
- Be sure that foods and water are safe to avoid contamination.
- Manage stress levels using complementary and integrative therapies, such as relaxation and meditation techniques.
- Stop smoking or using other forms of tobacco.
- Protect yourself against exposure to toxic substances in the workplace, such as lead and nickel.
- Seek medical treatment if you are experiencing symptoms of esophageal reflux.

2. *Chronic gastritis* is an inflammatory process that persists until the mucosal lining becomes thin and atrophies, the parietal (acid-secreting) cells decrease function, and the source of intrinsic factor needed for vitamin B_{12} absorption is lost.
    *   The most common form of chronic gastritis is type B gastritis, caused by *H. pylori* **infection**.
    *   Chronic gastritis is associated with an increased risk for gastric cancer. The persistent **inflammation** extends deep into the mucosa, causing gastric gland destruction and cellular changes (Rogers, 2023).

Interprofessional Collaborative Care
Recognize Cues: Assessment
*   Assess and document signs and symptoms:
    1. Epigastric discomfort, pain, or cramping
    2. Anorexia, dyspepsia, nausea, and vomiting
    3. Hematemesis, melena
*   Gastritis or food poisoning caused by endotoxins, such as staphylococcal endotoxin, has an abrupt onset. Severe nausea and vomiting often occur within 5 hours of ingestion of the contaminated food. *In some cases gastric hemorrhage, which is a life-threatening emergency, is the presenting symptom.*
*   *Chronic gastritis* causes few symptoms unless ulceration occurs. Patients may report nausea, vomiting, or upper abdominal discomfort. Periodic epigastric **pain** may occur after a meal. Some patients have anorexia.

Take Actions: Interventions
*   Gastritis is a very common health problem in the United States. A balanced diet, regular exercise, and stress-reduction techniques can help prevent it.
*   Acute gastritis is treated symptomatically and supportively.
*   Eliminating the causative factor, such as *H. pylori* infection if present, is the primary treatment approach.
* H_2-receptor antagonists, such as famotidine, are typically used to block gastric secretions.
*   Proton pump inhibitors (PPIs), such as omeprazole, may be prescribed to reduce gastric acid secretion.
*   Antacids are used as buffering agents.
*   Instruct the patient to avoid using drugs associated with gastric irritation, including corticosteroids and NSAIDs, or provide gastroprotective agents when irritants are used therapeutically.
*   If the patient experienced bleeding with symptomatic blood loss, blood transfusion may be needed. Fluid replacement is indicated

G

for less severe blood loss or symptoms of hypovolemia from low oral intake.

- Diet and lifestyle therapy to avoid tobacco, alcohol, and foods that contribute to gastric irritation, such as those with caffeine, high levels of acid (e.g., tomatoes, citrus fruits), "hot" spices, and large volumes during a meal.

- Teach techniques to reduce stress and discomfort, such as progressive relaxation, cutaneous stimulation, guided imagery, and distraction.

 See Chapter 47 in the main text for more information on gastritis.

GASTROENTERITIS

- **Gastroenteritis** is a very common health problem worldwide that causes diarrhea and/or vomiting related to *inflammation* of the mucous membranes of the stomach and intestinal tract. The small bowel is most commonly affected. Gastroenteritis can be caused by either viral (more common) or bacterial *infection*.

Common Types of Gastroenteritis and Their Characteristics

Type	Characteristics
Viral Gastroenteritis	
Epidemic viral	Caused by many parvovirus-type organisms Transmitted by the fecal-oral route in food and water Incubation period 10–51 hr Communicable during acute illness
Norovirus (Norwalk viruses)	Transmitted by the fecal-oral route and possibly the respiratory route (vomitus) Incubation in 48 hr Affects adults of all ages Older adults can become hypovolemic and experience electrolyte imbalances
Bacterial Gastroenteritis	
Campylobacter enteritis	Transmitted by the fecal-oral route or by contact with infected animals or infants Incubation period 1–10 days Communicable for 2–7 weeks
Escherichia coli diarrhea	Transmitted by fecal contamination of food, water, or fomites

Common Types of Gastroenteritis and Their Characteristics—cont'd	
Type	**Characteristics**
Shigellosis	Transmitted by direct and indirect fecal-oral routes Incubation period 1–7 days Communicable during the acute illness to 4 weeks after the illness Humans possibly carriers for months

- Gastroenteritis is an increase in the frequency and water content of stools and vomiting as a result of inflammation of the mucous membranes of the stomach and intestines, primarily affecting the small bowel.

Interprofessional Collaborative Care
Recognize Cues: Assessment
- Patient history can provide information about potential cause.
  1. Recent travel outside the United States or a recent meal at a restaurant associated with an outbreak of gastroenteritis
  2. Nausea and vomiting

> ## ! NURSING SAFETY PRIORITY
> ### *Action Alert*
>
> For patients with gastroenteritis, note any abdominal distention and listen for hyperactive bowel sounds. Depending on the amount of fluids and electrolytes lost through diarrhea and vomiting, patients may have varying degrees of dehydration manifested by:
> - Weight loss (unintentional)
> - Poor skin turgor
> - Fever (not common in older adults)
> - Dry mucous membranes
> - Orthostatic blood pressure changes (which can cause a fall, especially for older adults)
> - Hypotension
> - Oliguria (decreased or absent urinary output)
>
> In some cases, dehydration may be severe. It can occur very rapidly in older adults. Monitor mental status changes, such as acute confusion, that result from hypoxia due to dehydration in the older adult. These changes may be the only initial signs and symptoms of dehydration in older adults.

Take Actions: Interventions

For any type of gastroenteritis, encourage fluid replacement. The amount and route of fluid administration are determined by the patient's hydration status and overall health condition. Teach patients to drink extra fluids to replace fluid lost through vomiting and diarrhea. Oral rehydration therapy (ORT) may be needed for some patients to replace fluids and electrolytes. Examples of ORT solutions include sports drinks and Pedialyte. Depending on the patient's age and severity of dehydration, the patient may be treated in the hospital with IV fluids to restore hydration.

- Provide drug therapy as prescribed.
  1. Antibacterials are given for bacterial causes of gastroenteritis caused by an organism susceptible to therapy. Viral gastroenteritis, characterized by a shorter duration of illness (less than 72 hours), is treated symptomatically.
  2. Drugs that suppress intestinal motility may not be given for bacterial or viral gastroenteritis. *Use of these drugs can prevent the infecting organisms from being eliminated from the body.* If the primary health care provider determines that antiperistaltic/antidiarrheal agents are necessary, loperamide may be recommended.

◖ NURSING SAFETY PRIORITY

Drug Alert

Diphenoxylate hydrochloride with atropine sulfate reduces GI motility but is used sparingly because of its habit-forming ability. *The drug should not be used for older adults because it also causes drowsiness and could contribute to falls.*

- Promote skin protection from stool. Teach the patient to:
  1. Avoid toilet paper and harsh soaps and to gently clean the area with warm water and absorbent material, followed by thorough, gentle drying.
  2. Apply cream, oil, or gel to a damp, warm washcloth or flushable wipe to remove stool that sticks to open skin.
- Teach the patient to avoid transmission of the infecting microbe.
  1. Wash hands after each bowel movement for at least 30 seconds.
  2. Do not share eating utensils, glasses, and dishes.
  3. Do not prepare or handle food that will be consumed by others; the public health department can advise about return to employment if it includes food handling.

4. Maintain clean bathroom facilities to avoid exposure to stool.
5. Inform the health care provider if symptoms persist beyond 3 days.

See Chapter 49 in the main text for more information on gastro-enteritis.

GASTROESOPHAGEAL REFLUX DISEASE: NUTRITION CONCEPT EXEMPLAR

Overview

- **Gastroesophageal reflux disease (GERD)**, the most common upper gastrointestinal disorder in the United States, occurs most often in middle-age and older adults. **Gastroesophageal reflux (GER)** occurs as a result of backward flow of stomach contents into the esophagus, known as **regurgitation**. GERD is the chronic and more serious condition that arises from persistent GER.
- Reflux exposes the esophageal mucosa to the irritating effects of acidic gastric contents, resulting in i*nflammation*.
- A patient with acute symptoms of ***inflammation*** is often described as having mild or severe **reflux esophagitis** (Rogers, 2023). When the lower esophageal sphincter (LES) is compromised (relaxed), gastric contents reflux into the esophagus. Eating large meals, certain foods, drugs, smoking, and alcohol use influence the tone function of the LES.

Factors Contributing to Decreased Lower Esophageal Sphincter Pressure	
• Caffeinated beverages • Coffee, tea, and cola • Chocolate • Nitrates • Citrus fruits • Tomatoes and tomato products • Alcohol • Peppermint, spearmint	• Smoking and use of other tobacco products • Calcium channel blockers • Anticholinergic drugs • High levels of estrogen and progesterone • Nasogastric tube placement

Interprofessional Collaborative Care

Recognize Cues: Assessment

- Ask the patient about a history of heartburn or atypical chest pain associated with the reflux of GI contents. Ask whether the patient has been newly diagnosed with asthma, has experienced morning hoarseness, or has coughing or wheezing, especially at night. These symptoms may indicate severe reflux reaching the pharynx or mouth or pulmonary aspiration.

- Ask about dysphagia and **odynophagia** (painful swallowing), which can accompany chronic GERD.
  1. **Dyspepsia,** also known as *indigestion,* and regurgitation are the main symptoms of GERD, although symptoms may vary in severity.

KEY FEATURES

Gastroesophageal Reflux Disease

- Dyspepsia (indigestion)
- Regurgitation (may lead to aspiration or bronchitis)
- Water brash (hypersalivation)
- Dental caries (severe cases)
- Dysphagia
- Odynophagia (painful swallowing)
- Globus (feeling of something in back of throat)
- Pharyngitis
- Coughing, hoarseness, or wheezing at night
- Chest pain
- Pyrosis (heartburn)
- Epigastric **pain**
- Generalized abdominal **pain**
- Belching
- Flatulence
- Nausea

Analyze Cues and Prioritize Hypotheses: Analysis

- The priority collaborative problems for the patient with GERD include:
  1. Potential for compromised **nutrition** status due to dietary selection
  2. Acute **pain** due to reflux of gastric contents

Generate Solutions and Take Actions: Planning and Implementation

Balancing Nutrition

- Interventions are designed to optimize **nutrition** status, decrease symptoms experienced with GERD, and prevent complications. Nursing care priorities focus on teaching the patient about proper dietary selections that provide optimum nutrients and that do not contribute to reflux.

- Balance nutrition in collaboration with the patient and dietitian.
  1. Explore the patient's meal plan and food preferences.
  2. Plan diet modifications to reduce GERD symptoms by limiting or eliminating food that decreases the pressure of the lower esophageal sphincter (LES) and irritates inflamed tissue, including the following:
     - Avoid chocolate, peppermint, fatty (especially fried) foods, and carbonated beverages.
     - Eat small meals that are not spicy or acidic.
     - Avoid eating for 3 hours (or more) before bedtime.
     - Limit or eliminate alcohol and tobacco.

Minimizing Pain
- Nursing care priorities focus on teaching the patient about lifestyle modifications that will improve comfort.
  1. Encourage lifestyle changes.
     - If the patient is obese, examine approaches to weight reduction with the patient.
     - Promote smoking cessation and reduced alcohol intake.
     - Instruct the patient to elevate the head of the bed to prevent nighttime reflux.
     - Encourage the patient to avoid wearing tight-fitting clothing and working in a bent-over or stooped position.
  2. Drug therapy for GERD management includes three major types: antacids, histamine blockers, and proton pump inhibitors.

G

PATIENT-CENTERED CARE: OLDER ADULT HEALTH

Proton Pump Inhibitors

Research has found that long-term use of proton pump inhibitors (PPIs) may increase the risk for hip fracture, especially in older adults. PPIs can interfere with calcium absorption and protein digestion and therefore reduce available calcium to bone tissue. Decreased calcium makes bones more brittle and likely to fracture, especially as adults get older (Lins Vieira et al., 2021).

Endoscopic Therapies
- The Stretta procedure, a nonsurgical method, can replace surgery for GERD when other measures are ineffective.
- Patients with obesity or who have severe symptoms may not be candidates for this procedure.
- In the Stretta procedure, the health care provider applies radiofrequency (RF) energy through the endoscope using needles placed near the gastroesophageal junction. The RF energy decreases vagus nerve activity, thus reducing discomfort for the patient.

Surgical Management
- Laparoscopic Nissen fundoplication is a minimally invasive surgery that is the standard surgical approach for treatment of severe GERD.
- A very small percentage of patients with GERD require antireflux surgery.
- The LINX Reflux Management System is a device that augments the LES with a ring composed of rare earth magnets (Schwaitzberg, 2021). The magnets attract to increase the closure pressure of the LES yet still allow food passage with swallowing. The LINX can be effective for patients with typical GERD symptoms who have an abnormal pH study, only partially respond to PPI therapy, and do not have a hiatal hernia or severe esophagitis

---

! NURSING SAFETY PRIORITY

Action Alert

When caring for a patient who has had LINX device insertion, emphasize the importance of telling each health care provider about this procedure. If an MRI is recommended, only certain patients with more recent LINX devices *may* be eligible to undergo scanning. Patients with older LINX devices (which contain magnets) should *never* undergo MRI scanning. The health care provider can determine whether MRI is acceptable for the patient, given the date of LINX device insertion.

Care Coordination and Transition Management
- Remind the patient to make appropriate dietary selections that enhance nutrition and decrease symptoms associated with GERD.
- For patients with nonsurgical GERD, teach about signs and symptoms of more serious complications, such as esophageal stricture and Barrett's esophagus.

Evaluate Outcomes: Evaluation
- Evaluate the care of the patient with GERD based on the identified priority patient problem. The expected outcomes include that the patient will:
  1. Adhere to appropriate dietary selections, medication therapy, and lifestyle modifications, which decrease signs and symptoms of GERD.
  2. Experience minimized or absence of ***pain.***

See Chapter 46 in the main text for more information on gastroesophageal reflux disease.

GENDER CONSIDERATIONS

- People of minority sexual and gender identities are often grouped under one umbrella population category described by an acronym such as **LGBTQ**—lesbian, gay, bisexual, transgender, and queer/questioning individuals (people who do not feel they belong in one of the other subgroups). Another similar acronym used is **LGBTQIA2+**, encompassing lesbian, gay, bisexual, transgender, queer (or questioning), intersexual, asexual, and two-spirited people, as well as other sexualities, sexes, and genders not included in the acronym. Some literature includes only the letters "LGBT."

- Gender is a social construct—an idea created by people to help explain the world around them (The Trevor Project, 2021). Historically, it has been categorized by one of two terms: *male* and *female.* When babies are born, the child's gender is determined by the genitalia present, but there is no way of knowing the child's true sense of gender. Transgender people report feeling a mismatch between their gender identity and sex assigned at birth, often extending back into early childhood, and nonbinary people report having a gender identity that doesn't fall within the historical binary system.

- The word *transgender* is often used as an umbrella term under which other terminology falls, such as *transmen*, *transwomen*, and *nonbinary.*

G

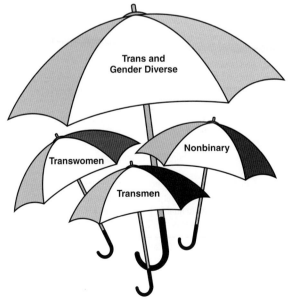

Umbrella terminology.

- Using appropriate terminology is essential to demonstrating respect.
  1. Congruence: The feeling of harmony with one's gender
  2. Cisgender: Gender identity is congruent with the patient's sex assigned at birth (the genital anatomy present at birth).
  3. Intersex: People born with a chromosomal pattern, a reproductive system, or sexual anatomy that does not fit the binary of male or female bodies
  4. Transgender: People who have gender identities that are not exclusively male or female, or are between and beyond genders, or who are without a gender (agender)
  5. Gender expression: The ways in which all people present themselves to the world
  6. Transition: Some people pursue ways of making their physical body and appearance affirm their identity. This may be based on clothing selection, mannerisms, hormones, or via gender affirmation surgery (GAS).
  7. Androgynous: People who present themselves as neither distinguishably male nor female

---

The Joint Commission Recommendations for Creating a Safe, Welcoming Environment for LGBTQ Patients

- Post the *Patients' Bill of Rights* and nondiscrimination policies in a visible place.
- Make waiting rooms inclusive for LGBTQ patients and families, such as posting *Safe Zone*, rainbow, or pink triangle signs.
- Designate unisex or single-stall restrooms.
- Ensure that visitation policies are equitable for families of LGBTQ patients.
- Avoid assumptions about any patient's sexual orientation and gender identity.
- Include gender-neutral language on all medical forms and documents (e.g., "partnered" in addition to married, single, or divorced categories).
- Do not limit gender options on medical forms to "male" and "female."
- Reflect the patient's choice of terminology in communication and documentation.
- Provide information on special health concerns for LGBTQ patients.
- Become knowledgeable about LGBTQ health needs and care.
- Refer LGBTQ patients to qualified health care professionals as needed.
- Provide community resources for LGBTQ information and support as needed.

Adapted from The Joint Commission (TJC). (2011). Advancing effective communication, cultural competence, and patient- and family-centered care for the lesbian, gay, bisexual, and transgender community. www.jointcommission.org/lgbt.

- People who were born with anatomically male genitalia (known as assigned male at birth, or AMAB) but whose gender identity is female are known as **male-to-female (MtF)**. Male-to-female people are also known as "transwomen," with the gender descriptor indicating the lived gender identity. **Female-to-male (FtM)** individuals are people who were born with anatomically female genitalia (known as **assigned female at birth**, or **AFAB**) and whose lived gender identity is male. They are also known as "transmen."

Interprofessional Collaborative Care
Recognize Cues: Assessment
- As with any patient, ask during the nursing history and physical assessment how they prefer to be addressed.
- In addition to preferred names, correct pronoun usage is also important. Each patient has pronouns that they use.
  1. Some patients may request the use of gender-neutral pronouns, or they may use these pronouns in the nurse's presence.

Examples of Gender Pronouns

Subjective	Objective	Possessive	Reflexive	Example
She	Her	Hers	Herself	She is speaking. I listened to her. The backpack is hers.
He	Him	His	Himself	He is speaking. I listened to him. The backpack is his.
They	Them	Theirs	Themself	They are speaking. I listened to them. The backpack is theirs.
Ze	Hir/Zir	Hirs/Zirs	Hirself/Zirself	Ze is speaking. I listened to hir. The backpack is zirs.

Gender pronouns. (Modified from Trans Student Educational Resources. Gender pronouns. https://transstudent.org/graphics/pronouns101/.)

Take Actions: Interventions
- Nurses may care for transgender or nonbinary patients of any age who may be transitioning or have completed gender affirmation. They may care for them for health problems related to their transition process or for problems that are unrelated to the patient's *sexuality* or gender identity.

- In general, care for transgender patients with most health problems is the same as for any other patient. However, some interventions such as hormone therapy may affect nursing assessment and care.

Nonsurgical Management

- The primary nonsurgical interventions for transgender patients include drug (hormone) therapy, counseling about **reproduction** and reproductive health, and vocal therapy. The type of intervention depends on whether the patient is MtF or FtM.
- Nonbinary patients may also choose to use nonsurgical interventions, such as hormone therapy in microdoses, to achieve a specific degree of transition.

Surgical Management

- **Gender affirming surgery (GAS)** is also known as gender-confirming or gender reassignment surgery
- Genital surgeries "below the waist" (often called "bottom surgery") are the most invasive procedures. The criteria for genital surgery depend on the type of surgery being requested.
  1. Most surgeons (usually gynecologic, urologic, and plastic surgeons) require 12 months of hormone therapy plus one or two referrals from qualified psychotherapists for male-to-female (MtF) patients who desire an orchiectomy (removal of testes). The same requirement may be needed for FtM patients who desire a hysterectomy (uterus removal) and bilateral salpingo-oophorectomy (BSO), or removal of both fallopian tubes and ovaries.
  2. Feminizing surgeries are performed for MtF patients to create a functional and/or aesthetic (cosmetic) female anatomy, including:
     - Breast/chest surgeries, such as breast augmentation (mammoplasty to increase breast tissue)
     - Genital surgeries, such as partial penectomy (removal of the penis), orchiectomy (removal of the testes), vaginoplasty and labiaplasty-vulvoplasty (creation of a vagina and labia/vulva), and clitoroplasty (creation of a clitoris)
     - Other surgeries, such as facial feminizing surgery (to achieve feminine facial contour), liposuction (fatty tissue removal), often from the waist or abdominal area, vocal feminizing surgery, and other body-contouring procedures
  3. Masculinizing surgeries are performed for FtM patients to create a functional and/or aesthetic male anatomy, including:
     - Breast/chest surgeries, usually a bilateral mastectomy (removal of both breasts) and chest reconstruction

- Genital surgeries, such as a hysterectomy and BSO, vaginectomy (removal of the vagina), phalloplasty (creation of an average-size male penis) with ureteroplasty (creation of a urethra), or metoidioplasty (creation of a small penis using hormone-enhanced clitoral tissue), and scrotoplasty (creation of a scrotum) with insertion of testicular prostheses
- Other surgeries, such as liposuction, pectoral muscle implants, and other body-contouring procedures

4. Pre- and postoperative care includes the following:
   - Use culturally sensitive and accurate language when communicating with transgender patients; use pronouns that match the patient's physical appearance and dress unless the patient requests a specific term.
   - Provide preoperative care for a patient having a vaginoplasty or other GAS procedures, including teaching about bowel preparation, food and fluid intake, hair removal methods, and the need for informed consent.
   - Monitor for potentially life-threatening complications of gender affirming surgery, such as fistula development, bleeding, and wound infection.

See Chapter 5 in the main text for more information on gender considerations.

G

✳ GLAUCOMA: SENSORY PERCEPTION EXEMPLAR

Overview

- Glaucoma is a group of eye disorders resulting in increased intraocular pressure (IOP) that can result in loss of visual *sensory perception.*
- The normal IOP is 8 to 21 mm Hg, maintained when there is a balance between production and outflow of aqueous humor.
- If the IOP becomes too high, pressure on blood vessels results in poorly oxygenated photoreceptors; combined with compression on nerve fibers, IOP can lead to ischemic injury and permanent blindness.
- In most types of glaucoma, vision is lost gradually and painlessly from the periphery to the central area.
- Types of glaucoma:
  1. *Open-angle glaucoma (OAG),* also known as primary open-angle glaucoma (POAG), has reduced outflow of aqueous humor through the chamber angle. Because the fluid cannot leave the eye at the same rate it is produced, IOP gradually increases.

2. *Angle-closure glaucoma (ACG),* also known as primary angle-closure glaucoma (PACG), has a sudden onset and is a ***medical emergency***.
3. *Secondary:* Glaucoma results from other problems within the eye, such as uveitis, iritis, trauma, and ocular surgeries.

Interprofessional Collaborative Care
Recognize Cues: Assessment
* Assess for signs and symptoms of early glaucoma.
  1. Ophthalmoscopic examination shows cupping and atrophy of the optic disc. It becomes wider and deeper and turns white or gray.
  2. In OAG the visual fields first show a small loss of peripheral vision that gradually progresses to a larger loss.
  3. Symptoms of angle-closure glaucoma include a sudden, severe pain around the eyes that radiates over the face. Headache or brow pain, nausea, and vomiting may occur.
     * Other symptoms include seeing colored halos around lights and sudden blurred vision with decreased light perception. The sclera may appear reddened, and the cornea foggy. Ophthalmoscopic examination reveals a shallow anterior chamber, a cloudy aqueous humor, and a moderately dilated, nonreactive pupil.
  4. Increased ocular pressure measured by tonometry.
     * Normal is 8 to 21 mm Hg

Analyze Cues and Prioritize Hypotheses: Analysis
* The priority collaborative problems for patients with glaucoma include:
  1. Impaired visual ***sensory perception*** due to glaucoma
  2. Need for health teaching due to treatment regimen for glaucoma

Generate Solutions and Take Actions: Planning and Implementation
Supporting Visual Acuity Via Health Teaching
* Teach the patient that loss of visual ***sensory perception*** from glaucoma can be prevented by early detection, lifelong treatment, and close monitoring.
* Use of ophthalmic drugs that reduce ocular pressure can delay or prevent damage.
* Drug therapy for glaucoma focuses on reducing IOP with eye drops; drug therapy does not improve lost vision.

Common Examples of Drug Therapy (Eye Drops)

Glaucoma

Drug Category	Nursing Implications

Adrenergic Agonists

Apraclonidine
Brimonidine tartrate

Ask whether the patient is taking any antidepressants from the MAO inhibitor class. *These enzyme inhibitors increase blood pressure, as do the adrenergic agonists. When taken together, the patient may experience hypertensive crisis.*

Teach the patient to wear dark glasses outdoors and to avoid too much sunlight exposure. *This type of drug can cause the eyes to become sensitive to light.*

Teach the patient not to use the eye drops with contact lenses in place and to wait 15 minutes after using the drug to put in contact lenses, if worn. *These drugs are absorbed by the contact lenses, which can become discolored or cloudy.*

Beta-Adrenergic Blockers

Betaxolol hydrochloride
Carteolol
Levobunolol
Timolol

Ask whether the patient has moderate to severe asthma or COPD. *If these drugs are absorbed systemically, they constrict pulmonary smooth muscle and narrow airways.*

Teach patients with diabetes to check their blood glucose levels more often when taking these drugs. *These drugs induce hypoglycemia and can mask the hypoglycemic symptoms.*

Teach patients who also take oral beta blockers to check their pulse at least twice a day and to notify the primary health care and eye care providers if the pulse is consistently below 60 beats/min. *These drugs potentiate the effects of systemic beta blockers and can cause an unsafe decrease in heart rate and blood pressure.*

Carbonic Anhydrase Inhibitors

Brinzolamide
Dorzolamide

Ask whether the patient has an allergy to sulfonamide antibacterial drugs. *Drugs are similar to the sulfonamides; if a patient is allergic to the sulfonamides, an allergy is possible with these drugs.*

Teach the patient to shake the drug before applying. *Drug separates on standing.*

Teach the patient not to use the eye drops with contact lenses in place and to wait 15 minutes after using the drug to put in the lenses. *These drugs are absorbed by the contact lenses, which can become discolored or cloudy.*

G

Continued

Common Examples of Drug Therapy (Eye Drops)—cont'd

Glaucoma

Drug Category	Nursing Implications

Cholinergic Agonists

Carbachol
Echothiophate
Pilocarpine

Teach not to administer more eye drops than are prescribed and to report increased salivation or drooling to the primary health care and eye care providers. *These drugs are readily absorbed by conjunctival mucous membranes and can cause systemic side effects of headache, flushing, increased saliva, and sweating.*

Teach to use good light when reading and to turn lights on in rooms. *The pupil of the eye will not open more to let in more light, and it may be harder to see objects in dim light. This can increase the risk for falls.*

Nitric Oxides

Latanoprostene bunod

Teach to refrain from driving and using machinery while using this medication. *This drug can cause blurred vision.*

Prostaglandin Agonists

Bimatoprost
Latanoprost
Tafluprost
Travoprost

Teach to check the cornea for abrasions or trauma. *Drugs should not be used when the cornea is not intact.*

Teach that eye color may darken, and eyelashes elongate, over time in the eye receiving one of these drugs. *Knowing the side effects in advance reassures the patient that their presence is expected and normal.*

If only one eye is to be treated, teach *not* to place drops in the other eye to try to make the eye colors similar. *Using the drug in an eye with normal IOP can cause a **lower**-than-normal IOP, which reduces vision.*

Caution that using more drops than prescribed can reduce drug effectiveness. *Drug action is based on blocking receptors, which can increase in number when the drug is overused.*

Rho Kinase Inhibitor

Netarsudil

If the patient is dispensed a multiple-dose container, caution about cross-contamination. *Reports of bacterial keratitis have arisen when patients with other disorders (e.g., a concurrent corneal disorder) have accidentally contaminated the medication.*

Combination Drug

Brimonidine tartrate and timolol maleate

Same as for each drug alone.

- Teach the patient:
  1. The importance of instilling the drops on time and not skipping doses
  2. To wait 5 to 10 minutes between drug instillations when more than one drug is prescribed to prevent one drug from "washing out" or diluting another drug
  3. The technique of punctal occlusion (placing pressure on the corner of the eye near the nose) immediately after eye drop instillation to prevent systemic absorption of the drug
  4. About the need for good handwashing, keeping the eye drop container tip clean, and avoiding touching the tip to any part of the eye

---

🔵 NURSING SAFETY PRIORITY

Drug Alert

Most eye drops used for glaucoma therapy can be absorbed systemically and cause systemic problems. It is critical to teach punctal occlusion to patients using eye drops for glaucoma therapy.

Parts of the eye

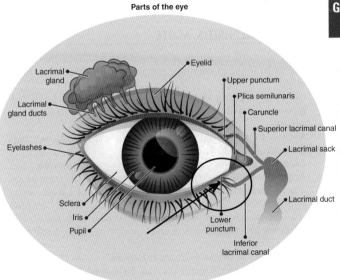

Apply punctal occlusion in the circled area to prevent systemic absorption of eyedrops. (Used with permission from istockphoto.com, 2020, VectorMine.)

- Surgery is used when drugs for the patient with open-angle glaucoma are ineffective in controlling IOP. The two most common procedures are laser trabeculoplasty and trabeculectomy to improve the outflow of aqueous fluid.

Care Coordination and Transition Management
- Reinforce teaching about self-management, especially the techniques for eye drop instillation.
- For the patient who has had surgery, teach the signs and symptoms of choroidal detachment and hemorrhage. These can occur after coughing, sneezing, straining at stools, or Valsalva maneuver.
- Refer to community agencies and resources for assistance in adapting to vision impairment.

Evaluate Outcomes: Evaluation
- Evaluate the care of the patient with glaucoma based on the identified priority patient problem. The primary expected outcomes are that the patient will have optimum visual acuity as long as possible as demonstrated by adherence to the treatment regimen.

 See Chapter 39 in the main text for more information on glaucoma.

GLOMERULONEPHRITIS, ACUTE

- Acute glomerulonephritis is a group of conditions that injure and inflame the glomerulus, the part of the kidney that filters blood.
- Glomerulonephritis is associated with high blood pressure, progressive kidney damage (leading to chronic kidney disease), and edema.
- Anemia from reduced production of erythropoietin and high cholesterol often co-occur.
- Glomerulonephritis can cause altered urinary *elimination*.
- **Acute glomerulonephritis** (GN) develops suddenly from an excess *immunity* response within the kidney tissues. Usually an infection is noticed before kidney symptoms of acute GN are present. The onset of symptoms is about 10 days from the time of infection. Usually patients recover quickly and completely from acute GN.
- Many causes of primary GN are infectious.
- Secondary glomerulonephritis can be caused by multisystem diseases and can manifest as acute or chronic disease.

Infectious Agents Associated With Glomerulonephritis

- Group A beta-hemolytic *Streptococcus*
- Staphylococcal or gram-negative bacteremia or sepsis
- Pneumococcal, *Mycoplasma*, or *Klebsiella* pneumonia
- Syphilis
- Dengue
- Hantavirus
- Varicella
- Parvovirus
- Hepatitis B and C
- Cytomegalovirus
- Parvovirus
- Epstein-Barr virus
- Human immunodeficiency virus

Adapted from Patel, N.P. (2018, November 28). Infection-induced kidney diseases. Retrieved from U.S. National Library of Medicine, National Institutes of Health. https://www.ncbi.nlm.nih.gov/pmc/articles/PMC6282040/.

Interprofessional Collaborative Care
Recognize Cues: Assessment

G

- Assess and document the following:
  1. History of recent infections, particularly skin and upper respiratory infections
  2. Recent travel or activities with exposure to viruses, bacteria, fungi, or parasites
  3. Diagnosis of systemic diseases, especially those that alter *immunity*, such as systemic lupus erythematosus (SLE)
- Assessment findings include:
  1. Presence of symptoms indicating systemic volume overload: extra heart sound (i.e., S_3 gallop), neck vein distention, edema, and crackles in the lungs with tachypnea and dyspnea or orthopnea
  2. Changes in urine color (typically smoky, reddish brown, or cola-colored urine), clarity, or odor; and altered patterns of urination such as dysuria, urgency, and incontinence
  3. Decreased urine output
  4. Mild to moderate hypertension
  5. Changes in weight
  6. Fatigue, malaise, and activity intolerance
  7. Abnormal urinalysis, including leukocyte esterase, nitrogen, red blood cells (RBCs), white blood cells (WBCs), low creatinine, and presence of protein, casts, or cells

8. Increased blood urea nitrogen (BUN) and serum creatinine levels
9. Results of percutaneous needle biopsy of the kidney to provide a precise diagnosis

Take Actions: Interventions

- Manage infection by administering antibiotic therapy as prescribed.
- Balance intake and output; fluid intake may be restricted to the previous 24-hour urinary output plus 500 to 600 mL for insensible fluid loss.
- Hypertension, fluid overload, and edema may be managed with diuretics or fluid and sodium restrictions.
- Avoid electrolyte imbalance and protein overload during kidney dysfunction with dietary adjustments in collaboration with the dietitian.
- Support education and blood pressure management for dialysis or plasmapheresis used to filter out antigen-antibody complexes and manage uremia or fluid and electrolyte imbalances.
- Provide health teaching, including:
  1. Reviewing prescribed drug instructions, including purpose, timing, frequency, duration, and side effects
  2. Ensuring that the patient and family understand dietary and fluid modifications. Offer assistance with coping with fluid restrictions, such as a mouth moisturizer or mouth swabs. In some situations ice chips or hard candy may be used to offer relief from a dry mouth.
  3. Advising the patient to measure weight and blood pressure daily and to notify the health care provider of any sudden changes

See Chapter 59 in the main text for more information on acute glomerulonephritis.

GLOMERULONEPHRITIS, CHRONIC

- Chronic glomerulonephritis, or *chronic nephritic syndrome*, is the diagnostic name given to changes in kidney tissue that develop over decades of infection, hypertension, *inflammation*, or poor kidney blood flow.
- Nephrons become damaged and are lost; proteinuria occurs; kidney tissue atrophies, and the ability to filter blood is reduced.
- The process eventually results in end-stage kidney disease (ESKD) and uremia, requiring dialysis or transplantation.

Interprofessional Collaborative Care

Recognize Cues: Assessment

- Record the patient's history regarding health problems, including systemic disease, kidney or urologic problems, and infectious diseases, especially streptococcal infections and recent exposure to infection.
- Assess for:
  1. Presence of symptoms indicating systemic volume overload: the cardiac extra sound of an S_3 gallop, neck vein engorgement, edema, and crackles in the lungs with tachypnea
  2. Uremic symptoms such as changes in concentration, slurred speech, ataxia, tremors, bruising, and rash or itching
  3. Changes in urine and elimination, including amount, frequency of voiding, and changes in urine color, clarity, and odor
  4. Skin changes, including a yellowish color, texture changes, bruises, rashes, or eruptions
  5. Abnormal urinalysis, especially proteinuria
  6. Elevated BUN and serum creatinine, and decreased glomerular filtration rate (GFR)
  7. Abnormal electrolyte values
  8. Ultrasound or radiographic findings of kidney size (usually small)

Take Actions: Interventions

- Management of chronic glomerulonephritis is similar to management for CKD, including dialysis when kidneys fail to adequately filter the blood.
- Treatment consists of dietary modification, fluid intake sufficient to prevent reduced blood flow volume to the kidneys, and drug therapy to temporarily control the symptoms of uremia.

See Chapter 59 in the main text for more information on chronic glomerulonephritis.

GONORRHEA

- Gonorrhea is a sexually transmitted bacterial infection caused by *Neisseria gonorrhoeae*.
- It is transmitted by direct sexual contact with mucosal surfaces (vaginal intercourse, orogenital contact, or anogenital contact).
- The first symptoms of gonorrhea may appear within a week after sexual contact with an infected person.
- The disease can be present without symptoms and can be transmitted or progress without warning.

- In women, ascending spread of the organism can cause pelvic infection (pelvic inflammatory disease [PID]), ectopic pregnancy, miscarriage, premature labor or birth, neonate eye infection, ongoing pelvic pain, and sepsis (if left untreated).
- In men, gonorrhea can cause fertility reduction, proctitis, and sepsis (if untreated).

Interprofessional Collaborative Care
Recognize Cues: Assessment
- Assess and document:
  1. Sexual history that includes sites of sexual exposure or intercourse, as gonorrhea can affect the genitals, rectum, and throat
  2. Allergies to antibiotics
  3. The *infection* can be asymptomatic in both men and women, but women have asymptomatic, or "silent," infections more often than do men.
  4. Symptoms in men:
     - Dysuria
     - Penile discharge (profuse, yellowish-green fluid or scant, clear fluid)
     - Urethritis
     - Pain or discomfort in the prostate, seminal vesicles, or epididymal regions
  5. Symptoms in women:
     - Vaginal discharge (yellow, green, profuse, odorous)
     - Urinary frequency
     - Dysuria and urethral discharge
  6. Anal manifestations (in men or women)
     - Itching and irritation
     - Rectal discharge or bleeding
     - Diarrhea
     - Painful defecation
  7. Oral cavity manifestations
     - Reddened throat
     - Ulcerated lips
     - Tender gingivae
     - Lesions in the throat
- Diagnostic testing may include:
  1. Nucleic acid amplification test (NAAT) using samples from vagina or male urethra
  2. Gram staining and cultures from a smear from penile discharge or from a vaginal swab

NURSING SAFETY PRIORITY

Critical Rescue

All patients with gonorrhea should be tested for syphilis, chlamydia, hepatitis B and hepatitis C, and HIV infection and, if possible, examined for HSV and HPV because they may have been exposed to these STIs as well. Sexual partners who have been exposed in the past 30 days should be examined, and specimens should be obtained.

Take Actions: Interventions

- Uncomplicated gonorrhea is treated with antibiotics. Chlamydia *infection*, which is four times more common, is frequently found in patients with gonorrhea. Because of this, patients treated for gonorrhea should also be managed with drugs that treat chlamydia infection.
- Drug therapy recommended by the CDC for uncomplicated gonorrhea of the pharynx, cervix, rectum, or urethra is IM ceftriaxone in a single dose at the time of visit.
- A coinfection with chlamydia is treated also with doxycycline.
- Sexual partners also must be treated.
- A test of cure is not required, but the patient should be advised to return for a follow-up examination if symptoms persist after treatment.
- Teach the patient about:
  1. Transmission and treatment of gonorrhea
  2. Prevention of reinfection
  3. Complications of chronic gonorrhea
  4. Avoiding sexual activity until the antibiotic therapy is completed
  5. The need for use of condoms at all times
  6. The need for all sexual contacts to be examined for STI
- Encourage patients to express their feelings during assessments and teaching sessions.
- Provide privacy for teaching, and maintain confidentiality of medical records.

 See Chapter 65 in the main text for more information on gonorrhea.

G

HEADACHE, MIGRAINE

- A migraine headache is a common clinical syndrome of recurrent episodic head pain that can last 4 to 72 hours, characterized by throbbing, intense unilateral pain that can be accompanied by nausea and sensitivity to light, sound, or head movement.
- The cause of migraine headaches is likely a combination of neuronal hyperexcitability and vascular, genetic, hormonal, and environmental factors that result in cerebral vasodilation followed by a sterile brain tissue inflammation.

Interprofessional Collaborative Care
Recognize Cues: Assessment

- Migraines fall into two major categories: migraines with aura and migraines without aura.
    1. An *aura* is a sensation (such as visual changes) that signals the onset of a headache or seizure. In a migraine, the aura occurs immediately before the migraine episode.

 KEY FEATURES

Migraine Headaches

Phases of Migraine With Aura (Classic Migraine)
Prodromal Phase
- Occurs 1 to 2 days prior to onset of migraine
- Subtle changes such as yawning excessively, constipation, emotional alterations, and food cravings
- Aura, which includes two or more of the following temporary central nervous system symptoms that last 5 to 60 minutes. Symptoms are generally unilateral. Visual disturbances include:
  - Flashing lights
  - Lines or spots
  - Shimmering or zigzag lights
- A variety of other neurologic changes may occur, including:
  - Numbness, tingling of the lips or tongue
  - Acute confusional state
  - Aphasia
  - Vertigo
  - Unilateral weakness
  - Drowsiness

KEY FEATURES—cont'd

Migraine Headaches

Migraine Phase
- Headache accompanied by nausea or vomiting
- Unilateral, frontotemporal, throbbing *pain* in the head that is often worse behind one eye or ear
- Also includes photophobia and or phonophobia

Migraine Without Aura (Common Migraine)
- Migraine beginning without an aura before the onset of the headache
- *Pain* aggravated by performing routine physical activities
- *Pain* that is unilateral and pulsating
- One of these symptoms is present:
  - Nausea or vomiting
  - *Photophobia* (light sensitivity)
  - *Phonophobia* (sound sensitivity)
  - Headache lasting 4 to 72 hours
  - Migraine often occurring in the early morning, during periods of stress, or in those with premenstrual tension or fluid retention

Take Actions: Interventions

- The priority of care is *pain* management.
  1. Prevention includes interventions and education to reduce migraine episodes.
     - Drugs may be used when migraine occurs more than twice per week, interferes with activities of daily living (ADLs), or is not relieved with acute treatment.
     - Migraine-preventive drugs include nonsteroidal antiinflammatory drugs (NSAIDs), beta-adrenergic blockers, calcium channel blockers, or antiepileptics.
  2. Abortive therapy is aimed at alleviating *pain* during the aura phase or soon after a headache starts. Examples of migraine abortive drugs are:
     - Acetaminophen and NSAIDs; the addition of caffeine to these drugs in some over-the-counter (OTC) agents results in vasoconstriction to enhance symptom relief
     - Antiemetics or prokinetics to relieve nausea and vomiting
     - For more *severe* migraines, drugs such as triptans, ditans, ergotamine derivatives, and isometheptene combinations are often needed. A potential side effect of these drugs is *rebound* headache.
  3. Trigger avoidance and management can reduce the frequency or severity of migraines by identifying and stopping exposure

H

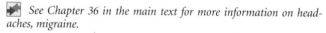

NURSING SAFETY PRIORITY

Drug Alert

Teach patients taking triptan drugs to take them as soon as migraine symptoms develop. Instruct patients to report angina (chest **pain**) or chest discomfort to their health care providers immediately to prevent cardiac damage from myocardial ischemia. Remind them to use contraception (birth control) while taking the drugs because the drugs may not be safe for women who are pregnant. Teach them to expect common side effects that include flushing, tingling, and a hot sensation. These annoying sensations tend to subside after the patient's body gets used to the drug. Triptan drugs should not be taken with selective serotonin reuptake inhibitor (SSRI) antidepressants or St. John's wort, an herb used commonly for depression.

to dietary and environmental factors that contribute to migraines.
- Instruct the patient to keep a diary to link exposures to migraine symptoms.
4. Complementary and integrative health therapies associated with symptom relief include acupressure and acupuncture, yoga, meditation, massage, exercise, yoga, and biofeedback. Vitamin B_2 (riboflavin) and magnesium supplement to maintain normal serum values have a role in migraine prevention.

See Chapter 36 in the main text for more information on headaches, migraine.

HEARING LOSS: SENSORY PERCEPTION CONCEPT EXEMPLAR

Overview
- Hearing loss, an auditory **sensory perception** impairment or loss, is common and may be conductive, sensorineural, or a combination of the two.
  1. *Conductive hearing loss* occurs when sound waves are blocked from contact with the inner ear nerve fibers because of external or middle ear disorders.
  2. *Sensorineural hearing loss* is a result of damage to the inner ear sensory nerve that leads to the brain.
     - **Presbycusis** is a sensorineural hearing loss that occurs with aging (Rogers, 2023). It is caused by degeneration of cochlear nerve cells, loss of elasticity of the basilar membrane, or a decreased blood supply to the inner ear.

Comparison of Features for Conductive, Sensorineural, and Mixed Hearing Loss

Conductive Hearing Loss	Sensorineural Hearing Loss	Mixed Hearing Loss
Causes		
Allergies Cerumen Eustachian tube dysfunction External otitis Fluid presence Foreign body Otitis media Perforation of the tympanic membrane	Aging Auditory tumors Genetic hearing problems Head injury Health disorders (e.g., diabetes, Ménière disease, meningitis, stroke) Ototoxic drugs Prolonged noise exposure	Combination of causes of conductive and sensorineural hearing loss (e.g., the patient has fluid in the ear, and the patient is exposed to prolonged noise in the work environment)
Assessment Findings		
Cerumen Hears better out of one ear Narrowing of ear canal Obstruction with a foreign body Otosclerosis Otitis externa Pain in the ear Report that one's own voice sounds strange Rupture of tympanic membrane Rinne test: bone conduction greater than air conduction in affected ear (will not hear fork at ear), and air conduction greater than bone conduction in unaffected ear. Weber test: lateralization to affected ear	Difficulty following conversations Dizziness Ear structures appear normal Hearing poorly in a loud environment Reports that speech of others is mumbled Tinnitus Rinne test: air conduction greater than bone conduction in most patients; some with severe loss may report bone conduction greater than air conduction if one ear functions better than the other. Weber test: lateralization to unaffected or better-hearing ear	Combination of any assessment findings associated with conductive and sensorineural hearing loss

H

Data from American Speech-Language-Hearing Association. (2023). Conductive hearing loss. https://www.asha.org/public/hearing/conductive-hearing-loss/; American Speech-Language-Hearing Association. (2023). Mixed hearing loss. https://www.asha.org/public/hearing/mixed-hearing-loss/; American Speech-Language-Hearing Association. (2023). Sensorineural hearing loss. https://www.asha.org/public/hearing/sensorineural-hearing-loss/; Weber, P. (2022). Evaluation of hearing loss in adults. *UpToDate*. Retrieved April 2, 2023, from https://www.uptodate.com/contents/evaluation-of-hearing-loss-in-adults.

Interprofessional Collaborative Care
Recognize Cues: Assessment
- Obtain patient information about:
    1. Any differences in the ears or hearing and whether the changes occurred suddenly or gradually, including:
        - Feeling of ear fullness or congestion
        - Dizziness or vertigo
        - Tinnitus
        - Difficulty hearing sounds or understanding conversations, especially in a noisy room
    2. Exposure to loud or continuous noises
    3. Current or previous use of ototoxic drugs
    4. History of head or ear trauma or surgery
    5. Number of past ear infections or perforations
    6. Presence of excessive cerumen
    7. Type and pattern of ear hygiene
    8. Air travel (especially in unpressurized aircraft)
    9. Recent upper respiratory infection and allergies affecting the nose and sinuses
- Assess for and document:
    1. External ear features (pinna), including size and position
    2. Abnormal otoscopic and Rinne or Weber (tuning fork) test findings by the provider
    3. Psychosocial issues
        - Social isolation
        - Depression, fear, and despair
- Diagnostic studies include audiometry to determine the type and extent of hearing loss and imaging to determine possible causes.

Analyze Cues and Prioritize Hypotheses: Analysis
- The priority collaborative problems for the patient with any degree of hearing impairment include:
    1. Decreased hearing ability due to obstruction, *infection*, damage to the middle ear, or damage to the auditory nerve
    2. Decreased communication due to difficulty hearing

Generate Solutions and Take Actions: Planning and Implementation
Increasing Hearing
- Interventions include early detection of impaired auditory *sensory perception,* use of appropriate therapy, and use of assistive devices to augment the patient's usable hearing.
    1. Promote early detection to help correct reversible problems causing the hearing loss.

2. Administer drug therapy, including antibiotic therapy for infection, to correct an underlying pathologic change or to reduce side effects of problems occurring with hearing loss.
3. Administer antivertiginous drugs to decrease dizziness when this symptom accompanies hearing loss.
4. Apply hearing-assistive devices:
   - Portable audio amplifiers
   - Collaborate with the audiologist to promote safe, effective use of a hearing aid.

Surgical Management

- The type of operative procedure selected depends on the cause of the hearing loss.
  1. *Tympanoplasty* reconstructs the middle ear. The procedures vary from simple reconstruction of the eardrum (myringoplasty) to replacement of the ossicles within the middle ear (ossiculoplasty).
     - Systemic antibiotics are required before surgery to decrease the risk of infection.
     - Hearing loss immediately after surgery is normal because of canal packing.
  2. *Stapedectomy* is the removal of the head and neck of the stapes and, less often, the footplate. After removal of the bone, a small hole is drilled or made with a laser in the footplate, and a prosthesis in the shape of a piston is connected between the incus and the footplate.
     - Improvement in hearing may not occur until 6 weeks after surgery.
     - The surgery is performed near cranial nerves VII, VIII, and X. Assess for facial nerve damage or muscle weakness.
  3. A totally implanted device is placed to treat bilateral moderate to severe sensorineural hearing loss.

H

! NURSING SAFETY PRIORITY

Action Alert

Prevent injury by assisting the patient with ambulation during the first 1 to 2 days after stapedectomy. Keep top bed side rails up, and remind the patient to move the head slowly to avoid vertigo.

PATIENT AND FAMILY EDUCATION

Prevention of Ear Infection or Trauma

- Do not use small objects, such as cotton-tipped applicators, matches, toothpicks, keys, or hairpins, to clean your external ear canal.
- Wash your external ear and canal daily in the shower or while washing your hair.
- Blow your nose gently.
- Do not block one nostril while blowing your nose.
- Sneeze with your mouth open.
- Wear sound protection around loud or continuous noises.
- Avoid or wear head and ear protection during activities with high risk for head or ear trauma, such as wrestling, boxing, motorcycle riding, and skateboarding.
- Keep the volume on head receivers at the lowest setting that allows you to hear.
- Frequently clean objects that come into contact with your ear (e.g., headphones, telephone receivers).
- Avoid environmental conditions with rapid changes in air pressure.

Maximizing Communication
- Use best practices for communicating with a hearing-impaired patient, including:
  1. Positioning yourself directly in front of the patient
  2. Making sure that the room is well lighted
  3. Getting the patient's attention before you begin to speak
  4. Moving closer to the better hearing ear
  5. Speaking clearly and slowly
  6. Not shouting (shouting often makes understanding more difficult)
  7. Keeping hands and other objects away from your mouth when talking to the patient
  8. Attempting to have conversations in a quiet room with minimal distractions
  9. Having the patient repeat your statements rather than just indicating assent
  10. Rephrasing sentences and repeating information to aid in understanding
  11. Using appropriate hand motions
  12. Writing messages on paper if the patient is able to read
- Have the patient use hearing-assistive devices described earlier.

- Manage anxiety and promote social interaction by:
  1. Enhancing communication, as described earlier
  2. Working with the patient to identify the patient's most satisfying activities and social interactions and to determine the amount of effort necessary to continue them
  3. Suggesting the use of closed captioning for television programming

Care Coordination and Transition Management

- Patients with ear and hearing disorders rarely are hospitalized.
- Surgery, if needed, is often performed in an ambulatory surgery center. Follow-up hearing tests may be scheduled routinely or after surgical lesions are well healed in about 12 weeks.
- Give patients written instructions about how to take drugs and when to return for follow-up care.
- Teach patients how to instill eardrops and irrigate the ears, and obtain a return demonstration.
- Teach patients with hearing aids how to effectively use and care for them. Remember that costs associated with hearing devices can be extensive. Refer patients to appropriate agencies that specialize in working with patients with disorders affecting auditory *sensory perception.*

Evaluate Outcomes: Evaluation

- Evaluate the care of the patient who needs maximization of communication based on the identified priority patient problems. The expected outcomes include that the patient will:
  1. Maintain as much hearing as possible and/or use appropriate hearing compensation behaviors
  2. Successfully use (a) method(s) of communication that works best for the individual
  3. Successfully use assistive devices as needed

See Chapter 40 in the main text for more information on hearing loss.

❋ HEART FAILURE: PERFUSION CONCEPT EXEMPLAR

Overview

- Heart failure (HF), also called *pump failure*, is a general term for the inability of the heart to work effectively as a pump. Heart failure is a common, chronic health problem that leads to frequent hospitalization.

- The major types of HF are:
  1. *Left-sided HF*, which is characterized by decreased perfusion from low cardiac output and pulmonary congestion. This type is further subdivided into systolic HF and diastolic HF:
     - *Systolic HF* with reduced ejection fraction (HFrEF) results when the heart is unable to contract forcefully enough during systole to eject adequate amounts of blood into the circulation.
     - *Diastolic HF* with preserved ejection fraction (HFpEF) occurs when the left ventricle is unable to relax adequately during diastole, preventing the ventricle from filling with sufficient blood to ensure an adequate cardiac output.
  2. *Right-sided HF,* which occurs when the right ventricle is unable to empty completely. Right HF in the absence of left HF is most often the result of pulmonary problems. Increased volume and pressure develop in the systemic veins, resulting in peripheral edema.
  3. *High-output failure,* which can occur when cardiac output remains normal or above normal and is caused by increased metabolic needs or hyperkinetic conditions such as septicemia, anemia, and hyperthyroidism.

👤 PATIENT-CENTERED CARE: OLDER ADULT HEALTH
Exacerbation of Heart Failure

> Heart failure is a common problem among older adults. The use of certain drugs can contribute to the development or exacerbation of the problem in this population. For example, long-term use of NSAIDs for arthritis and other persistent (chronic) pain can cause fluid and sodium retention. NSAIDs may cause peripheral vasoconstriction and increase the toxicity of diuretics and angiotensin-converting enzyme inhibitors (ACEIs).

- When cardiac output is insufficient to meet the demands of the body, compensatory mechanisms operate to improve cardiac output. Although these mechanisms may initially increase cardiac output, they eventually have a damaging effect on pump function. Compensatory mechanisms contribute to increased myocardial oxygen consumption, leading to worsening signs and symptoms of HF. Compensatory mechanisms include:
  1. Sympathetic nervous system stimulation
  2. Renin-angiotensin system (RAS) activation
  3. Other chemical responses
  4. Myocardial hypertrophy

H

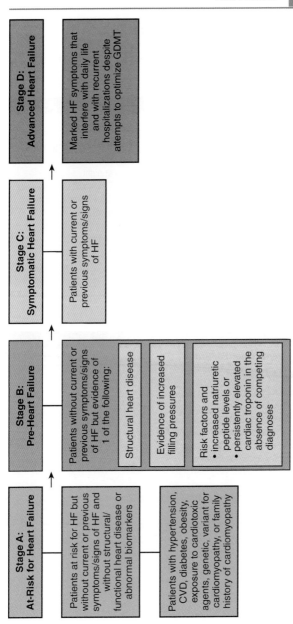

Stages of heart failure *(HF)*. *CVD,* Cardiovascular disease; *GDMT,* guideline-directed medical therapy. (Reprinted with permission from *Circulation.* 2022;145:e895-e1032 ©2022 American Heart Association, Inc.)

Interprofessional Collaborative Care
Recognize Cues: Assessment
- Assess for key symptoms of right- and left-sided heart failure.

 KEY FEATURES

Left Ventricular Failure

Decreased Cardiac Output
- Fatigue
- Weakness
- Oliguria during the day (nocturia at night)
- Angina
- Confusion, restlessness
- Dizziness
- Tachycardia, palpitations
- Pallor/ash gray skin
- Weak peripheral pulses
- Cool extremities

Pulmonary Congestion
- Hacking cough, worse at night
- Dyspnea/breathlessness
- Crackles or wheezes in lungs
- Frothy, pink-tinged sputum
- Tachypnea
- S_3/S_4 summation gallop

 KEY FEATURES

Right Ventricular Failure

- Systemic congestion
- Jugular (neck vein) distention
- Enlarged liver and spleen
- Anorexia and nausea
- Dependent edema (legs and sacrum)
- Distended abdomen
- Swollen hands and fingers
- Polyuria at night
- Weight gain
- Increased blood pressure (from excess volume) or decreased blood pressure (from failure)

⚠ NURSING SAFETY PRIORITY
Action Alert

> Edema is an extremely unreliable sign of HF. Be sure that accurate daily weights are taken to document fluid retention. Assessing weight at the same time of the morning using the same scale is important. *Weight is the most reliable indicator of fluid gain and loss!*

- Arterial blood gas values may reveal hypoxemia. Chest x-rays may show cardiomegaly, representing hypertrophy or dilation. Hemodynamic monitoring can be used for direct assessment of cardiac function for acutely ill patients.

Analyze Cues and Prioritize Hypotheses: Analysis
- The priority collaborative problems for most patients with HF include:
  1. Decreased *gas exchange* due to ventilation/perfusion imbalance
  2. Potential for decreased *perfusion* due to inadequate cardiac output
  3. Potential for pulmonary edema due to left-sided HF

Generate Solutions and Take Actions: Planning and Implementation
Increasing Gas Exchange
- The purpose of collaborative care is to help promote gas exchange.
- Interventions include:
  1. Monitoring for decreased gas exchange by assessing respiratory rate, rhythm, and character with breath sounds and cognitive status every 1 to 4 hours
  2. Providing supplemental oxygen to maintain Spo$_2$ at 90% or greater
  3. Placing the patient experiencing respiratory difficulty in a high Fowler's position, with pillows under each arm to maximize chest expansion and improve oxygenation
  4. Encouraging the patient to deep breathe and reposition every 2 hours while awake and in bed

Increasing Perfusion
- Collaborative care begins with nonsurgical interventions, but the patient may need surgery if these are unsuccessful in meeting optimal outcomes.

H

Nonsurgical Management
- Administer drug therapy to improve perfusion by enhancing cardiac output. Monitor for therapeutic and adverse effects.
  1. Drugs that reduce afterload (relax arterioles):
     - Angiotensin-converting enzyme inhibitors (ACEIs) or angiotensin receptor blockers (ARBs) reduce arterial constriction.
     - Because of the significant clinical experience with ACE inhibitors, this drug class is the drug of choice in the treatment of HF (Burchum & Rosenthal, 2022).
     - Monitor for the possibility of hyperkalemia, an adverse drug effect in patients who have renal dysfunction. Be aware that there is a risk of angioedema as well; while the risk is low, angioedema is a potentially lethal side effect (Burchum & Rosenthal, 2022).
     - A combination drug (angiotensin receptor neprilysin inhibitor [ARNI]), sacubitril/valsartan, has demonstrated a reduction in death and hospitalization in patients with chronic Class II to IV heart failure with a decreased ejection fraction. Valsartan is an ARB that is combined with sacubitril, which inhibits neprilysin. Together these drugs increase natriuretic peptides while suppressing the RAAS (Burchum & Rosenthal, 2022).

! NURSING SAFETY PRIORITY

Action Alert

ACEIs and ARBs are started slowly and cautiously. The first dose may be associated with a rapid drop in BP. Patients at risk for hypotension usually have an initial systolic BP of less than 100 mm Hg, are older than 75 years, have a serum sodium level of less than 135 mEq/L, or are volume depleted. Monitor BP every hour for several hours after the initial dose and each time the dose is increased. Immediately report to the health care provider and document a systolic blood pressure of less than 90 mm Hg (or designated protocol level). If this problem occurs, place the patient flat and elevate legs to increase cerebral perfusion and promote venous return.

  2. Interventions that reduce preload:
     - Ventricular fibers contract less forcefully when they are overstretched, such as in a failing heart. Interventions aimed at reducing preload attempt to decrease volume and pressure in the left ventricle, increasing ventricular muscle stretch and contraction.

- Nutritional therapy: Reduce sodium and water retention. Many patients need to omit table salt from their diet (reducing sodium intake to about 3 g daily). Weigh the patient daily, and remember that 1 kg of weight gain or loss equals 1 L of retained or lost fluid.
- Drug therapy: Diuretics are the first-line drug of choice in older adults with HF and fluid overload. These drugs enhance the renal excretion of sodium and water by reducing circulating blood volume, decreasing preload, and reducing systemic and pulmonary congestion.

PATIENT-CENTERED CARE: OLDER ADULT HEALTH
Diuretics and Dehydration

Loop diuretics continue to work even after excess fluid is removed. As a result, some patients, especially older adults, can become dehydrated. Observe for signs of dehydration in the older adult, especially acute confusion, decreased urinary output, and dizziness. Provide evidence-based interventions to reduce the risk for falls.

3. To enhance contractility, positive inotropic drugs are most commonly used, but vasodilators and beta-adrenergic blockers may also be administered. For *chronic* HF, low-dose beta blockers are most commonly used. Digoxin may be prescribed to improve symptoms, thereby decreasing dyspnea and improving functional activity.

NURSING SAFETY PRIORITY
Drug Alert

Increased cardiac automaticity occurs with toxic digoxin levels or in the presence of hypokalemia, resulting in ectopic beats (e.g., premature ventricular contractions [PVCs]). Changes in potassium level, especially a decrease, cause patients to be more sensitive to the drug and cause toxicity.

The signs and symptoms of digoxin toxicity are often vague and nonspecific and include anorexia, fatigue, blurred vision, and changes in mental status, especially in older adults. Toxicity may cause nearly any dysrhythmia, but PVCs are most commonly noted. Assess for early signs of toxicity such as bradycardia, heart block, and loss of the P wave on the ECG. Carefully monitor the apical pulse rate and heart rhythm of patients receiving digoxin.

Continued

> ### 💊 NURSING SAFETY PRIORITY—cont'd
>
> **Drug Alert**
>
> The health care provider determines the desirable heart rate (HR) to achieve. Current evidence indicates that a heart rate greater than 70 beats/min is a risk factor for increased mortality and has negative clinical effects (Prasun & Albert, 2018). Report the development of either an irregular rhythm in a patient with a previously regular rhythm or a regular rhythm in a patient with a previously irregular one. Monitor serum digoxin and potassium levels (hypokalemia potentiates digoxin toxicity) to identify toxicity. Older adults are more likely than other patients to become toxic because of decreased renal excretion.
>
> Any drug that increases the workload of the failing heart also increases its oxygen requirement. Be alert for the possibility that the patient may experience angina (chest pain) in response to digoxin.

4. Other positive inotropes used during acute exacerbation of HF include milrinone and dobutamine.

5. Beta-adrenergic blockers (commonly referred to as beta blockers) improve the condition of some patients in HF. *Beta blockers must be started slowly for HF.* Patients in acute HF should not be started on these drugs. Carvedilol, extended-release metoprolol succinate, and bisoprolol are approved for treatment of chronic HF.

6. Aldosterone antagonists (spironolactone or eplerenone) can reduce symptoms associated with HF and may be added to HF therapy in patients who remain symptomatic while taking an ACE inhibitor and a beta blocker (Burchum & Rosenthal, 2022).

7. Ivabradine is a first-in-class, hyperpolarization-activated cyclic nucleotide-gated (HCN) channel blocker, which slows the heart rate by inhibiting a specific channel in the sinus node. This medication is used for patients who are on the maximally tolerated dose of beta-blocker therapy or have a contraindication to beta-blocker therapy

8. Sodium-glucose cotranporter-2 inhibitor (SGLT2i) drugs (canagliflozin, empagliflozin) were included in the most recent heart failure guidelines due to a reduction in mortality as well as improved renal function.

- For patients with *diastolic* HF, drug therapy has not been as effective. Calcium channel blockers, ACEIs, and beta blockers have been used with various degrees of success.
- Monitor patient responses to other options to treat HF.
  1. Continuous positive airway pressure (CPAP) improves sleep apnea (oxygen desaturation) and supports cardiac output and ejection fraction.
  2. Cardiac resynchronization therapy (CRT) uses a permanent pacemaker alone or in combination with an implantable cardioverter-defibrillator to provide biventricular pacing.
  3. *CardioMems implantable monitoring system* can be inserted into the pulmonary artery and allows the patient to take a daily reading of the pulmonary artery pressure. These data are transmitted to the provider's office and allow for the management and adjustment of medications.
  4. Investigative gene therapy replaces damaged myocytes or genes by a series of injections into the left ventricle.
- Heart transplantation is the most definitive surgical option for patients with refractory end-stage HF. However, donor availability is limited, and candidacy for heart transplantation is often complicated by comorbidities that exist in the HF patient.

Preventing or Managing Pulmonary Edema

- Monitor for signs of acute pulmonary edema, a life-threatening event that can result from severe HF (with fluid overload), acute myocardial infarction (MI), mitral valve disease, and possibly dysrhythmias.

H

KEY FEATURES

Pulmonary Edema

- Crackles
- Dyspnea at rest
- Disorientation or acute confusion (especially in older adults as an early symptom)
- Tachycardia
- Hypertension or hypotension
- Reduced urinary output
- Cough with frothy, pink-tinged sputum
- Premature ventricular contractions and other dysrhythmias
- Anxiety
- Restlessness
- Lethargy

NURSING SAFETY PRIORITY

Critical Rescue

Assess for and report early symptoms such as crackles in the lung bases, dyspnea at rest, disorientation, and confusion, especially in older patients. Document the precise location of the crackles because the level of the fluid progresses from the bases to higher levels in the lungs as the condition worsens. The patient in acute pulmonary edema is typically extremely anxious, tachycardic, and struggling for air. As pulmonary edema becomes more severe, the patient may have a moist cough productive of frothy, blood-tinged sputum, and the patient's skin may be cold, clammy, or cyanotic.

+ NURSING SAFETY PRIORITY

Critical Rescue

If the patient is not hypotensive, place in a sitting (high-Fowler's) position with the legs down to decrease venous return to the heart. The *priority nursing action* is to administer oxygen therapy at 5 to 12 L/min by simple face mask or at 6 to 10 L/min by nonrebreathing mask with reservoir (which may deliver up to 100% oxygen) to promote **gas exchange** and **perfusion**. Apply a pulse oximeter and titrate the oxygen flow to keep the patient's oxygen saturation above 90%. If supplemental oxygen does not resolve the patient's respiratory distress, collaborate with the respiratory therapist, physician, advanced practice nurse, or physician associate for more aggressive therapy, such as continuous positive airway pressure (CPAP) or bilevel positive airway pressure (BiPAP) ventilation. Intubation and mechanical ventilation may be needed for some patients.

Care Coordination and Transition Management

- Collaborate with the case manager or social worker to assess the patient's needs for health care resources (e.g., home care nurse) and social support (family and friends to help with care if needed), and facilitate appropriate placement.
- Encourage the patient to stay as active as possible and develop a regular exercise program; investigate the possibility of a rehabilitation program referral.
- Instruct the patient to watch for and report to the primary health care provider:
  1. Rapid weight gain (5 lb in a week or 2 to 3 lb in 24-hour period)
  2. Decrease in exercise tolerance lasting 2 to 3 days
  3. Cold symptoms (cough) lasting more than 3 to 5 days
  4. Excessive awakening at night to urinate
  5. Development of dyspnea or angina at rest or worsening angina
  6. Increased swelling in the feet, ankles, or hands

- Provide oral and written instructions concerning drugs.
- Teach the patient and caregiver how to take and record the pulse rate and BP to help monitor response to drug and exercise regimens.
- Instruct the patient to weigh each day in the morning.
- Review the signs and symptoms of dehydration and hyper- and hypokalemia for patients taking diuretics, and provide information on foods high in potassium.
- Recommend that the patient restrict dietary sodium. Provide written instructions on low-salt diets, and identify food flavorings to use as a substitute for salt, such as lemon, garlic, and herbs.
- Discuss the importance of advance directives with the patient or family. If resuscitation is desired, the family should know how to activate the Emergency Medical System and how to provide CPR until an ambulance arrives. If CPR is not desired, the patient and family should be given resources on what to do and how to respond in the event of declining patient condition.

Evaluate Outcomes: Evaluation

- Evaluate the care of the patient with HF on the basis of the identified patient problems. The expected outcomes include that the patient will:
    1. Have adequate pulmonary tissue *perfusion*
    2. Have increased cardiac pump effectiveness
    3. Be free of pulmonary edema

H

See Chapter 29 in the main text for more information on heart failure.

HEMATOPOIETIC STEM CELL TRANSPLANTATION

- Hematopoietic stem cell transplantation (HSCT) is used to treat various kinds of leukemia.
- HSCT is used also for lymphoma, multiple myeloma, aplastic anemia, sickle cell disease, and many solid tumors.
- Transplantation has five phases: stem cell obtainment, conditioning regimen, transplantation, engraftment, and posttransplantation recovery.
    1. Obtaining stem cells: Stem cells are taken either from the patient directly (*autologous stem cells*), an HLA-identical twin (*syngeneic stem cells*), or from an HLA-matched person (*allogeneic stem cells*).
    2. The conditioning regimen "wipes out" the patient's own bone marrow in preparation for its replacement with a new immune system.

- Adverse effects from high-dose chemotherapy are common.
- Severe immunosuppression from the regimen leaves the patient vulnerable to infection.

3. The transplantation of thawed marrow, peripheral blood stem cells (PBSCs), or umbilical cord blood cells is infused through the patient's central catheter like an ordinary blood transfusion.

> ### ! NURSING SAFETY PRIORITY
> **Action Alert**
>
> Do not use blood administration tubing to infuse stems cells because the cells may be trapped in the filter, resulting in the transfer of fewer stem cells to the patient. Usually, standard, larger-bore IV administration tubing is used.

4. Engraftment, or the successful "take," of the transplanted cells in the patient's bone marrow occurs after the transfused PBSCs and marrow cells circulate briefly in the peripheral blood. The stem cells find their way to the marrow-forming sites of the patient's bones and establish residency there.
   - Monitoring of engraftment involves checking the patient's blood for "*chimerism*," which is the presence of blood cells that show a different genetic profile or marker from those of the patient. Mixed chimerism is the presence of both the patient's cells and those from the donor. Regressive chimerism with increasing percentages of the patient's cells indicates graft failure.
   - When engraftment is successful, only the donor's cells are present.

5. Posttransplant recovery can be difficult, with potential complications, which include:
   - **Infection** and poor **clotting** with bleeding are severe problems because the patient remains without bone marrow cells to provide white blood cells (WBCs) and platelets until the transfused cells grow and engraft.
   - Other complications of HSCT include failure to engraft, development of graft-versus-host disease (GVHD), and sinusoidal obstructive syndrome (SOS).

See Chapter 34 in the main text for more information on hematopoietic stem cell transplantation.

HEMORRHOIDS

- Hemorrhoids are unnaturally swollen or distended veins in the anorectal region. The condition is common and not significant unless the hemorrhoids cause prolonged **pain** or bleeding.
- Internal hemorrhoids cannot be seen on inspection of the perianal area and lie above the anal sphincter.
- External hemorrhoids can be seen on inspection and lie below the anal sphincter.
- Prolapsed hemorrhoids can become thrombosed or inflamed, or they can bleed.
- Common causes are increased abdominal pressure associated with pregnancy, constipation with straining, obesity, HF, prolonged sitting or standing, strenuous exercise, and weight lifting.

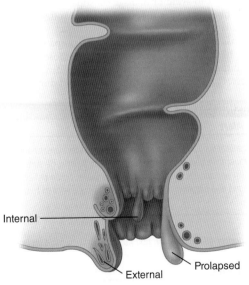

Internal, external, and prolapsed hemorrhoids. *Internal hemorrhoids* lie above the anal sphincter and cannot be seen on inspection of the anal area. *External hemorrhoids* lie below the anal sphincter and can be seen on inspection of the anal region. Hemorrhoids that enlarge, fall down, and protrude through the anus are called *prolapsed hemorrhoids.*

Interprofessional Collaborative Care

- The most common symptoms of hemorrhoids are bleeding, swelling, and prolapse (bulging).
  1. Blood is characteristically bright red and is present on toilet tissue or streaked in the stool.
  2. *Pain* is a common symptom and is often associated with thrombosis, especially if thrombosis occurs suddenly.
  3. Other symptoms include itching and a mucous discharge.
- Diagnosis is usually made by inspection and digital examination.
- Interventions are typically conservative and are aimed at reducing symptoms with minimal discomfort, cost, and time lost from usual activities.
  1. Cold packs applied to the anorectal region for a few minutes at a time beginning with the onset of pain and tepid sitz baths three or four times a day are often enough to relieve discomfort, even if the hemorrhoids are thrombosed.
  2. Topical anesthetics, such as lidocaine, are useful for severe pain.
  3. Treatment to avoid or manage constipation includes fluids, a high-fiber diet, fiber supplements, stool softeners, and bowel stimulants.
  4. Ultrasound, laser removal, or other outpatient procedures may be indicated for prolapsed or thrombosed hemorrhoids. Monitor for bleeding and pain postoperatively. Warm compresses or a sitz bath can promote comfort during recovery.

> **! NURSING SAFETY PRIORITY**
> *Action Alert*
>
> Tell the patient who has had surgical intervention for hemorrhoids that the first postoperative bowel movement may be very painful. Be sure that someone is with or near the patient when this happens. Some patients become light-headed and diaphoretic and may have syncope related to a vasovagal response.

 See Chapter 48 in the main text for more information on hemorrhoids.

HEMOTHORAX

- Hemothorax is blood loss into the chest cavity and is a common result of blunt chest trauma or penetrating injuries. It can be combined with a pneumothorax.
  1. A simple hemothorax is a blood loss of less than 1000 mL.
  2. A massive hemothorax is a blood loss of more than 1000 mL.
- Bleeding can occur with rib and sternal fractures, causing lung contusions and lacerations in addition to the hemothorax.

Interprofessional Collaborative Care
Recognize Cues: Assessment
- Physical assessment findings depend on the size of the hemothorax and include:
  1. Respiratory distress
  2. Reduced breath sounds
  3. Blood in the pleural space (seen on a chest x-ray and confirmed by diagnostic thoracentesis)

Take Actions: Interventions
- Interventions for hemothorax include chest tube placement to remove the blood in the pleural space to normalize breathing and prevent infection.
- A hemothorax may require an open thoracotomy to repair torn vessels and to evacuate the chest cavity.
- Nursing interventions include:
  1. Monitoring vital signs and reporting when signs of hypoperfusion or hypotension occur
  2. Carefully monitoring chest tube drainage for blood loss
  3. Measuring intake and output and replacing output with IV fluids or blood products as ordered

See Chapter 26 in the main text for more information on hemothorax.

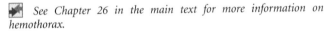

✳ HEPATITIS: INFECTION CONCEPT EXEMPLAR

H

Overview
- Hepatitis is the widespread *inflammation* and *infection* of liver cells. *Viral* hepatitis, which can be acute or chronic, is the most common type.
- The five major types of acute viral hepatitis vary by etiology, mode of transmission, manner of onset, and incubation periods. Hepatitis cases must be reported to the local public health department, which then notifies the Centers for Disease Control and Prevention (CDC).
  1. Hepatitis A virus (HAV)
     - HAV is spread by the fecal-oral route, by consuming contaminated food, or by person-to-person contact (e.g., oral-anal sexual activity). Unsanitary water, shellfish caught in contaminated water, and food contaminated by food handlers infected with HAV are all potential sources of infection.

- Characterized by a mild course and often goes unrecognized. HAV is the most common type of viral hepatitis.
- The incubation period is usually 15 to 50 days.

2. Hepatitis B virus (HBV)
   - HBV is transmitted through broken skin or mucous membranes by infected blood and body fluids.
   - HBV is spread by:
     - Unprotected sexual intercourse with an infected partner
     - Sharing needles, syringes, or other drug-injection equipment
     - Sharing razors or toothbrushes with an infected individual
     - Accidental needlesticks or injuries from sharp instruments, primarily in health care workers (low incidence)
     - Blood transfusions (that have not been screened for the virus, before 1992)
     - Hemodialysis
     - Direct contact with the blood or open sores of an infected individual
     - Birth (spread from an infected mother to baby during birth)
   - The clinical course is varied, with an insidious onset and mild symptoms
   - The incubation period is generally between 25 and 180 days, and blood tests confirm the disease.

3. Hepatitis C virus (HCV)
   - HCV is spread by contaminated items, such as illicit IV drug needles, blood and blood products, and transplanted organs received before 1992; needlestick injury with HCV-contaminated blood; or sharing of drug paraphernalia.
   - It is not transmitted by casual contact or intimate household contacts. However, those infected should not share razors, toothbrushes, or pierced earrings because there may be microscopic blood on these items.
   - The incubation period ranges from 2 weeks to 6 months, and it can lead to cirrhosis.

4. Hepatitis D virus (HDV)
   - Incubation period is 14 to 56 days.
   - HDV is transmitted primarily by parenteral routes.

5. Hepatitis E virus (HEV)
   - HEV is caused by fecal contamination of food or water.
   - The incubation period is 15 to 64 days.

Interprofessional Collaborative Care

- Prevention of hepatitis includes administration of hepatitis A and B vaccination.
- Care of the patient with hepatitis includes preventing immunity-related complications.

Recognize Cues: Assessment

- Record patient information:
  1. Known exposure to persons with hepatitis infection or a contaminated water source
  2. For the patient who presents with few or no symptoms of liver disease but has abnormal laboratory tests (e.g., elevated alanine aminotransferase [ALT] or aspartate aminotransferase [AST] level), the history may need to include additional questions regarding risk factors.
- Assess for key features of viral hepatitis. Remember, HCV may be asymptomatic.

 KEY FEATURES

Viral Hepatitis

- Abdominal pain
- Yellowish sclera (**icterus**)
- Arthralgia (joint pain) or myalgia (muscle pain)
- Diarrhea/constipation
- Light clay-colored stools
- Dark yellow to brownish urine
- **Jaundice**
- Fever
- Fatigue
- Malaise
- Anorexia
- Nausea and vomiting
- Dry skin
- Pruritus (itching)

- Patients may be angry about being sick and being fatigued; may feel guilty about having exposed others to the disease; may be embarrassed by the isolation and hygiene precautions that are necessary; and may be worried about the loss of wages, cost of hospitalization, and general financial issues.
- Family members may be afraid of contracting the disease and therefore distance themselves from the patient.
- Liver biopsy may be used to confirm the diagnosis of hepatitis and to establish the stage and grade of liver damage.

Analyze Cues and Prioritize Hypotheses: Analysis

- The priority collaborative problems for patients with hepatitis include:
  1. Weight loss due to complications associated with *inflammation* of the liver
  2. Fatigue due to *infection* and decreased metabolic energy production

Generate Solutions and Take Actions: Planning and Implementation

- The patient with viral hepatitis can be mildly or acutely ill, depending on the severity of the inflammation. Most patients are not hospitalized, although older adults and those with dehydration may be admitted for a short-term stay. The plan of care for all patients with viral hepatitis is based on measures to rest the liver, promote hepatic regeneration, strengthen *immunity*, and prevent complications, if possible.

Promoting Nutrition

- The patient with hepatitis may decline food due to general malaise, anorexia, abdominal discomfort, or nausea.
  1. Determine food preferences that are high in calories and carbohydrates.
  2. Provide small, frequent meals and high-calorie snacks as needed.

Managing Fatigue

- Maintain physical rest alternating with periods of activity to promote liver cell regeneration by reducing the liver's metabolic needs.
- Individualize the patient's plan of care, and adjust it to reflect the severity of symptoms, fatigue, and the results of liver function tests and enzyme determinations.
- Drugs of any kind are used sparingly for patients with hepatitis to allow the liver to rest. An antiemetic to relieve nausea may be prescribed. However, due to the life-threatening nature of chronic hepatitis B and hepatitis C, a number of drugs are given, including antiviral and immunomodulating drugs.

Care Coordination and Transition Management

- A primary focus in any case is to prevent the spread of the infection. For hepatitis transmitted by the fecal-oral route, careful handwashing and sanitary disposal of feces are important.
- Provide health teaching.

> **! NURSING SAFETY PRIORITY**
>
> *Action Alert*
>
> Teach the patient with viral hepatitis and the family to use measures to prevent infection transmission. In addition, instruct the patient to avoid alcohol and to check with the primary health care provider before taking any medication or vitamin, supplement, or herbal preparation. Encourage the patient to increase activity gradually to prevent fatigue. Suggest that the patient eat small, frequent meals of high-carbohydrate foods and plan frequent rest periods.
>
> Collaborate with the certified infection control practitioner and infectious disease specialist if needed in caring for these patients. These experts can suggest appropriate resources for the patient and family.

Evaluate Outcomes: Evaluation

- Evaluate the care of the patient with hepatitis based on the identified priority patient problems. The expected outcomes include that the patient will:
    1. Maintain nutritional status adequate for body requirements
    2. Report increasing energy levels as the liver rests

 See Chapter 50 in the main text for more information on hepatitis.

HERNIATION

- A hernia is a weakness in the abdominal muscle wall through which a segment of bowel or other abdominal structure protrudes. Hernias can also penetrate through any other defect in the abdominal wall, through the diaphragm, or through other structures in the abdominal cavity.
- Congenital or acquired muscle weakness and increased intraabdominal pressure contribute to hernia formation.
- Hernias are labeled by anatomic location, combined with the severity of protrusion.
    1. An *indirect inguinal hernia* is a sac formed from the peritoneum that contains a portion of the intestine or omentum; in males, indirect hernias can become large and descend into the scrotum.
    2. A *direct inguinal hernia* passes through a weak point in the abdominal wall.
    3. A *femoral hernia* occurs through the femoral ring as a plug of fat in the femoral canal that enlarges and pulls the peritoneum and the bladder into the sac.

4. An *umbilical hernia* is congenital or acquired as a result of increased intra-abdominal pressure, most often in people who are obese.
5. An *incisional (ventral) hernia* occurs at the site of a previous surgical incision as a result of inadequate healing, postoperative wound infection, inadequate nutrition, or obesity.

- Hernias may also be classified as reducible, irreducible (incarcerated), or strangulated.
  1. A *reducible hernia* allows the contents of the hernia sac to be reduced or placed back into the abdominal cavity.
  2. An *irreducible,* or *incarcerated, hernia* cannot be reduced or placed back into the abdominal cavity. It requires immediate surgical evaluation.
  3. A *strangulated hernia* results when the blood supply to the herniated segment of the bowel is cut off by pressure from the hernia ring, causing ischemia and obstruction of the bowel loop; this can lead to bowel necrosis and perforation, which are surgical emergencies.

Interprofessional Collaborative Care
Recognize Cues: Assessment

- Assess for a hernia when the patient is lying down and again when the patient is standing. If a hernia is reducible, it may disappear when the patient is lying flat.
- Listen for bowel sounds (absence may indicate gastrointestinal [GI] obstruction or strangulation, which is considered a medical emergency).

Take Actions: Interventions

- A truss (a pad with firm support) may be used for patients who are poor surgical risks.
- Herniorrhaphy, the surgical treatment of choice, involves replacing the contents of the hernia sac into the abdominal cavity and closing the opening.
- Hernioplasty reinforces the weakened muscular wall with a mesh patch.
- Provide preoperative and postoperative care, and instruct the patient to:
  1. Avoid coughing but encourage deep breathing
  2. For inguinal hernia repair, wear a scrotal support and elevate the scrotum with a soft pillow when in bed
  3. Avoid bladder and bowel distention by:
     - Using techniques to stimulate voiding, such as assisting a male to stand

- Avoiding constipation and avoiding straining with stool during healing
- Teach the patient:
  1. How to care for the incision if surgery corrects the muscle defect
  2. To limit activity, including avoiding lifting and straining, for several weeks after surgery
  3. To report to the health care provider symptoms such as fever and chills, wound drainage, redness/hyperpigmentation or separation of the incision, or increasing incisional pain

 See Chapter 48 in the main text for more information on herniation.

HERNIA, HIATAL

- Hiatal hernias, also called *diaphragmatic hernias*, involve the protrusion of the stomach through the esophageal hiatus (opening) of the diaphragm into the chest.
- Hiatal hernias are classified as type I (*sliding* hernias, which are most common) or types II through IV (paraesophageal, or *rolling,* hernias).
  1. Type I: *Sliding hernias, which are most common,* occur when the esophagogastric junction and a portion of the fundus of the stomach slide upward through the esophageal hiatus into the chest, usually as a result of weakening of the diaphragm.
  2. Types II through IV: *Paraesophageal,* or *rolling, hernias* are characterized as follows:
     - Type II: The gastroesophageal junction remains in its normal intra-abdominal location, but the fundus (and possibly portions of the stomach's greater curvature) rolls through the esophageal hiatus and into the chest beside the esophagus.
     - Type III: The gastroesophageal junction and the fundus both herniate through the hiatus, with the fundus lying above the gastroesophageal junction.
     - Type IV: The colon, spleen, pancreas, or small intestine (instead of the stomach) is found in the hernia sac.

Interprofessional Collaborative Care
Recognize Cues: Assessment
- Assess for key features of hiatal hernias. Many patients are asymptomatic.

H

KEY FEATURES

Hiatal Hernias

Sliding Hiatal Hernias	Paraesophageal Hernias
• Heartburn	• Feeling of fullness (after eating)
• Regurgitation	• Breathlessness (after eating)
• Chest pain	• Feeling of suffocation (after eating)
• Dysphagia	• Chest pain that mimics angina
• Belching	• Worsening of symptoms in a recumbent position

Take Actions: Interventions

Nonsurgical Management

- Drug therapy includes the use of a proton pump inhibitor to control esophageal reflux and its symptoms.
- Diet therapy includes avoiding fatty foods, caffeine, carbonation, chocolate, alcohol, spicy foods, and acidic foods such as orange juice.
- Encourage the patient to eat small-volume meals and to consume liquids between meals to avoid abdominal distention.
- Lifestyle therapy includes attaining or sustaining ideal body weight because obesity increases intra-abdominal pressure.

! NURSING SAFETY PRIORITY

Action Alert

When caring for a patient with hiatal hernia, education is one of the most important parts of nursing care. Follow health teaching as described for patients with GERD.

Surgical Management

- Elective surgery is indicated when the risk of complications such as aspiration is high or damage from chronic reflux is severe.
- Surgical approaches for sliding hernias involve reinforcement of the lower esophageal sphincter (LES) to prevent reflux through fundoplication, or the wrapping of a portion of the stomach fundus around the distal esophagus to anchor it and reinforce the LES.
- Provide preoperative and postoperative care.
  1. Provide safe and effective care for the patient with a chest tube if a transthoracic approach was used.

2. Assess for complications of surgery, such as temporary dysphagia, gas bloat syndrome, atelectasis or pneumonia, and obstruction of the NG tube.

>> **BEST PRACTICE FOR PATIENT SAFETY AND QUALITY CARE**

Assessment of Postoperative Complications Related to Fundoplication Procedures

Complication	Assessment Findings
Temporary dysphagia	Difficulty swallowing when oral feeding begins
Gas bloat syndrome	Difficulty belching to relieve distention
Atelectasis, pneumonia	Dyspnea, chest pain, or fever
Obstructed nasogastric tube	Nausea, vomiting, or abdominal distention, and/or a nondraining nasogastric tube

3. Prevent aspiration and respiratory complications with positioning, early ambulation, and the use of incentive spirometry and deep breathing while providing adequate pain relief.
4. Elevate the head of the bed at least 30 degrees.
5. Teach the patient to support the incisional area during coughing and deep breathing.
6. Ensure correct placement and patency of the NG tube.
7. Reinforce dietary restrictions and nutritional goals.

Care Coordination and Transition Management

- Advise the patient:
  1. To avoid lifting and restrict stair climbing for 3 to 6 weeks after open surgical repair. For those who had laparoscopic surgery, activity is typically restricted for a shorter time, usually about a week
  2. To inspect the surgical wound daily and report the incidence of swelling, redness/hyperpigmentation, tenderness, or discharge to the physician
  3. About the importance of reporting fever or other signs of infection to the surgeon
  4. To avoid people with respiratory infection, because prolonged coughing can cause the incision to break open (dehisce)
  5. About diet modifications, including weight goals, eating small portions, avoiding irritating foods and liquids, and reporting recurrence of reflux symptoms to the physician
  6. To avoid straining and prevent constipation; stool softeners or bulk laxatives may be needed

 See Chapter 46 in the main text for more information on hiatal hernia.

HERPES, GENITAL

- Genital herpes (GH) is a common acute, recurring viral disease. Although preventative and therapeutic vaccines are still under investigation, at this time GH is still considered incurable (American Sexual Health Association, 2022).
- The two types of herpes simplex virus (HSV) are diagnosed and treated with the same interventions.
  1. Type 1 (HSV-1) causes most nongenital lesions, such as cold sores. It can also produce genital lesions through oral-genital or genital-genital contact with an infected person.
  2. Type 2 (HSV-2) causes most of the genital lesions.
- The incubation period is 2 to 20 days, with the average period being 1 week; many people do not have symptoms during this time.
- The virus can become dormant and recur periodically, even if the patient is asymptomatic. Recurrences are not caused by reinfection; they are related to *viral shedding, and the patient is infectious.*
- Long-term complications of GH include the risk of neonatal transmission and an increased risk for acquiring HIV infection.

Interprofessional Collaborative Care
Recognize Cues: Assessment

Assessing the Patient With a Sexually Transmitted Infection

Assess History of Present Illness
- Chief concern
- Time of onset
- Symptoms by quality and quantity, precipitating and palliative factors
- Any treatments taken (self-prescribed or over-the-counter products), and whether they have been helpful

Assess Past Medical History
- Major health problems, including any history of STIs, PID, or immuno-suppression
- Surgeries: obstetric and gynecologic; circumcision

Assess Current Health Status
- Menstrual history for irregularities
- Sexual history:
  - Type and frequency of sexual activity
  - Number of sexual contacts/partners, lifetime and past 6 months; or monogamous
  - Sexual orientation
  - Contraception history

Assessing the Patient With a Sexually Transmitted Infection—cont'd

- Medications
- Allergies
- Lifestyle risks: drugs, alcohol, tobacco

Assess Preventive Health Care Practices
- Papanicolaou (Pap) tests
- Regular STI screening
- Use of barrier contraceptives to prevent STIs and/or pregnancy

Assess Physical Examination Findings
- Vital signs
- Oropharyngeal findings
- Abdominal findings
- Genital or pelvic findings
- Anorectal findings

Assess Laboratory Data
- Urinalysis
- Hematology
- ESR or CRP if PID is being considered
- Cervical, urethral, oral, rectal specimens
- Lesion samples for microbiology and virology
- Pregnancy testing

CRP, C-reactive protein; *ESR*, erythrocyte sedimentation rate; *PID*, pelvic inflammatory disease; *STI*, sexually transmitted infection

H

- Obtain patient information about:
  1. The sensation of itching or tingling felt in the skin 1 to 2 days before the outbreak
- Assess for and document:
  1. The presence of *vesicles* (blisters) or painful erosions in a typical cluster on the penis, scrotum, vulva, vagina, cervix, or perianal region
  2. Swelling of inguinal lymph nodes or other symptoms of infection such as headache, malaise, or fever
- GH is usually confirmed through a viral culture or polymerase chain reaction (PCR) assays of the lesions (Albrecht, 2022).

Take Actions: Interventions
- GH is treated with oral antiviral medications such as acyclovir, famciclovir, or valacyclovir.

- The drugs decrease the severity, promote healing, and decrease the frequency of recurrent outbreaks, but do not cure the **infection**.
- Emphasize the risk for neonatal infection to all patients, both male and female.
- Teach patients to avoid transmission by:
  1. Adhering to suppressive therapy
  2. Abstaining from sexual activity while lesions are present
  3. Using latex or polyurethane condoms during all sexual exposures

---

! NURSING SAFETY PRIORITY

Action Alert

Remind patients to abstain from sexual activity while GH lesions are present. Sexual activity can cause **pain,** and the likelihood of viral transmission is higher. Urge condom use during all sexual encounters because of the increased risk for HSV transmission from viral shedding, which can occur even when lesions are not present. Teach the patient about how to properly use condoms.

---

  4. Keeping the skin in the genital region clean and dry
  5. Washing hands thoroughly after contact with lesions and laundering towels that have had direct contact with lesions
  6. Wearing gloves when applying ointments or making direct contact with lesions
- Help patients and their partners cope with the diagnosis by assessing the patient's and partner's emotional responses to the diagnosis of GH.

See Chapter 65 in the main text for more information on herpes, genital.

HUMAN IMMUNODEFICIENCY VIRUS (HIV): IMMUNITY ✳ CONCEPT EXEMPLAR

Overview

- The human immunodeficiency virus (HIV) causes **infection** and disease that can progress along a continuum known as *HIV disease*.
- The continuum of HIV disease has three identified stages.
  1. Stage HIV-I begins with the onset of acute infection responses after an initial invasion by the virus causes overt symptoms.
  2. Stage II: Chronic HIV infection
  3. Stage III: AIDS (acquired immunodeficiency syndrome).
- A diagnosis of AIDS (HIV-III) requires that the adult be HIV positive and have either a CD4+ T-cell count of less than 200 cells/mm^3 or an opportunistic infection.

- Everyone who has Stage III has an HIV infection; however, not everyone who has an HIV infection has progressed to Stage III.

PATIENT-CENTERED CARE: GENDER HEALTH

HIV Transmission in Women

HIV is easily transmitted from an infected male to an uninfected female when infected body fluids come into contact with mucous membranes or nonintact skin. A vagina has more mucous membrane surface area compared to a penile urethra. Teach all people the importance of always using a condom when engaging in any type of sexual activity.

Interprofessional Collaborative Care
Recognize Cues: Assessment

- The adult who has HIV disease at stages HIV-II or HIV-III is monitored on a regular basis for changes in *immunity* or health status that indicate disease progression and the need for intervention. The frequency of monitoring varies from every 2 to 6 months based on disease progression and responses to treatment. Continuing assessment is crucial to ensure that the drugs continue to work optimally, because the patient may have medication issues or problems related to disease in many organ systems. Assess for subtle changes so that any problems can be found early and treated.
  1. Determine the risk for HIV by asking focused questions about sexual history and drug-injecting activities.
  2. Remain objective, nonjudgmental, and supportive while talking with the patient, focusing on five P's: **P**artners, **P**ractices, **P**rotection (from STIs), **P**ast history, and **P**revention of pregnancy (Sexuality Information and Education Council of the United States, 2018).
  3. Ask the patient about when the HIV infection was diagnosed and what symptoms led to that diagnosis.

Laboratory Assessment

- Patients in Stage III are often leukopenic, with a WBC count of less than 4000 cells/mm^3 (4×10^9/L), and lymphopenic (<1500 lymphocytes/mm^3 [<1.5×10^9/L]) (Pagana et al., 2022).
- HIV serologic and virologic tests detect infection. Prior to any testing, it is important to let patients know that there is a 3-week "seroconversion window" following HIV exposure in which a test may produce a false-negative result.
- Viral load testing directly measures the actual amount of HIV viral RNA particles present in 1 mL of blood. An uninfected adult has no viral load for HIV. The higher the viral load, the greater the risk for transmission.

H

Analyze Cues and Prioritize Hypotheses: Analysis

- The priority problems for patients with HIV infection are:
  1. Potential to transmit infection due to lack of health education and/or risky behaviors (Stages I, II, and III)
  2. Potential for infection and life-threatening complications due to reduced immunity associated with HIV infection (Stages II and III)

Generate Solutions and Take Actions: Planning and Implementation

Preventing Transmission of Infection

- Instruct about modes of transmission and preventive behaviors (e.g., guidelines for safer sex; not sharing toothbrushes, razors, and other potentially blood-contaminated articles).
- Discuss treatment as prevention (TasP) and determine adherence.

Preventing Infections and Life-Threatening Complications

- The patient in any stage of HIV disease is susceptible to infection. Initial management focuses on supporting the patient's *immunity* by controlling the HIV infection with antiretroviral therapy, reducing the viral load, and preventing infection.
  1. Identification of infection early reduces the risk for development of sepsis.
  2. Patients with leukopenia may not demonstrate traditional signs and symptoms of infection.
  3. Use best practices to prevent infection in the care of the patient with HIV who is hospitalized.

> ### ⫸ BEST PRACTICE FOR PATIENT SAFETY AND QUALITY CARE
>
> *Care of the Patient With Reduced Immunity Who Is Hospitalized*
>
> **Room**
> - Place the patient in a private room whenever possible.
> - Limit the number of personnel entering the patient's room.
> - Use evidence-based handwashing techniques or alcohol-based hand rubs before touching the patient or any of the patient's belongings. Perform hand hygiene again upon exiting the room.
> - Limit visitors to healthy adults.
> - Ensure that the patient's room and bathroom are cleaned at least once a day.
>
> **Equipment and Supplies**
> - Keep frequently used equipment in the room for use with this patient only (e.g., blood pressure cuff, stethoscope, thermometer).
> - Do not use supplies from common areas.

BEST PRACTICE FOR PATIENT SAFETY AND QUALITY CARE—cont'd

Care of the Patient With Reduced Immunity Who Is Hospitalized

- Keep a dedicated box of disposable gloves in the patient's room, and do not share this box with other patients.
- Use individually wrapped supplies (e.g., gauze).
- Provide single-use food products when possible.

Assessment and Care
- Monitor vital signs, including temperature, every 4 hours or more as needed.
- Inspect the mouth, skin, and mucous membranes (including the anal area) for fissures and abscesses at least once per shift.
- Inspect open areas such as IV sites every 4 hours for signs of infection.
- Change gauze-containing wound dressings daily.
- Obtain specimens of all suspicious areas for culture (as specified by the agency), and promptly notify the primary health care provider.
- Demonstrate and encourage coughing and deep-breathing exercises.
- Use strict aseptic technique for all invasive procedures.

- Approved antiretroviral drugs have excellent activity against HIV replication. These drugs do not cure or kill the virus; they only control replication.
  1. Treatment may involve multiple drugs from different classes used together in combinations, known as combination antiretroviral therapy (cART). This approach helps reduce viral load, improve CD4+ T-cell counts, and slow disease progression.
  2. Patients must take drug therapy exactly as prescribed to realize the most benefits.

NURSING SAFETY PRIORITY

Drug Alert

Teach patients the importance of taking the cART drugs as prescribed to maintain the highest medication benefits. It is important that patients attempt to avoid missing or delaying doses, and to resume and continue their prescribed therapy as soon as they discover a missed dose. Ongoing missed doses can promote drug resistance.

  3. Drug therapy to address gas exchange complications is started immediately when an infection that affects the respiratory system is identified. For patients in Stage III, prophylaxis against *Pneumocystis jiroveci* pneumonia (PCP) is often used.

4. Drugs for pain management may be required related to peripheral neuropathy or from advanced disease progression in Stage III.
5. Nutritional support may be required, especially for patients in Stage III who can develop HIV-associated wasting syndrome (unintentional weight loss and decreased endurance).
6. Drugs for persistent diarrhea may be required for patients in Stage III due to opportunistic infections. Assess the perineum regularly, and keep this area clean and dry.

Care Coordination and Transition Management

- The management of HIV disease as a chronic progressive disease occurs in many settings, most often at home.
- Hospitalizations occur during periods of severe *infection* or other acute exacerbations of symptoms.
- As the illness becomes more severe, the patient may need referral to a long-term care facility, home care agency, or hospice.
- In collaboration with the social worker, dietitian, and others, work with patients to plan what will be needed and how they will manage at home with self-care and ADLs.
- Teach the patient, family, and significant others about:
  1. Modes of HIV transmission and preventive behaviors
  2. Guidelines for safer sex; urge all patients who are HIV positive to use condoms and other precautions during sexual intimacy, even if the partner is also HIV positive
  3. Not sharing toothbrushes, razors, and other potentially blood-contaminated articles
  4. Signs of infection and when to seek medical help
  5. Teach patients with protein-calorie malnutrition what foods to include in the diet to promote better *nutrition*.
  6. Protection against infection transmission by:
     - Avoiding crowds and other large gatherings of people where someone may be ill
     - Not sharing personal toilet articles, such as toothbrushes or razors, with others
     - Washing hands thoroughly with an antimicrobial soap before eating or drinking, after touching a pet, after shaking hands with anyone, returning home from any outing, and after using the toilet
     - Washing dishes between uses with hot sudsy water or using a dishwasher
     - Not changing pet litter boxes; if unavoidable, using gloves and washing hands immediately
     - Avoiding turtles and reptiles as pets

7. Support psychosocial integrity.
   - Urge all patients who are HIV positive to inform their sexual partners of their HIV status.
   - Respect the patient's right to inform or not to inform family members about personal HIV status.
   - Ensure the confidentiality of the patient's HIV status.
   - Use a nonjudgmental approach when discussing sexual practices, sexual behaviors, and recreational drug use.

Evaluate Outcomes: Evaluation
- The overall outcomes for care of patients living with HIV (PLWH) are to maintain the highest possible level of function for as long as possible during the course of this chronic condition. Evaluate the care of the patient with HIV-III (AIDS) on the basis of the identified priority problems. Expected outcomes include that they will be adherent to the prescribed drug therapy, use safe sexual practices, and maintain a self-perceived high quality of life by:
  1. Refraining from spreading the HIV virus to others
  2. Avoiding acute infections
  3. Avoiding development of opportunistic infections

 See Chapter 17 in the main text for more information on HIV and AIDS.

HYDROCELE

H

- A hydrocele is a swelling in the scrotum where fluid has collected on or around both testicles.

Interprofessional Collaborative Care
- Treatment is usually not needed unless the condition becomes painful or too large for comfort; at that time, surgery may be recommended.
- If pain does occur, acetaminophen or ibuprofen can be taken.
- Report any changes involving pain, fever, redness/hyperpigmentation, or swelling.

 See Chapter 64 in the main text for more information on hydrocele.

HYDRONEPHROSIS AND HYDROURETER

- Hydronephrosis and hydroureter are problems of urinary *elimination* with outflow obstruction. Urethral strictures obstruct urine outflow and may contribute to bladder distention, hydroureter, and hydronephrosis. Prompt recognition and treatment are crucial to prevent permanent kidney damage.

- In hydronephrosis, the kidney becomes enlarged as urine accumulates in the renal pelvis and the calyces. Obstruction within the pelvis or ureteropelvic junction results in renal pelvic distention, and extensive damage to the vasculature and renal tubules can result.
- Hydroureter is the obstruction of the ureter and obstruction of urine outflow to the bladder.
- Urinary obstruction causes damage when pressure builds up directly on kidney tissue.
- Common causes of urinary obstruction include kidney stones, tumors, fibrosis, structural abnormalities, trauma, abscess, or cysts.

Interprofessional Collaborative Care
Recognize Cues: Assessment
- Record history of kidney or urologic disorders, including pelvic radiation or surgery.
- Document pattern of urination, including amount and frequency.
- Assess urine, including color, clarity, and odor.
- Assess symptoms, including flank or abdominal pain, chills, fever, and malaise.

Take Actions: Interventions
- Urinary retention and potential for infection are the primary problems. Failure to treat the cause of obstruction leads to infection and acute kidney injury (AKI).
    1. If obstruction is caused by a kidney stone (calculus), it can be located and removed using cystoscopic or retrograde urogram procedures.
    2. When an abnormal narrowing of the urinary tract (**stricture**) causes hydronephrosis and cannot be corrected with urologic procedures, a **nephrostomy** is performed.

✚ NURSING SAFETY PRIORITY
Critical Rescue

After nephrostomy, monitor the patient for indications of complications (i.e., decreased or absent drainage, cloudy or foul-smelling drainage, leakage of blood or urine from the nephrostomy site, back pain) (Martin & Baker, 2019). If any indications are present, respond by notifying the surgeon immediately.

See Chapter 59 in the main text for more information on hydronephrosis and hydroureter.

HYPERALDOSTERONISM

- Hyperaldosteronism is increased secretion of aldosterone (mineralocorticoid excess) by the adrenal glands.
- Primary hyperaldosteronism (Conn syndrome) results from excessive secretion of aldosterone from one or both adrenal glands and is most often caused by a benign adrenal tumor (adrenal adenoma).
- Secondary hyperaldosteronism is caused by high levels of angiotensin II that are stimulated by high plasma renin levels. Kidney hypoxemia, diabetic nephropathy, and excessive use of some diuretics can result in secondary hyperaldosteronism.
- Regardless of the cause, hyperaldosteronism is manifested by hypernatremia, hypokalemia, metabolic alkalosis, hypervolemia, and hypertension.

Interprofessional Collaborative Care

- Surgery is a common treatment for hyperaldosteronism, and one or both adrenal glands may be removed.
  1. The patient's potassium level must be corrected before surgery. Drugs used to increase potassium levels include spironolactone, a potassium-sparing diuretic and aldosterone antagonist.
  2. The patient who has undergone a unilateral adrenalectomy may need temporary glucocorticoid replacement, and replacement is lifelong when both adrenal glands are removed. Glucocorticoids are given before surgery to prevent adrenal crisis.
  3. When surgery cannot be performed, spironolactone therapy is continued to control hypokalemia and hypertension. Because spironolactone is a potassium-sparing diuretic, hyperkalemia can occur in patients who have impaired kidney function or excessive potassium intake. Teach the patient the following:
     - Avoid potassium supplements and food rich in potassium.
     - An increase in dietary sodium may be required.
     - Report symptoms of hyponatremia (muscle weakness, dizziness, lethargy, or drowsiness).
     - Report side effects of spironolactone therapy, including gynecomastia, diarrhea, headache, rash, urticaria, confusion, erectile dysfunction, hirsutism, and amenorrhea.

H

See Chapter 54 in the main text for more information on hyperaldosteronism.

HYPERCALCEMIA

- Hypercalcemia is a total serum calcium level above 10.5 mg/dL or 2.62 mmol/L.
- Because the normal range for serum calcium is so narrow, even small increases have severe effects, and all systems are affected.

Common Causes of Hypercalcemia

Actual Calcium Excesses
- Excessive oral intake of calcium
- Excessive oral intake of vitamin D
- Kidney failure
- Use of thiazide diuretics

Relative Calcium Excesses
- Hyperparathyroidism
- Malignancy
- Hyperthyroidism
- Immobility
- Use of glucocorticoids
- Dehydration

Interprofessional Collaborative Care
Recognize Cues: Assessment

- Assess for and document:
  1. Cardiovascular changes, which are the most serious and life-threatening
     - Increased heart rate and BP (early)
     - Slow heart rate (late or severe)
     - Cyanosis and pallor/ash gray skin from impaired blood flow and hypercoagulation
  2. Neuromuscular changes, which include:
     - Severe muscle weakness
     - Decreased deep tendon reflexes without paresthesia
     - Altered level of consciousness (confusion, lethargy, coma)
  3. Intestinal changes, which include:
     - Constipation, anorexia, nausea, vomiting, and abdominal pain
     - Hypoactive or absent bowel sounds
     - Increased abdominal size

Take Actions: Interventions

- Restore calcium balance and prevent additional increases in calcium by:
  1. Discontinuing IV solutions containing calcium (lactated Ringer's solution)
  2. Discontinuing oral drugs containing calcium or vitamin D (e.g., calcium-based antacids, OTC vitamin supplements)
  3. Discontinuing thiazide diuretics that increase kidney calcium resorption

4. Administering drug therapy to reduce circulating calcium and monitoring its effect on serum calcium levels:
   - IV normal saline (0.9% sodium chloride) to dilute serum levels and promote elimination
   - Diuretics that enhance calcium excretion, such as furosemide
   - Drugs that inhibit calcium resorption from bone such as calcitonin and bisphosphonates
5. *Cardiac monitoring* of patients with hypercalcemia is needed to identify dysrhythmias and decreased cardiac output.

See Chapter 13 in the main text for more information on hypercalcemia.

HYPERKALEMIA

- Hyperkalemia is a serum potassium level greater than 5 mEq/L (5 mmol/L). Even small increases above normal values can affect excitable tissues, especially the heart.

Common Causes of Hyperkalemia	
Actual Potassium Excesses	**Relative Potassium Excesses**

• Overingestion of potassium-containing foods or medications:
  • Salt substitutes
  • Potassium chloride
• Rapid infusion of potassium-containing IV solution
• Bolus IV potassium injections
• Transfusions of whole blood or packed cells
• Adrenal insufficiency
• Kidney failure
• Potassium-sparing diuretics
• Angiotensin-converting enzyme inhibitors (ACEIs)
	• Tissue damage
	• Acidosis
	• Hyperuricemia
	• Uncontrolled diabetes mellitus

- The problems that occur with hyperkalemia are related to how rapidly extracellular fluid (ECF) potassium levels increase. Sudden rises in serum potassium cause severe problems at potassium levels between 6 and 7 mEq/L. When serum potassium rises slowly, problems may not occur until potassium levels reach 8 mEq/L or higher.

Interprofessional Collaborative Care
Recognize Cues: Assessment

- Obtain patient information about:
  1. Age
  2. Chronic illnesses (particularly kidney disease and diabetes mellitus)
  3. Recent medical or surgical treatment
  4. Urine output, including the frequency and amount of voiding
  5. Drug use, particularly potassium-sparing diuretics and ACE inhibitors (ACEIs)
  6. Nutritional history to determine the intake of potassium-rich foods or the use of salt substitutes that contain potassium
  7. Palpitations, skipped heartbeats, and other cardiac irregularities
  8. Muscle twitching and weakness in the leg muscles
  9. Unusual tingling or numbness in the hands, feet, or face
  10. Recent changes in bowel habits, especially diarrhea
- Assess for and document:
  1. Cardiovascular changes: Cardiovascular changes are the most severe problems from hyperkalemia and are the most common cause of death in patients with hyperkalemia.
     - Bradycardia
     - Hypotension
     - ECG changes (peaked T waves, prolonged PR intervals, wide QRS complexes, flat or absent P waves)
  2. Neuromuscular changes, early
     - Skeletal muscle twitches
     - Tingling and burning sensations followed by numbness in the hands and feet and around the mouth
  3. Neuromuscular changes, late
     - Muscle weakness
     - Flaccid paralysis first in hands and feet, then moving higher
  4. Intestinal changes
     - Increased motility
     - Hyperactive bowel sounds
     - Frequent watery bowel movements
  5. Laboratory data: serum potassium level greater than 5 mEq/L

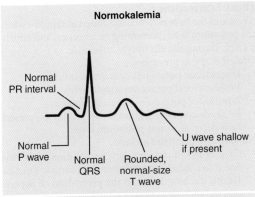

Normokalemia

Normal PR interval

Normal P wave

Normal QRS

Rounded, normal-size T wave

U wave shallow if present

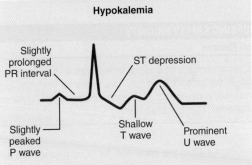

Hypokalemia

Slightly prolonged PR interval

ST depression

Slightly peaked P wave

Shallow T wave

Prominent U wave

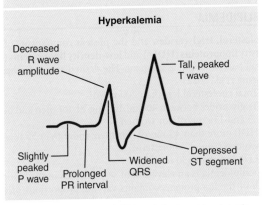

Hyperkalemia

Decreased R wave amplitude

Tall, peaked T wave

Slightly peaked P wave

Prolonged PR interval

Widened QRS

Depressed ST segment

Electrocardiogram changes with hyperkalemia and hypokalemia.

H

Take Actions: Interventions

- Interventions for hyperkalemia are aimed at rapidly reducing the serum potassium level, preventing recurrences, and ensuring patient safety during the electrolyte imbalance.
  1. Drug therapy as prescribed
     - Discontinue potassium-containing infusions
     - Withhold oral potassium supplements
     - Administer potassium-excreting diuretics
     - IV fluids containing glucose and insulin are prescribed to help decrease serum potassium levels
  2. Nursing care priorities include:
     - Cardiac monitoring for early recognition of dysrhythmias and other signs of hyperkalemia on cardiac function
     - Health teaching is key to the prevention of hyperkalemia and the early detection of complications.

NURSING SAFETY PRIORITY
Critical Rescue

Assess anyone who has or is at risk for hyperkalemia to recognize cardiac changes. If the patient's heart rate falls below 60 beats/min or if the T waves become spiked, both of which accompany hyperkalemia, respond by notifying the Rapid Response Team.

See Chapter 13 in the main text for more information on hyperkalemia.

HYPERLIPIDEMIA

- **Cholesterol**, **triglycerides**, and the protein components of **high-density lipoproteins (HDLs)** and **low-density lipoproteins (LDLs)** are all part of a lipid assessment. The desired ranges for lipids are (Pagana et al., 2022):
  1. Total cholesterol less than 200 mg/dL
  2. Triglycerides between 40 and 160 mg/dL for men and between 35 and 135 mg/dL for women
  3. HDL more than 45 mg/dL for men; more than 55 mg/dL for women ("good" cholesterol)
  4. LDL less than 130 mg/dL
- Hyperlipidemia is an elevation of serum lipids in the blood.
- Each of the lipoproteins contains varying proportions of cholesterol, triglyceride, protein, and phospholipid. HDL contains mainly protein and 20% cholesterol, whereas LDL is mainly cholesterol.

- Elevated LDL levels are positively correlated with coronary artery disease (CAD), whereas elevated HDL levels are negatively correlated and appear to be protective for heart disease.
- Elevated lipids are considered a risk factor for CAD.

Interprofessional Collaborative Care

- Hyperlipidemia is treated with lifestyle interventions (e.g., diet, exercise) and cholesterol-lowering drugs, typically statins (e.g. lovastatin and simvastatin).

See Chapter 27 in the main text for more information on hyperlipidemia.

HYPERMAGNESEMIA

- *Hypermagnesemia* is a serum magnesium level above 2.1 mEq/L or 1.05 mmol/L.
- Magnesium is a membrane stabilizer; therefore, symptoms of hypermagnesemia occur as a result of reduced membrane excitability when serum magnesium levels exceed 4 mEq/L (2 mmol/L).
- Common causes of hypermagnesemia include magnesium-containing antacids and laxatives, IV magnesium replacement, and decreased kidney excretion of magnesium in kidney disease.
- *Cardiac changes* include bradycardia, peripheral vasodilation, and hypotension.
    1. ECG changes show a prolonged PR interval with a widened QRS complex.
    2. Bradycardia can be severe, and cardiac arrest is possible. Hypotension is also severe, with a diastolic pressure lower than normal.
    3. Patients with severe hypermagnesemia are in grave danger of cardiac arrest.

Interprofessional Collaborative Care
Recognize Cues: Assessment
- Assess for:
    1. Cardiac changes of bradycardia, peripheral vasodilation, and hypotension
    2. CNS changes of drowsiness, lethargy, or coma
    3. Neuromuscular changes of reduced or absent deep tendon reflexes and weak or absent voluntary skeletal muscle contractions

Take Actions: Interventions
- Restore magnesium balance by:
    1. Stopping magnesium oral and parental supplementation as prescribed

2. Administering magnesium-free IV fluids and diuretic drugs as prescribed to excrete this mineral
3. When cardiac problems are severe, giving calcium as prescribed may reverse the cardiac effects of hypermagnesemia

See Chapter 13 in the main text for more information on hypermagnesemia.

HYPERNATREMIA

- Hypernatremia is a serum sodium level greater than 145 mEq/L and is often accompanied by changes in fluid volume.
- It makes excitable tissues more easily excited, a condition known as irritability, and leads to cellular dehydration.

Common Causes of Hypernatremia	
Actual Sodium Excesses	**Relative Sodium Excesses**
• Hyperaldosteronism	• Dehydration
• Kidney failure	• Increased rate of metabolism
• Corticosteroids	• Fever
• Cushing syndrome or disease	• Hyperventilation
• Excessive oral sodium ingestion	• Infection
• Excessive administration of sodium-containing IV fluids	• Excessive diaphoresis
	• Watery diarrhea

Interprofessional Collaborative Care
Recognize Cues: Assessment
- Assess for and document:
  1. Nervous system changes
     - Altered cognition, such as decreased attention span or recall of recent events
     - Agitation or confusion
     - Lethargy, drowsiness, stupor, or coma (when accompanied by fluid overload)
  2. Musculoskeletal changes
     - Muscle twitching and irregular muscle contractions (mild hypernatremia)
     - Muscle weakness and reduced hand grip strength
  3. Cardiovascular changes that differ with fluid status
     - High sodium with hypovolemia leads to increased pulse rate, hypotension, and reduced quality of peripheral pulses.

- High sodium with euvolemia or hypervolemia leads to normal or bounding pulses, neck vein distention, and elevated diastolic BP.

Take Actions: Interventions

- Nursing care priorities for the patient with hypernatremia include monitoring the response to therapy and ensuring patient safety by preventing hyponatremia and dehydration.
- *Drug therapy* is used to restore fluid balance when hypernatremia is caused by fluid loss.
  1. Isotonic saline (0.9%) and dextrose 5% in 0.45% sodium chloride are most often prescribed.
- Hypernatremia caused by reduced kidney sodium excretion requires drug therapy with diuretics that promote sodium loss, such as furosemide or bumetanide.
  1. Assess the patient hourly for indications of excessive losses of fluid, sodium, or potassium.
- *Nutrition therapy* to prevent or correct mild hypernatremia involves ensuring adequate water intake, especially among older adults.
- Dietary sodium restriction may be needed to prevent sodium excess when kidney problems are present.

See Chapter 13 in the main text for more information on hypernatremia.

HYPERPARATHYROIDISM

- Hyperparathyroidism is a disorder in which parathyroid secretion of parathyroid hormone (PTH) is increased, resulting in *hypercalcemia* (excessive serum calcium levels) and *hypophosphatemia* (inadequate serum phosphorus levels).
  1. Primary hyperparathyroidism results when one or more parathyroid glands do not respond to the normal feedback mechanisms for serum calcium levels. The most common cause is a benign tumor in the parathyroid gland.
  2. Secondary hyperparathyroidism is a response to the hypocalcemia associated with chronic kidney disease (CKD) or vitamin D deficiency, which leads to hyperplasia of the parathyroid glands.
- In bone, excessive PTH levels increase bone *resorption* (bone loss of calcium) by decreasing *osteoblastic* (bone production) activity and increasing *osteoclastic* (bone destruction) activity. This process releases calcium and phosphorus into the blood and reduces bone density.

Interprofessional Collaborative Care
Recognize Cues: Assessment
- Obtain patient information about:
  1. Bone fractures; joint, bone, and muscle pain
  2. GI problems of anorexia, nausea, vomiting, epigastric pain, constipation, and weight loss
  3. History of radiation treatment to the head or neck
  4. History of kidney stones
- Assess for and document:
  1. Waxy pallor/ash gray appearance of the skin
  2. Bone deformities in the extremities and back
  3. GI problems such as anorexia, nausea, vomiting, epigastric pain, or constipation
  4. Fatigue and lethargy
  5. Confusion, coma (severe hyperparathyroidism)
  6. Diagnostic studies that include results for:
     - Serum electrolyte levels, especially calcium and phosphorus
     - Serum PTH and urine cyclic adenosine monophosphate (cAMP) levels
     - X-rays with calcium deposits in joints or blood vessels, renal stones, or bone loss or abnormal lesions
     - CT with or without arteriography
     - Loss of bone density in a DEXA scan

Take Actions: Interventions
Nonsurgical Management
- Intravenous fluids followed by a loop diuretic (furosemide) are used most often for reducing symptomatic serum calcium levels in patients.
- When symptoms are severe or related to parathyroid cancer, drug therapy includes:
  1. Cinacalcet to decrease serum calcium
  2. Oral phosphates to interfere with dietary calcium absorption
- Interventions to manage symptoms and complications from hyperparathyroidism include:
  1. Evaluating cardiac rate, rhythm, and waveforms with continuous ECG monitoring
  2. Measuring intake and output 2 to 4 hours during hydration therapy
  3. Closely monitoring serum calcium levels for return to safe range
  4. Assessing for tingling and numbness in the hands, feet, and around the mouth to detect hypocalcemia early
  5. Preventing injury by implementing fall precautions to avoid fracture and injury to hypodense bones

Surgical Management
- Surgical management of hyperparathyroidism is parathyroidectomy.
  1. All four parathyroid glands are examined for enlargement.
  2. If a tumor is present on one side but the other side is normal, the surgeon removes the glands containing tumor and leaves the remaining glands on the opposite side intact.
  3. If all four glands are diseased, they are all removed.
  4. Nursing care before and after surgical removal of the parathyroid glands is the same as that for thyroidectomy.
  5. A hypocalcemic crisis can occur during this critical period, and the serum calcium level is assessed frequently after surgery.
     - Check serum calcium levels immediately after surgery and every 4 hours thereafter until calcium levels stabilize.
     - Monitor for manifestations of hypocalcemia.
       - Tingling and twitching in the extremities and face indicating onset of tetany
       - Positive Trousseau or Chvostek sign (tetany; see *Hypocalcemia*)
  6. Assess for damage to the recurrent laryngeal nerve with changes in voice patterns and hoarseness.
- If all four parathyroid glands are removed, the patient will need lifelong treatment with calcium and vitamin D because the resulting *hypoparathyroidism* is permanent.

See Chapter 55 in the main text for more information on hyperparathyroidism.

H

HYPERPITUITARISM

- Hyperpituitarism is hormone oversecretion that occurs with pituitary tumors or hyperplasia.
- Tumors occur most often in the anterior pituitary cells that produce growth hormone (GH), prolactin (PRL), and adrenocorticotropic hormone (ACTH).
  1. Overproduction of growth hormone results in acromegaly, with symptoms such as increased skeletal thickness, hypertrophy of the skin, and enlargement of all visceral organs.
  2. Excessive PRL inhibits secretion of sex hormones in men and women and results in galactorrhea, amenorrhea, and infertility.
  3. Excess ACTH overstimulates the adrenal cortex, resulting in excessive production of corticosteroids, mineralocorticoids, and androgens, which leads to the development of Cushing disease or syndrome.

PATIENT-CENTERED CARE: GENETICS/GENOMICS
MEN1

One cause of hyperpituitarism is multiple endocrine neoplasia, type 1 (MEN1), in which there is inactivation of the suppressor gene *MEN1* (Online Mendelian Inheritance in Man [OMIM], 2017). MEN1 has an autosomal dominant inheritance pattern and may result in a benign tumor of the pituitary, parathyroid glands, or pancreas. In the pituitary, excessive production of growth hormone occurs and leads to acromegaly. Ask a patient with acromegaly whether either parent also has this problem or has had a tumor of the pancreas or parathyroid glands.

Interprofessional Collaborative Care
Recognize Cues: Assessment

- Obtain patient information about changes in appearance and target organ function:
  1. Family history of endocrine problems
  2. Change in appearance: gain or change in hat, glove, ring, or shoe size
  3. Fatigue and lethargy
  4. Arthralgias (joint pain)
  5. Headaches and changes in vision
  6. Menstrual changes (e.g., amenorrhea, irregular menses, difficulty in becoming pregnant)
  7. Changes in sexual functioning (e.g., decreased libido, painful intercourse, impotence)
  8. Loss of or change in secondary sexual characteristics
  9. Weight gain or loss (unplanned)
- Assess for and document:
  1. Changes in the facial features (e.g., increases in lip and nose sizes; prominent brow ridge; increases in head, hand, and foot sizes); moon face
  2. Extremity muscle wasting
  3. Acne
  4. Hirsutism
  5. Striae
  6. Hypertension
  7. Areas of uneven pigmentation or hyperpigmentation
  8. Dysrhythmias, including tachycardia or bradycardia
- Diagnostic testing may include:
  1. Blood test for hormone levels (any or all may be elevated)
  2. Hormone suppression tests

Take Actions: Interventions

Nonsurgical Management

- Drug therapy may be used alone or in combination with surgery and/or radiation.
  1. Dopamine agonists bromocriptine and cabergoline stimulate dopamine receptors in the brain and inhibit the release of growth hormone and PRL.

🔲 NURSING SAFETY PRIORITY

Drug Alert

Teach patients taking bromocriptine to seek medical care immediately if chest pain, dizziness, or watery nasal discharge occurs because of the possibility of serious side effects, including cardiac dysrhythmias, coronary artery spasms, and cerebrospinal fluid leakage.

---

  2. Other agents used for acromegaly are the somatostatin analogs, especially octreotide and lanreotide, and a growth hormone receptor blocker, pegvisomant.
- Gamma knife or stereotactic radiation therapy may be used to manage some conditions.

Surgical Management

- Surgical removal of the pituitary gland and tumor (hypophysectomy) is the most common treatment for hyperpituitarism.
- A minimally invasive transnasal or a transsphenoidal hypophysectomy is the most commonly used surgical approach. With a transsphenoidal approach, the surgeon makes an incision just above the upper lip and reaches the pituitary gland through the sphenoid sinus.
- A craniotomy may be needed if the tumor cannot be reached by a transsphenoidal approach.
- Provide preoperative care and:
  1. Explain that because nasal packing is present for 2 to 3 days after surgery, it will be necessary to breathe through the mouth, and a "mustache dressing" ("drip pad") will be placed under the nose.
  2. Instruct the patient not to cough, sneeze, blow the nose, or bend forward after surgery.
- Provide postoperative care and:
  1. Monitor neurologic responses hourly for the first 24 hours and then every 4 hours and document any changes in vision,

H

mental status, altered level of consciousness, or decreased strength of the extremities.

2. Observe for complications such as transient diabetes insipidus, cerebrospinal fluid (CSF) leakage, infection, and increased intracranial pressure (ICP).
   - Excess urine output may indicate onset of diabetes insipidus.
   - Any postnasal drip may indicate leakage of CSF.
   - Assess nasal drainage for quantity, quality, and odor; send a sample to the laboratory for testing because the presence of glucose may confirm CSF drainage.
3. Keep the head of the bed elevated.
4. Instruct the patient to avoid transient elevated ICP from coughing, straining, or placing head below heart (bending at waist).
5. Perform frequent oral rinses and apply lip moisturizer.
6. Assess for manifestations of meningitis:
   - Headache
   - Fever
   - Nuchal (neck) rigidity
7. Teach the patient self-administration of the prescribed hormones.

See Chapter 54 in the main text for more information on hyperpituitarism.

✴ HEART FAILURE: PERFUSION CONCEPT EXEMPLAR

Overview

- Hypertension, or high blood pressure (BP), is the most common health problem seen in primary care settings and can cause stroke, myocardial infarction (MI) (heart attack), kidney failure, and death if not treated early and effectively.
- Current guidelines from the American College of Cardiology (ACC) and the American Heart Association (AHA) recommend a BP below 130/80 mm Hg in all people. This BP recommendation is lower than the guidance provided by the Eighth Joint National Committee (JNC 8) on Prevention, Detection, Evaluation, and Treatment of High Blood Pressure.
- According to JNC 8, in the general population ages 60 years and older, the desired BP is below 150/90 mm Hg. For people younger than 60 years, the desired BP is below 140/90 mm Hg. Patients with a BP above these goals should be treated with medication (James et al., 2014).
- Hypertension reduces perfusion to heart, brain, kidney, eyes (retinal; vision), and tissues in the periphery.

Categories of Blood Pressure in Adults

Guidelines From Eighth Joint National Committee (JNC-8) on Prevention, Detection, Evaluation, and Treatment of High Blood Pressure Guidelines and From American College of Cardiology (ACC)/American Heart Association (AHA)

Blood Pressure Category	Systolic Blood Pressure		Diastolic Blood Pressure
Normal (ACC/AHA)	<120 mm Hg	and	<80 mm Hg
Elevated (ACC/AHA)	120–129 mm Hg	and	<80 mm Hg
Prehypertension (JNC-8)	120–139 mm Hg	or	80–89 mm Hg
Hypertension			
Stage 1			
ACC/AHA	130–139 mm Hg	or	80–89 mm Hg
JNC-8	140–159 mm Hg	or	90–99 mm Hg
Stage 2			
ACC/AHA	≥140 mm Hg	or	≥90 mm Hg
JNC-8	>160 mm Hg	or	>100 mm Hg

Data from Whelton, P. K., Carey, R. M., Aronow, W. S., et al. (2017). CC/AHA/AAPA/ABC/ACPM/AGS/APhA/ASH/ASPC/NMA/PCNA guideline for the prevention, detection, evaluation, and management of high blood pressure in adults: Executive summary. A report of the American College of Cardiology/American Heart Association Task Force on Clinical Practice Guidelines. *Hypertension*, Nov 13; and James, P. A., Oparil, S., Carter, B. L., et al. (2014). 2014 Evidence-based guidelines for the management of high blood pressure in adults: Report from the panel members appointed to the Eighth National Committee (JNC 8). *JAMA: The Journal of the American Medical Association, 311*(5), 507–520.

Etiology of Hypertension

Primary
- Family history of hypertension
- Black race
- Hyperlipidemia
- Smoking
- Older than 60 years or postmenopausal
- Excessive sodium and caffeine intake
- Overweight/obesity
- Physical inactivity
- Excessive alcohol intake
- Low potassium, calcium, or magnesium intake
- Excessive and continuous stress

Secondary
- Kidney disease
- Primary aldosteronism
- Pheochromocytoma
- Cushing disease
- Coarctation of the aorta
- Brain tumors
- Encephalitis
- Pregnancy
- Drugs:
  - Estrogen (e.g., oral contraceptives)
  - Glucocorticoids
  - Mineralocorticoids
  - Sympathomimetics

![icon] **PATIENT-CENTERED CARE: HEALTH EQUITY**

Hypertension and Black Americans

The prevalence of hypertension in Black people in the United States is among the highest in the world and is increasing. Black people develop more severe high blood pressure earlier in life, making them much more likely to die from strokes, heart disease, and kidney disease (Tsao et al., 2022). Because of this prevalence in the Black population, JNC-8 guidelines, as well as ACC/AHA guidelines, provide population-specific recommendations for treatment (Whelton et al., 2017; James et al., 2014).

Interprofessional Collaborative Care

Recognize Cues: Assessment

- Record patient information
  1. BP in both arms while sitting
  2. Age
  3. Race or ethnic origin
  4. Family history of hypertension
  5. Dietary intake pattern, including alcohol
  6. Smoking
  7. Exercise habits
  8. Past and present history of cardiovascular, kidney disease, and diabetes
  9. Drug use (prescribed, OTC, and illicit)
- Assess for hypertensive symptoms
  1. When a diagnosis of hypertension is made, most people have no symptoms.
  2. Headache, dizziness, facial flushing, or fainting
  3. Vision changes or retinal changes on funduscopic examination
  4. Signs of kidney injury, such as elevated BUN or creatinine levels or low urine output
  5. Physical findings related to vascular damage, including atherosclerosis, acute coronary syndrome, peripheral arterial disease, stroke, chronic kidney disease, blindness, and HF
     - Abdominal, carotid, or femoral bruits
     - Dysrhythmias, tachycardia, sweating, and pallor/ash gray skin
     - Decreased or absent peripheral pulses
     - Cardiomegaly or left ventricular hypertrophy
  6. Diagnostic assessment
     - No laboratory tests are diagnostic of essential hypertension; several laboratory tests can assess possible causes of secondary hypertension.
     - An ECG can determine atrial and ventricular hypertrophy, which is one of the first ECG signs of heart disease resulting from hypertension.

Analyze Cues and Prioritize Hypotheses: Analysis

- The priority collaborative problems for most patients with hypertension are:
  1. Need for health teaching due to the plan of care for hypertension management
  2. Potential for decreased adherence due to side effects of drug therapy and necessary changes in lifestyle

Generate Solutions and Take Actions: Planning and Implementation

Health Teaching

- Assist with planning and implementing lifestyle changes, including the regular evaluation of BP outside of office visits.
- In collaboration with the health care team, teach the patient to:
  1. Restrict sodium intake in the diet per the ACC/AHA guidelines.
  2. Reduce weight, if overweight or obese.
  3. Implement a heart-healthy diet, such as the DASH diet.
  4. Abstain or decrease alcohol consumption (no more than one drink a day for women and two drinks a day for men).
  5. Increase physical activity with a structured exercise program.
  6. Use relaxation techniques to decrease stress.
  7. Stop smoking and tobacco use.
- Drug therapy is individualized for each patient, with consideration given to culture, age, other existing illness, severity of BP elevation, and cost of drugs and follow-up.
  1. The most common drugs to control hypertension are:
     - Diuretics
     - Calcium channel blockers (CCBs)
     - Angiotensin-converting enzyme inhibitors (ACEIs)
     - Angiotensin II receptor blockers (ARBs)
     - Beta-adrenergic blockers
  2. Diuretics are the first type of drugs for managing hypertension. Three basic types of diuretics are used to decrease blood volume and lower blood pressure:
     - Thiazide diuretics, such as hydrochlorothiazide
     - Loop (high-ceiling) diuretics, such as furosemide
     - Potassium-sparing diuretics, such as spironolactone

H

👤 PATIENT-CENTERED CARE: OLDER ADULT HEALTH

Diuretic Therapy

Loop diuretics are not used commonly for older adults because they can cause dehydration and orthostatic hypotension. These complications increase the patient's risk for falls. Teach families to monitor for and report patient dizziness, falls, or confusion to the primary health care provider as soon as possible and discontinue the drug.

3. Calcium channel blockers (CCBs), such as verapamil, lower blood pressure by interfering with the transmembrane flux of calcium ions. This results in vasodilation, which decreases blood pressure.

4. Angiotensin-converting enzyme inhibitors (ACEIs), known as the "-pril" drugs, are also used as single or combination agents in the treatment of hypertension. These drugs block the action of the ACE as it attempts to convert angiotensin I to angiotensin II, one of the most powerful vasoconstrictors in the body. This action also decreases sodium and water retention and lowers peripheral vascular resistance, both of which lower blood pressure.

🔖 NURSING SAFETY PRIORITY

Drug Alert

Instruct the patient receiving an ACEI for the first time to get out of bed slowly to avoid the severe hypotensive effect that can occur with initial use. Orthostatic hypotension may occur with subsequent doses, but it is usually less severe. If dizziness continues or there is a significant decrease in the systolic blood pressure (more than a change of 20 mm Hg), notify the health care provider or teach the patient to notify the health care provider. *The older patient is at the greatest risk for orthostatic hypotension because of the cardiovascular changes associated with aging.*

---

5. Angiotensin II receptor blockers (ARBs) selectively block the binding of angiotensin II to receptor sites in the vascular smooth muscle and adrenal tissues by competing directly with angiotensin II but not inhibiting ACE. Examples of drugs in this group are candesartan, valsartan, losartan, and azilsartan.
   - ARBs can be used alone or in combination with other antihypertensive drugs.
   - These drugs provide an option for patients who report a nagging cough associated with ACEIs.

6. Beta-adrenergic blockers can also be used in the treatment of hypertension. Beta blockers are often the drug of choice for hypertensive patients with ischemic heart disease (IHD) because the heart is the most common target of end-organ damage with hypertension.

Promoting Adherence to the Plan of Care
- Patients who require medications to control primary hypertension usually need to take them for the rest of their lives.
- Patients who do not adhere to antihypertensive treatment are at high risk for target organ damage and hypertensive crisis.

Care Coordination and Transition Management
- Provide educational information for hypertension control, especially:
  1. Salt/sodium restriction
  2. Weight maintenance or reduction
  3. Self-awareness for healthy food selections, such as the DASH diet
  4. Stress reduction or coping strategies
  5. Alcohol restriction
  6. Exercise program
  7. Taking prescribed antihypertensive drugs even in the absence of symptoms
  8. Regular ongoing follow-up with health care provider
- Give oral and written information on drug therapy, including:
  1. Rationale for use, dose, and time of administration
  2. Side effects and vigilance for drug interactions
  3. The value of BP control to avoid serious adverse health consequences such as stroke
- Instruct the patient and family members in the technique of ambulatory BP, and record values to share with scheduled provider interactions.

 See Chapter 30 in the main text for more information on hypertension.

H

HYPERTHYROIDISM

- Hyperthyroidism is excessive thyroid hormone secretion from the thyroid gland.
- Thyroid hormones cause hypermetabolism and increased sympathetic nervous system activity.
- The most common cause is Graves disease, an autoimmune disorder.
- Hyperthyroidism caused by multiple thyroid nodules is termed *toxic multinodular goiter (TMNG)*.
- *Thyroid storm*, or *thyroid crisis*, is a life-threatening condition of extreme hyperthyroidism that occurs when the condition is uncontrolled or triggered by stressors such as trauma, infection, diabetic ketoacidosis, and pregnancy. Key signs include fever, tachycardia, and systolic hypertension.

KEY FEATURES

Hyperthyroidism

Cardiovascular Symptoms
- Palpitations
- Chest pain
- Increased systolic blood pressure
- Tachycardia
- Dysrhythmias
- Rapid, shallow respirations

Metabolic Symptoms
- Increased basal metabolic rate
- Heat intolerance
- Fatigue

Neuromuscular Symptoms
- Eyelid retraction, eyelid lag
- Hyperactive deep tendon reflexes
- Tremors
- Insomnia
- Muscle weakness

Integumentary Symptoms
- Diaphoresis (excessive sweating)
- Fine, soft, silky body hair
- Smooth, warm, moist skin
- Thinning of scalp hair

Gastrointestinal Symptoms
- Weight loss
- Increased appetite
- Increased stools

Reproductive Symptoms
- Amenorrhea
- Erectile dysfunction
- Gynecomastia

Psychosocial Symptoms
- Restlessness
- Anxiety
- Hyperactivity

Other Symptoms
- Goiter
- Wide-eyed or startled appearance (exophthalmos)[a]

[a]Present in Graves disease only.

Interprofessional Collaborative Care
Recognize Cues: Assessment
- Obtain patient information about:
  1. Heat intolerance: a hallmark of hyperthyroidism
  2. Age, usual weight, and any unplanned weight loss
  3. Increased appetite
  4. Increased number of daily bowel movements
  5. Palpitations or chest pain
  6. Dyspnea (with or without exertion)
  7. Changes in vision, especially exophthalmos (specific to Graves disease)
  8. Fatigue, weakness

9. Insomnia (common)
10. Irritability, depression
11. Amenorrhea or a decreased menstrual flow (common)
12. Changes in libido
13. Previous thyroid and neck surgery or radiation therapy to the neck
14. Past and current drugs, especially the use of thyroid hormone replacement or antithyroid drugs
- Assess for and document key features of hyperthyroidism.
- Observe the size and symmetry of the thyroid gland.
  1. If goiter is present, the thyroid gland may be up to four times its normal size.

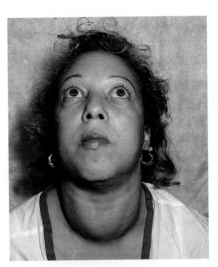

Goiter.

- Diagnostic assessment may include:
  1. Blood tests for:
     - Triiodothyronine (T_3)
     - Thyroxin (T_4)
     - TSH
     - Thyrotropin receptor antibodies (TRAb) (Graves disease)
  2. Thyroid scan (radionuclide)
  3. Ultrasonography of the thyroid gland
  4. ECG, usually with tachycardia

> **⚠ NURSING SAFETY PRIORITY**
> *Action Alert*
>
> Do not palpate a goiter or thyroid tissue in a patient with hyperthyroid symptoms. This action can stimulate the sudden release of excessive thyroid hormones and trigger a life-threatening episode of thyroid storm.

Take Actions: Interventions

- Interventions are described for Graves disease because it is the most common form of hyperthyroidism.
- The goals of management are to restore cellular regulation by decreasing the effect of thyroid hormone on cardiac function during the acute phase and, both acutely and for long-term, reduce thyroid hormone secretion.

Nonsurgical Management

- Monitoring, including:
  1. Measure apical pulse and BP at least every 4 hours, and report status changes in a timely manner.
  2. Instruct the patient to report palpitations, dyspnea, chest pain, or dizziness immediately.
  3. Check temperature at least every 4 hours and report fever in a timely manner. Even an increase of 1 degree should be reported.
  4. Immediately report hyperthermia and hypertension to the provider because these signs precede thyroid storm.
  5. Promote comfort by keeping the environment cool and linens dry.
  6. Administer drug therapy:
     - Antithyroid drugs such as methimazole

> **◆ NURSING SAFETY PRIORITY**
> *Drug Alert*
>
> Methimazole can cause birth defects and may need to be changed to a different medication during the first trimester of pregnancy. Instruct women to notify their primary health care provider if pregnancy occurs.

- Supportive drug therapy with propranolol to relieve diaphoresis, anxiety, tachycardia, and palpitations
- Radioactive iodine (RAI) therapy, typically administered in an outpatient setting as an oral drug
  - Do not use in pregnant women because RAI crosses the placenta and can damage the fetal thyroid gland.

- May take 6 to 8 weeks for results
- May cause some patients to experience hypothyroidism as a result of the treatment
- Some radioactivity is present in the patient's body fluids and stool for a few days after therapy; radiation precautions are needed to prevent exposure to family members and other people.

Surgical Management
- Surgery to remove all (total thyroidectomy) or part of the thyroid gland (subtotal thyroidectomy) is used to manage Graves disease, when a goiter compresses the trachea or esophagus, or when hyperthyroidism does not respond to therapy.
- A thyroidectomy is typically performed under general anesthesia using a minimally invasive approach.
- After a total thyroidectomy, patients must take lifelong thyroid hormone replacement.

PATIENT AND FAMILY EDUCATION

Safety Precautions for the Patient Receiving an Unsealed Radioactive Isotope

- Sit to urinate (males and females) to avoid splashing urine on the seat, walls, and floor.
- Flush the toilet (with the lid closed) two to three times after each use.
- Men with urinary incontinence should use condom catheters and a drainage bag rather than absorbent gel-filled briefs or pads.
- Women with urinary incontinence should use facial tissue layers in their clothing to catch the urine rather than absorbent gel-filled briefs or pads. These tissues should then be flushed.
- Avoid close contact with pregnant women, infants, and young children for the prescribed amount of time (usually at least a week) after therapy; this is dose-dependent. Remain at least 6 feet away from these people, and avoid sleeping in the same bed.
- Patients may need to delay travel or returning to work for a few days, depending on the dose of therapy given.
- Some radioactivity will be in the saliva during the first week after therapy. Precautions to avoid exposing others to this contamination include:
  - Not sharing toothbrushes or toothpaste tubes
  - Not preparing food or sharing beverages

- Provide preoperative care, including the following:
  1. Administer antithyroid drugs and iodine preparations to decrease the secretion of thyroid hormones and reduce thyroid size and vascularity.

2. Ensure that hypertension, dysrhythmias, and tachycardia are controlled before surgery.
- Provide postoperative care, including the following:
  1. Monitor closely for complications
  2. Use pillows to support the head and neck to avoid neck extension.
  3. Place the patient, while awake, in a semi-Fowler's position.
  4. Prevent complications from airway obstruction or respiratory distress by:
     - Listening for laryngeal stridor (harsh, high-pitched respiratory sounds)
     - Ensuring that oxygen and suctioning equipment are nearby and in working order
     - Assessing for laryngeal damage resulting in hoarseness or a weak voice

---

✚ NURSING SAFETY PRIORITY

Critical Rescue

Monitor the patient to identify symptoms of obstruction and poor **gas exchange** (stridor, dyspnea, falling oxygen saturation, inability to swallow, drooling) after thyroid surgery. If any indications are present, respond by immediately initiating the Rapid Response Team.

---

  5. Monitor for hemorrhage.
     - Inspect the neck dressing and behind the patient's neck for blood.
     - Assess drainage for amount, color, and character.
  6. Avoid injury from concurrent parathyroid removal or injury resulting in hypocalcemia and tetany.
     - Ask the patient about any tingling around the mouth or of the toes and fingers.
     - Assess for muscle twitching.
     - Ensure that calcium gluconate is available.
- Thyroid storm or thyroid crisis requires emergency management; even with optimal management, it can result in death.
  1. A life-threatening, uncontrolled hyperthyroidism can result in a rapid onset of symptoms and life-threatening complications.
  2. Stressors such as trauma, infection, diabetic ketoacidosis, and pregnancy can cause thyroid storm. Thyroid crisis can also occur after thyroid surgery if thyroid hormone reduction drug therapy was not used.

3. *Key symptoms include fever and tachycardia.* The patient may have abdominal pain, nausea, vomiting, and diarrhea. Often anxiety and tremors are reported.
4. Emergency measures to prevent death from thyroid storm vary with the intensity and type of changes. Interventions focus on maintaining airway patency, providing adequate ventilation, reducing fever, and stabilizing the hemodynamic status.

✚ NURSING SAFETY PRIORITY

Critical Rescue

When caring for a patient with hyperthyroidism, even after a thyroidectomy, assess temperature often because an increase of even 1°F (1.8°C) may indicate an impending thyroid crisis. If a temperature increase occurs, respond by reporting it immediately to the primary health care provider.

» BEST PRACTICE FOR PATIENT SAFETY AND QUALITY CARE

Emergency Care of the Patient During Thyroid Storm

- Maintain a patent airway and adequate ventilation.
- Give oral antithyroid drugs as prescribed: methimazole or propylthiouracil.
- If antithyroid drugs cannot be used, a bile acid sequestrant such as cholestyramine may be ordered to help reduce thyroid levels.
- Administer iodide solution, nonsalicylate antipyretic drugs, and glucocorticoids as prescribed.
- Give oral propranolol as prescribed to control heart rate.
- Monitor continually for cardiac dysrhythmias.
- Monitor vital signs every 15 to 30 minutes.
- Provide comfort measures, including a cooling blanket.
- Correct dehydration with normal saline infusions per orders.
- Apply a cooling blanket or ice packs to reduce fever.

H

- Teach the patient and family about:
    1. The signs of hyperthyroidism, and instruct them to report an increase or recurrence of symptoms
    2. The signs of hypothyroidism and the need for thyroid hormone replacement
    3. The need for regular follow-up because hypothyroidism can occur several years after RAI therapy

See Chapter 55 in the main text for more information on hyperthyroidism.

HYPOCALCEMIA

- Hypocalcemia is a total serum calcium (Ca^{2+}) level less than 9 mg/dL or 2.25 mmol/L. Because the normal blood level of calcium is so low, any change in calcium levels has major effects on function.

Common Causes of Hypocalcemia

Actual Calcium Deficits
- Inadequate oral intake of calcium
- Lactose intolerance
- Malabsorption syndromes:
  - Celiac sprue
  - Crohn's disease
- Inadequate intake of vitamin D
- End-stage kidney disease
- Diarrhea
- Steatorrhea
- Wound drainage (especially GI)

Relative Calcium Deficits
- Hyperproteinemia
- Alkalosis
- Acute pancreatitis
- Hyperphosphatemia
- Immobility
- Removal or destruction of parathyroid glands

- Low serum calcium levels increase sodium movement across excitable membranes, allowing depolarization to occur more easily and at inappropriate times.

PATIENT-CENTERED CARE: GENDER HEALTH

Calcium Loss

Postmenopausal women are at risk for chronic calcium loss. This problem is related to reduced weight-bearing activities and a decrease in estrogen levels. As they age, many women decrease weight-bearing activities such as running and walking, which allows osteoporosis to occur at a more rapid rate. In addition, the estrogen secretion that protects against osteoporosis diminishes. Teach older women to continue walking and other weight-bearing activities.

Interprofessional Collaborative Care
Recognize Cues: Assessment

- Assess for and document dietary intake of calcium or calcium supplement.
- Evaluate low serum calcium levels and related symptoms of:
  1. Neuromuscular changes (most common)
     - Paresthesias with sensations of tingling and numbness
     - Muscle twitches, painful cramps, and spasms
     - Anxiety, irritability

- Positive Trousseau's sign: Place a BP cuff around the upper arm, inflate the cuff to greater than the patient's systolic pressure, and keep the cuff inflated for 1 to 4 minutes. Under these hypoxic conditions, a positive Trousseau's sign occurs when the hand and fingers go into spasm in palmar flexion.
- Positive Chvostek sign: Tap the face just below and in front of the ear (over the facial nerve) to trigger facial twitching of one side of the mouth, nose, and cheek.

2. Cardiovascular changes
   - Bradycardia or tachycardia
   - Weak, thready pulse
   - Hypotension (severe hypocalcemia)
   - ECG changes (prolonged ST interval, prolonged QT interval)
3. GI changes
   - Hyperactive bowel sounds
   - Abdominal cramping
   - Diarrhea
4. Skeletal changes (thin, brittle, and fragile bones)
   - Overall loss of height
   - Unexplained bone pain

Take Actions: Interventions

- Restore calcium balance
  1. Administer drug therapy with:
     - Direct calcium replacement (oral and IV)
     - Drugs that enhance the absorption of calcium, such as vitamin D
  2. Collaborate with the registered dietitian nutritionist (RDN) to provide and teach about a high-calcium diet
- Promote safety during severe hypocalcemia by:
  1. Managing the environment to reduce stimulation, such as keeping the room quiet or adjusting lighting
  2. Instituting fall precautions and gentle handling when fragile bones occur with prolonged hypocalcemia

 See Chapter 13 in the main text for more information on hypocalcemia.

HYPOKALEMIA

- Hypokalemia is a serum potassium level less than 3.5 mEq/L (3.5 mmol/L).
- With hypokalemia, the cell membranes of all excitable tissues, such as nerve and muscle, are less responsive to normal stimuli.
- Rapid reduction of serum potassium levels results in dramatic changes in function, whereas gradual reductions may not show changes in function until the level is very low.

- Older adults are more vulnerable to hypokalemia because of the risk factors of chronic conditions and drug therapy, which may contribute to this electrolyte imbalance.

Common Causes of Hypokalemia

Actual Potassium Deficits
- Inappropriate or excessive use of drugs:
  - Diuretics
  - Corticosteroids
- Increased secretion of aldosterone
- Cushing syndrome
- Diarrhea
- Vomiting
- Wound drainage (especially GI)
- Prolonged nasogastric suction
- Heat-induced excessive diaphoresis
- Kidney disease impairing reabsorption of potassium

Relative Potassium Deficits
- Alkalosis
- Hyperinsulinism
- Hyperalimentation
- Total parenteral nutrition
- Water intoxication
- IV therapy with potassium-poor solutions

Interprofessional Collaborative Care
Recognize Cues: Assessment
- Obtain patient information about:
  1. Drugs, especially diuretics, corticosteroids, digoxin, and potassium supplements
  2. Presence of acute or chronic disease, especially cardiac or kidney conditions
  3. Diet history
- Assess for and document:
  1. Respiratory changes
     - Breath sounds
     - Respiratory effort, including rate and depth of respiration
     - Oxygen saturation
     - Color of nail beds and mucous membranes

! NURSING SAFETY PRIORITY
Action Alert

Assess the respiratory status of a patient who has hypokalemia at least every 2 hours because respiratory insufficiency is a major cause of death from hypokalemia.

  2. Musculoskeletal changes that indicate weakness
     - Weak hand grasps
     - Lethargy, inability to complete ADLs
     - Flaccid paralysis

3. Cardiovascular changes
   - Rapid, thready pulse that is difficult to palpate
   - Dysrhythmias and ECG changes (characteristic ST segment depression and prominent U wave)
   - Orthostatic hypotension
4. Neurologic changes
   - Altered mental status
   - Irritability and anxiety
   - Lethargy, acute confusion, coma
5. GI changes of reduced peristalsis, leading to:
   - Hypoactive or absent bowel sounds
   - Abdominal distention
   - Nausea, vomiting
   - Constipation

Take Actions: Interventions

- Interventions for hypokalemia focus on preventing potassium loss, increasing serum potassium levels, and ensuring patient safety.
  1. Administer potassium replacement therapy or drugs to reduce urinary loss of potassium.

NURSING SAFETY PRIORITY

Drug Alert

Potassium must be diluted for intravenous administration and must be administered slowly. The recommended infusion rate is 5 to 10 mEq/hr (mmol/hr). In accordance with National Patient Safety Goals (NPSGs), potassium is **not** given by IV push. **Do NOT administer potassium undiluted or by IV push as this can cause cardiac arrest (death).**

- Oral potassium preparations have a strong, unpleasant taste that is difficult to mask; give the drug during or after a meal or dilute it with nearly any patient-preferred liquid.
- Potassium-sparing diuretics such as spironolactone may be used to slow potassium loss.
  2. Monitor patient response to potassium replacement therapy, including cardiac and neurologic derangements from too rapid or delayed replacement therapy.

NURSING SAFETY PRIORITY

Action Alert

If infiltration of a solution containing potassium occurs, stop the IV solution immediately, remove the venous access, and notify the health care provider. Document these actions, and provide a complete description and photograph of the IV site.

H

3. Collaborate with the RDN for nutritional therapy to increase dietary potassium intake.
4. Institute fall precautions as a safety measure.
5. Perform respiratory monitoring at least hourly for severe hypokalemia.
    - Respiratory effort, including rate and depth (checking for increasing rate and decreasing depth)
    - Oxygen saturation by pulse oximetry

 See Chapter 13 in the main text for more information on hypokalemia.

HYPOMAGNESEMIA

- Hypomagnesemia is a serum magnesium (Mg^2) level below 1.3 mEq/L or 0.65 mmol/L. It is most often caused by decreased absorption of dietary magnesium or increased kidney magnesium excretion from thiazide diuretics.

Interprofessional Collaborative Care
Recognize Cues: Assessment
- Assess serum magnesium levels and symptoms of low magnesium.
    1. *Cardiovascular changes* associated with hypomagnesemia are serious. Low magnesium levels increase the risk for hypertension, atherosclerosis, hypertrophic left ventricle, and a variety of dysrhythmias (Rogers, 2023).
    2. Neuromuscular changes, including hyperactive deep tendon reflexes, numbness and tingling, and painful muscle contractions
        - Low magnesium often occurs with low calcium.
        - Positive Chvostek and Trousseau signs may be present when hypocalcemia co-occurs.
    3. Intestinal changes, including paralytic ileus from decreased intestinal smooth muscle contraction, anorexia, nausea, constipation, and abdominal distention, are common

Take Actions: Interventions
- Magnesium is replaced with oral or IV magnesium sulfate ($MgSO_4$).
    1. Assess deep tendon reflexes at least hourly in the patient receiving IV magnesium to monitor effectiveness and prevent hypermagnesemia.
    2. If hypocalcemia is also present, drug therapy to increase serum calcium levels is prescribed.
- Stop drugs that promote magnesium loss until balance is restored.

 See Chapter 13 in the main text for more information on hypomagnesemia.

HYPONATREMIA

- **Hyponatremia** is an electrolyte imbalance in which the serum sodium (Na^+) level is below 136 mEq/L (mmol/L). Sodium imbalances often occur with a fluid imbalance because the same hormones regulate both sodium and water balance.
- The problems caused by hyponatremia involve reduced excitable membrane depolarization and cellular swelling.
- The cells especially affected are those involved in cerebral, neuromuscular, intestinal smooth muscle, and cardiovascular functions.

Common Causes of Hyponatremia

Actual Sodium Deficits
- Gastrointestinal fluid loss
  - Vomiting
  - Diarrhea
- Excessive diaphoresis
- Diuretics
- Burns that affect a large portion of the body
- Decreased secretion of aldosterone
- Kidney disease
- Hyperglycemia

Relative Sodium Deficits (Dilution)
- Excessive ingestion of water
- Psychiatric disorders with polydipsia
- Kidney failure
- Irrigation with hypotonic fluids
- Syndrome of inappropriate antidiuretic hormone secretion
- Heart failure
- Liver cirrhosis

H

Interprofessional Collaborative Care
Recognize Cues: Assessment
- Assess for and document:
  1. Cerebral changes
     - Acute confusion
     - Reduced level of cognition
     - Seizure activity
  2. Neuromuscular changes
     - General muscle weakness, especially in arms and legs
     - Diminished deep tendon reflexes

! NURSING SAFETY PRIORITY
Action Alert

If muscle weakness is present, immediately check respiratory effectiveness because ventilation depends on adequate strength of respiratory muscles.

3. GI changes
   * Increased motility
   * Diarrhea
   * Abdominal cramping
   * Hyperactive bowel sounds
4. Cardiovascular changes
   * Hyponatremia with hypovolemia
     * Rapid, weak, thready pulse
     * Reduced peripheral pulses
     * Hypotension
   * Hyponatremia with hypervolemia
     * Full, bounding pulse
     * Normal or high BP
     * Edema

Take Actions: Interventions

* The priorities for nursing care of the patient with hyponatremia are to monitor the patient's response to therapy and prevent hypernatremia and fluid overload.
  1. Drug therapy
     * Discontinue or reduce drugs that increase sodium loss, such as most diuretics.
     * If hyponatremic with a fluid deficit, anticipate administering IV saline infusion to restore both sodium and fluid volume; severe hyponatremia may be treated with small-volume infusions of hypertonic (3%) saline.
     * If hyponatremic with fluid excess, drug therapy includes drugs that promote the excretion of water rather than sodium (e.g., vasopressin receptor antagonists such as conivaptan or tolvaptan) (Sterns, 2022).
     * If hyponatremia caused by inappropriate secretion of antidiuretic hormone (ADH), anticipate therapy that includes agents that antagonize ADH, such as lithium and demeclocycline.
  2. Monitor the amount and quality of oral and IV intake and urine output.
  3. Evaluate serum and urine lab results for electrolyte panel and osmolality.
  4. Weigh daily.
  5. Observe for signs and complications of electrolyte imbalance in neurologic, muscular, GI, and cardiovascular health, including ECG patterns.
  6. Collaborate with the registered dietitian nutritionist (RDN) to increase sodium intake and, if prescribed, restrict fluid intake.

See Chapter 13 in the main text for more information on hyponatremia.

HYPOPARATHYROIDISM

- **Hypoparathyroidism** is a rare disorder in which parathyroid function is decreased, serum calcium levels cannot be maintained, and *hypocalcemia* (low serum calcium level) results. Problems are directly related to a lack of parathyroid hormone (PTH) secretion or to decreased effectiveness of PTH on target tissue.
- Hypoparathyroidism occurs most often postsurgically after removal of the thyroid or parathyroid glands, or after surgery for head or neck cancers.

Interprofessional Collaborative Care
Recognize Cues: Assessment
- Obtain patient information about:
  1. Any head or neck surgery, injury, or radiation therapy
  2. Presence of mild tingling and numbness around the mouth or in the hands and feet
  3. Presence of muscle cramps and spasms of the hands and feet
- Assess for and document hypocalcemia signs or symptoms:
  1. Symptoms of tetany from hypocalcemia, including numbness or tingling (mild) or cramping and spasms (moderate or severe)
     - Positive Chvostek or Trousseau sign (see *Hypocalcemia*)
  2. Irritability, psychosis, or seizures
  3. Bands or pits encircling the crowns of the teeth indicating a loss of tooth calcium and enamel
- Diagnostic tests for hypoparathyroidism include:
  1. Serum electrolyte tests, vitamin D and PTH levels

Take Actions: Interventions
- Nonsurgical management of hypoparathyroidism focuses on correcting hypocalcemia and preventing kidney stones.
- Drug therapy includes the following:
  1. Oral calcitriol and calcium carbonate may also be given, depending on the severity of the hypocalcemia and with milder symptoms.
  2. Oral vitamin D supplementation may be given with mild hypocalcemia.
  3. Long-term oral therapy for hypocalcemia involves the intake of calcium (usually calcium carbonate), 1 to 2 g daily, in divided doses.
- Nursing management includes teaching:
  1. Inform the patient and family about the drug regimen and the need for ongoing monitoring and adjustments.
  2. Collaborate with the registered dietitian nutritionist (RDN) to identify and include foods high in calcium but low in

H

phosphorus (milk, yogurt, and processed cheeses are avoided because of their high phosphorus content).
3. Advise the patient to wear a medical alert bracelet.
4. Teach the patient that therapy for hypocalcemia is lifelong.

See Chapter 55 in the main text for more information on hypoparathyroidism.

HYPOPITUITARISM

* Hypopituitarism is a deficiency of one or more anterior pituitary hormones, resulting in metabolic problems that vary, depending on the undersecreted hormones.
* Decreased production of all anterior pituitary hormones is a rare condition known as panhypopituitarism.
* Usually, there is a decrease in the secretion of one hormone (selective hypopituitarism) and a lesser decrease in the other hormones.
* Deficiencies of ACTH and TSH are the most life-threatening because they result in a corresponding decrease in the secretion of vital hormones from the adrenal and thyroid glands.
* Other deficiencies include gonadotropins (luteinizing hormone [LH] and follicle-stimulating hormone [FSH]), and growth hormone.

KEY FEATURES
Pituitary Hypofunction

Deficient Hormone	Signs and Symptoms
Anterior Pituitary Hormones	
Adrenocorticotropic hormone (ACTH)	Anorexia
	Decreased axillary and pubic hair (women)
	Decreased serum cortisol levels
	Headache
	Hypoglycemia
	Hyponatremia
	Malaise and lethargy
	Pale/ash gray complexion
	Postural hypotension

KEY FEATURES—cont'd

Pituitary Hypofunction

Deficient Hormone	Signs and Symptoms
Gonadotropins • Luteinizing hormone (LH) • Follicle-stimulating hormone (FSH)	Women: • Amenorrhea • Anovulation • Breast atrophy • Decreased axillary and pubic hair • Decreased libido • Loss of bone density • Low estrogen levels Men: • Decreased body hair • Decreased facial hair • Decreased ejaculate volume • Decreased libido • Impotence • Loss of bone density • Reduced muscle mass
Growth hormone (GH)	Decreased bone density Decreased muscle strength Increased serum cholesterol levels Pathologic fractures
Thyroid-stimulating hormone (TSH, thyrotropin)	Alopecia Decreased libido Decreased thyroid hormone levels Hirsutism Intolerance to cold Lethargy Menstrual abnormalities Slowed cognition Weight gain

Posterior Pituitary Hormones

Vasopressin (antidiuretic hormone [ADH])	AVP-D (diabetes insipidus): • Dehydration • Greatly increased urine output • Hypotension • Increased plasma osmolarity • Increased plasma electrolyte levels, especially sodium • Increased thirst • Low urine specific gravity (<1.005) • Urine output that does not decrease when fluid intake decreases

H

Interprofessional Collaborative Care
Recognize Cues: Assessment
- Assess for and document changes noted in the key features of pituitary hypofunction
- Diagnostic assessment may include:
  1. Blood levels of pituitary hormones
  2. Hormone stimulation testing
  3. MRI of the head
  4. Angiography (brain)

Take Actions: Interventions
- Management of the patient with hypopituitarism focuses on replacement of deficient hormones.
- Instruct the patient about the hormone replacement method and regimen.
  1. Men with gonadotropin deficiency receive sex steroid replacement therapy with androgens (testosterone) parenterally or with transdermal testosterone patches.
     - High doses are used until virilization (presence of male secondary sex characteristics) occurs; then maintenance doses are used.
     - Side effects may include gynecomastia (development of breast tissue in men), acne, baldness, and prostate enlargement.
     - Fertility is difficult to achieve and requires additional therapy.
  2. Women who have gonadotropin deficiency receive hormone replacement with a combination of estrogen and progesterone.
     - Combined estrogen and progestin are used, usually orally or by transdermal patch.
     - Complications include hypertension and deep vein thrombosis.
     - Additional therapy is needed for fertility.
  3. Adult patients with growth hormone deficiency may be treated with injections of growth hormones.

See Chapter 54 in the main text for more information on hypopituitarism.

HYPOTHYROIDISM: CELLULAR REGULATION CONCEPT ✳ EXEMPLAR

Overview

- **Hypothyroidism** is reduced or absent hormone secretion from the thyroid gland that results in decreased metabolism from inadequate *cellular regulation*.
- Most cases of hypothyroidism in the United States occur as a result of an autoimmune problem resulting from Hashimoto thyroiditis (HT), thyroid surgery, or radioactive iodine (RAI) treatment of hyperthyroidism.
- Worldwide, hypothyroidism is common in areas where the soil and water have little natural iodide, a mineral essential to normal thyroid function.
- Myxedema coma is a rare, serious complication of untreated or poorly treated hypothyroidism.
    1. Myxedema is characterized by changes in the patient's appearance from the formation of nonpitting edema, especially around the eyes, hands, feet, and between the shoulder blades.

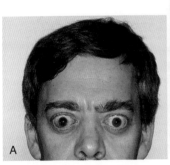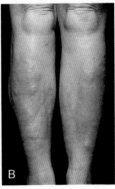

(A) Exophthalmos. (B) Pretibial myxedema. (From Belchetz, P., & Hammond, P. [2003]. *Mosby's color atlas and text of diabetes and endocrinology.* Edinburgh: Mosby.)

H

    2. Myxedema coma, sometimes called "hypothyroid crisis," is a rare, serious complication with a high mortality rate.
        - The decreased metabolism causes the heart muscle to become flabby and the chamber size to increase, similar to HF.
        - Decreased cardiac output and decreased perfusion to the brain and other vital organs make the already slowed cellular metabolism worse, resulting in multiple tissue and organ failure.

Interprofessional Collaborative Care
Recognize Cues: Assessment
- Obtain patient information about:
  1. Energy levels, including activity levels and amount of time sleeping now compared with the previous time period of assessment
  2. Generalized weakness, anorexia, muscle aches, and paresthesias
  3. Constipation
  4. Cold intolerance (use of more blankets at night or sweaters and extra clothing, even in warm weather)
  5. Change in libido
  6. Heavy, prolonged menses or amenorrhea
  7. Impotence and infertility
  8. Current or previous use of drugs known to interfere with thyroid function, such as lithium, amiodarone, aminoglutethimide, sodium or potassium perchlorate, thiocyanates, or cobalt
  9. Medical history, including prior treatment for hyperthyroidism and the specific treatment
  10. Recent weight gain
- Assess for and document:
  1. Key features of hypothyroidism
  2. Diagnostic blood and imaging results, including:
     - Triiodothyronine (T_3)
     - Thyroxin (T_4)
     - TSH levels

Analyze Cues and Prioritize Hypotheses: Analysis
- The priority problems for patients who have hypothyroidism are:
  1. Decreased *gas exchange* and oxygenation as a result of decreased energy, obesity, muscle weakness, and fatigue
  2. Reduced perfusion due to decreased heart rate
  3. Potential for the complication of myxedema coma

Generate Solutions and Take Actions: Planning and Implementation
Improving Gas Exchange
- Respiratory and cardiac problems are serious, and their management is a priority.
  1. Observe and record the rate and depth of respirations.
  2. Measure oxygen saturation by pulse oximetry.
  3. Apply oxygen if the patient has hypoxemia.
  4. Auscultate the lungs for a decrease in breath sounds or presence of crackles.
  5. If hypothyroidism is severe, the patient may require ventilatory support.
  6. Severe respiratory distress occurs with myxedema coma.

KEY FEATURES

Hypothyroidism

Cardiovascular Symptoms
- Bradycardia
- Decreased activity tolerance
- Diastolic hypertension
- Pericardial effusion

Respiratory Symptoms
- Dyspnea
- Hypoventilation
- Pleural effusion

Gastrointestinal Symptoms
- Abdominal distention/ascites
- Constipation
- Weight gain

Metabolic Symptoms
- Decreased basal metabolic rate
- Decreased body temperature
- Cold intolerance

Reproductive Symptoms
Women
- Anovulation
- Decreased libido
- Menstrual changes (amenorrhea or prolonged periods)

Men
- Decreased libido
- Impotence

Psychosocial Symptoms
- Apathy
- Depression

Integumentary Symptoms
- Cool, pale/ash gray, dry, coarse, scaly skin
- Decreased hair growth, with loss of eyebrow hair
- Dry, coarse, brittle hair
- Poor wound healing
- Thick, brittle nails

Neuromuscular Symptoms
- Confusion
- Decreased tendon reflexes
- Hearing loss
- Impaired memory
- Inattentiveness
- Lethargy or somnolence
- Muscle aches and pain
- Paresthesia of the extremities
- Slowing of intellectual functions
- Slowness or slurring of speech

Other Symptoms
- Facial puffiness
- Goiter (enlarged thyroid gland)
- Hoarseness
- Nonpitting edema of the hands and feet
- Periorbital edema
- Thick tongue
- Weakness, fatigue

H

- Drug therapy to restore cellular regulation is the mainstay of management for hypothyroidism.
- The patient requires lifelong thyroid hormone replacement; the most commonly used drug is levothyroxine.
  1. Therapy is started with a low dose that is gradually increased over a period of weeks.

2. The patient with more severe symptoms of hypothyroidism is started on the lowest dose of thyroid hormone replacement because starting at too high a dose or increasing the dose too rapidly can cause severe hypertension, HF, and myocardial infarction.

NURSING SAFETY PRIORITY
Drug Alert

Teach patients and families who are beginning thyroid replacement therapy to take the drug *exactly* as prescribed and not to change the dose or schedule without consulting the primary health care provider. Levothyroxine should be taken with water on an empty stomach, 30 to 60 minutes before a meal in the morning. Teach the patient that there are several drugs that can reduce the absorption of this medication, such as iron, calcium supplements, and antacids. These drugs should be taken separately from levothyroxine administration by at least 4 hours.

- Monitor for and teach the patient and family about the signs of hyperthyroidism including:
  1. Tachycardia
  2. Intolerance to heat
  3. Difficulty sleeping
  4. Diarrhea
  5. Excessive weight loss
  6. Fine tremors of the hands

Preventing Myxedema Coma
- *Myxedema coma* is a severe and life-threatening form of hypothyroidism in which the patient's overall metabolism slows to the point that cardiac and respiratory arrest can occur.
- Factors leading to myxedema coma include acute illness, surgery, chemotherapy, discontinuance of thyroid replacement therapy, and the use of sedatives or opioids.
- Signs and symptoms include:
  1. Respiratory failure
  2. Coma
  3. Hypotension
  4. Hyponatremia
  5. Hypothermia
  6. Hypoglycemia

- Emergency care of the patient with myxedema coma includes:
    1. Maintain a patent airway.
    2. Replace fluids with IV normal or hypertonic saline as per orders.
    3. Replace T_3 and/or T_4 via IV as per orders.
    4. Give glucose IV as per orders
    5. Administer corticosteroids as prescribed.
    6. Check the patient's temperature hourly.
    7. Monitor blood pressure hourly.
    8. Cover the patient with warm blankets.
    9. Monitor for changes in mental status.
    10. Turn every 2 hours.
    11. Institute aspiration precautions.

Care Coordination and Transition Management
- Hypothyroidism is usually a chronic condition, and the patient may live in any type of environment. Ensure that whoever is responsible for overseeing the patient's daily care is aware of the condition and understands its treatment.
- The patient may need help from family, friends, or a home care aide with the drug regimen.
- Develop a plan for drug therapy so that doses are neither missed nor duplicated.
- Teach the patient and family about hormone replacement therapy and its side effects.
    1. Emphasize the need for lifelong drugs.
    2. Review the signs and symptoms of both hyperthyroidism and hypothyroidism.
    3. Teach the patient to wear a medical alert bracelet and to sustain health provider contact, follow-up blood tests, and the need for periodic reevaluation during changes in health and with aging.
    4. Instruct the patient to carefully evaluate OTC drugs because thyroid hormone preparations interact with many other drugs.
- Teach the patient to monitor for therapy effectiveness by assessing the need for sleep and the frequency of bowel elimination.
    1. When the patient requires more sleep and is constipated, the dose of replacement hormone may need to be increased.
    2. When the patient has difficulty getting to sleep and has more bowel movements than normal, the dose may need to be decreased.

H

Evaluate Outcomes: Evaluation

- Evaluate the care of the patient with hypothyroidism based on the identified priority patient problems. The expected outcomes are that with proper management the patient should:
    1. Maintain normal cardiovascular function with a pulse above 60 beats/min and a blood pressure within normal limits for age and general health
    2. Maintain adequate respiratory function and **gas exchange** with SpO_2 above 92%
    3. Demonstrate improvement in cognition

See Chapter 55 in the main text for more information on hypothyroidism.

INFECTION

Overview

- *Infection* is the invasion of *pathogens* (harmful microorganisms) into the body that multiply and cause disease or illness.
- Infections can be communicable (transmitted from person to person [e.g., COVID-19]) or not communicable (e.g., peritonitis).
- Transmission of infection requires three factors:
  1. Reservoir (or source) of infectious agents
  2. Susceptible host with a portal of entry
  3. Route and method of transmission
- Immunity is the protection from illness or disease that is maintained by the body's physiologic defenses. Breakdown of these defense mechanisms may increase the susceptibility (risk) of the host for infection.
- The patient's immune status plays a large role in determining risk for infection.

Factors That May Increase Risk for Infection in the Older Patient	
Factor	**Aging-Associated Changes or Conditions**
Immune system	Decreased antibody production, lymphocytes, and fever response
Integumentary system	Thinning skin, decreased subcutaneous tissue, decreased vascularity, slower wound healing
Respiratory system	Decreased cough and gag reflexes
Gastrointestinal system	Decreased gastric acid and intestinal motility
Chronic illness	Diabetes mellitus, chronic obstructive pulmonary disease, neurologic impairments
Functional/cognitive impairments	Immobility, incontinence, dementia
Invasive devices	Urinary catheters, feeding tubes, IV devices, tracheostomy tubes
Institutionalization	Increased person-to-person contact and transmission

- Pathogens can enter the body through many routes of transmission, such as the respiratory tract, where microbes in droplets can be sprayed into the air when infected persons sneeze, talk, or cough. These droplets are then inhaled by a susceptible host, where the pathogens can localize in the lungs or distribute throughout the body via the lymphatic system or the bloodstream. Pathogens can also enter the body via the gastrointestinal (GI) tract, genitourinary tract, breaks in the skin, and the bloodstream.
- For infection to be transmitted from an infected source to a susceptible host, a transport mechanism is required:
  1. Contact transmission (indirect and direct)
  2. Droplet transmission
  3. Airborne transmission
- Prevention of infection and detecting signs and symptoms of infection as early as possible are integral elements of care.
- Infection acquired in the inpatient health care setting (not present or incubating at admission) is termed a health care–associated infection (HAI). HAIs can be endogenous (from a patient's flora) or exogenous (from outside the patient, often from the hands of health care workers, tubes, or implants).
- Health care workers' hands are the primary way in which infection is transmitted from patient to patient or staff to patient. Hand hygiene refers to both handwashing and alcohol-based hand rubs (ABHRs) ("hand sanitizers").
- Standard Precautions are based on the belief that all body excretions, secretions, and moist membranes and tissues, excluding perspiration, are potentially infectious.
  1. As barriers to potential or actual infections, personal protective equipment (PPE) is used. PPE refers to gloves, isolation gowns, face protection (masks, goggles, face shields), and powered air-purifying respirators (PAPRs) or N95 respirators.

Transmission-Based Infection Control Precautions

Precautions (in Addition to Standard Precautions)	Examples of Diseases in Category
Airborne Precautions	
1. Private room required with monitored negative airflow (with appropriate number of air exchanges and air discharge to outside or through HEPA filter); keep door(s) closed	Diseases that are known or suspected to be transmitted by air: • Measles (rubeola) • *Mycobacterium tuberculosis,* including multidrug-resistant TB (MDRTB) • Varicella (chicken pox)[b]; disseminated zoster (shingles)[b] • COVID-19 (likely spread as airborne)

Precautions (in Addition to Standard Precautions)	Examples of Diseases in Category

2. Special respiratory protection:
   - Wear PAPR for known or suspected TB.
   - Susceptible people not to enter room of patient with known or suspected measles or varicella unless immune caregivers are not available
   - Susceptible people who must enter room must wear PAPR or N95 HEPA filter.[a]
3. Transport: patient to leave room only for essential clinical reasons, wearing surgical mask

Droplet Precautions

1. Private room preferred: if not available, may cohort with patient with same active infection with same microorganisms if no other infection present; maintain distance of at least 3 feet from other patients if private room not available
2. Mask: required when working within 3 feet of patient
3. Transport: as for Airborne Precautions

Diseases that are known or suspected to be transmitted by droplets:
- Diphtheria (pharyngeal)
- Streptococcal pharyngitis
- Pneumonia
- Influenza
- COVID-19
- Rubella
- Invasive disease (meningitis, pneumonia, sepsis) caused by *Haemophilus influenzae* type B or *Neisseria meningitidis*
- Mumps
- Pertussis

Contact Precautions

1. Private room preferred: if not available, may cohort with patient with same active infection with same microorganisms if no other infection present
2. Wear gloves when entering room.
3. Wash hands with antimicrobial soap before leaving patient's room.
4. Wear gown to prevent contact with patient or contaminated items or if patient has uncontrolled body fluids; remove gown before leaving room.
5. Transport: patient to leave room only for essential clinical reasons; during transport, use needed precautions to prevent disease transmission
6. Dedicated equipment for this patient only (or disinfect after use before taking from room)

Diseases that are known or suspected to be transmitted by direct contact:
- *Clostridium difficile*
- Colonization or infection caused by multidrug-resistant organisms (e.g., MRSA, VRE)
- Pediculosis
- Scabies
- COVID-19 (possibly)

[a]Before use: training and fit testing required for personnel.
[b]Add Contact Precautions for draining lesions.
HEPA, High-efficiency particulate air; *MRSA*, methicillin-resistant *Staphylococcus aureus*; *PAPR*, powered air-purifying respirator; *TB*, tuberculosis; *VRE*, vancomycin-resistant *Enterococcus*.

> **⚠ NURSING SAFETY PRIORITY**
>
> ### Action Alert
>
> Remember that gloves are an essential part of infection control and should always be worn as part of Standard Precautions. Either handwashing or the use of ABHRs should be done before donning (putting on) and after removing gloves. The combination of hand hygiene and wearing gloves is the most effective strategy for preventing infection transmission!

Antimicrobial Resistance

- Antibiotics have been available for many years. These drugs were commonly prescribed for conditions that did not need them or were given at higher doses and for longer periods of time than were necessary. As a result, a number of microorganisms have become resistant to certain antibiotics; that is, drugs that were once useful no longer control these infectious agents (multidrug-resistant organisms [MDROs]). Common MDROs are:

1. Methicillin-resistant *Staphylococcus aureus* (MRSA)
   - MRSA is spread by direct contact and invades hospitalized patients through indwelling urinary catheters, vascular access devices, open wounds, and endotracheal tubes.
   - It is susceptible to only a few antibiotics, such as IV vancomycin and oral linezolid. IV ceftaroline is the first cephalosporin antibiotic approved to treat MRSA (Burchum & Rosenthal, 2022).
2. Vancomycin-resistant *Enterococcus* (VRE)
   - *Enterococci* are bacteria that live in the intestinal tract and are important for digestion. When they move to another area of the body, such as during surgery, they can cause an infection, which is usually treatable with vancomycin.
   - In recent years, many of these infections have become resistant to the drug, and VRE results. Risk factors for this infection include prolonged hospital stays, severe illness, abdominal surgery, enteral nutrition, and immunosuppression. Place patients with VRE infections on Contact Precautions to prevent contamination from body fluids.
3. Carbapenem-resistant *Enterobacteriaceae* (CRE)
   - CRE is a family of pathogens that are difficult to treat because they have a high level of resistance to carbapenem antibiotics caused by enzymes that break down the antibiotics.
   - Patients who are at high risk for CRE include those in ICUs or nursing homes and patients who are immunosuppressed, including older adults.

Interprofessional Collaborative Care

Recognize Cues: Assessment

- Assess and document patient history, including:
  1. Age, history of tobacco or alcohol use, current illness or disease, poor nutritional status, or current therapies such as chemotherapy or radiation that can alter *immunity*
  2. Ask patients whether they have recently been in a hospital or nursing home, or whether they have had any recent invasive testing (such as a colonoscopy).
  3. Travel history
  4. Sexual history
  5. Type and location of symptoms

Physical Assessment
- Common signs and symptoms are associated with specific sites of infection.
- Fever (generally above 101°F [38.3°C], chills, and malaise are primary indicators of systematic infection.
- Lymphadenopathy (enlarged lymph nodes), pharyngitis, and GI disturbance (usually diarrhea or vomiting) are often associated with infection.

Laboratory Assessment
- The definitive diagnosis of an infectious disease requires identification of a microorganism in the tissues of an infected patient.
- The best procedure for identifying a microorganism is culture, or isolation of the pathogen by cultivation in tissue cultures or artificial media.
- A white blood cell (WBC) count is often done for the patient with a suspected infection. The normal range for WBCs is 5000/mm^3 (5.0 × 10^9/L) to 10,000/mm^3 (10.0 × 10^9/L) (Pagana et al., 2022).

Analysis: Analyze Cues and Prioritize Hypotheses

- The priority collaborative problem for patients with an infection is fever due to the immune response triggered by the pathogen. In addition, the patient has a potential for developing severe sepsis and septic shock.

Generate Solutions and Take Actions: Planning and Implementation

Managing Fever
- The primary concern is to eliminate the underlying cause of the fever and destroy the causative microorganism.

Drug Therapy
- Antimicrobials (called antiinfective agents) are the cornerstone of drug therapy.
- Antipyretic drugs such as acetaminophen are often given to reduce fever. These drugs often mask fever, which makes it difficult to monitor the course of the disease. As a result, antipyretics are not always prescribed.

NURSING SAFETY PRIORITY
Drug Alert

Before administering an antimicrobial drug, check to see that the patient is not allergic to it. Be sure to take an accurate allergy history before drug therapy begins to prevent possible life-threatening reactions, such as anaphylaxis.

Other Interventions
- External cooling using hypothermia blankets or ice packs can be effective for reducing a high fever. Assess for shivering because this can be an indication that the patient is being cooled too quickly.
- Monitor fluid balance because fluid volume loss is increased in a patient with a fever.

Care Coordination and Transition Management
- Patients with infections may be cared for in the home (group or individual), hospital, nursing home, or ambulatory care setting, depending on the type and severity of the infection.
  1. Explaining the disease and making certain that the patient understands what is causing the illness are the primary purposes of health teaching.
  2. For the patient who is discharged to the home setting to complete a course of antimicrobial therapy, the importance of adherence to the planned drug regimen needs to be stressed. Explain the importance of both the timing of doses and the completion of the planned number of days of therapy.
  3. Many patients are discharged with an infusion device to continue drug therapy at home or in other inpatient facilities.

 See Chapter 19 in the main text for more information on infection.

INFLUENZA, SEASONAL

- Seasonal influenza, or "flu," is a highly contagious, acute viral respiratory infection that can occur at any age.
- Influenza infection can lead to complications of pneumonia or death, especially in older adults, those with heart failure or chronic lung disorders, and in immunocompromised patients.
  1. Seasonal influenza can be prevented or its severity reduced when adults receive an annual influenza vaccination.
     - The vaccine is changed every year based on which specific viral strains are most likely to cause illness during the influenza season (i.e., late fall and winter in the Northern Hemisphere).
  2. For adults aged over 65 years, a higher-dose, quadrivalent vaccine is available for increased protection for adults with age-related reduced *immunity* (Hibberd, 2023).
  3. Although annual vaccination is not 100% effective at preventing influenza, it is especially important for adults who:
     - Are older than 50 years
     - Have chronic illness or immune compromise
     - Reside in institutions
     - Live with or care for others with health problems that put them at risk for severe complications of influenza
     - Are health care personnel providing direct care to patients (CDC, 2021)

Interprofessional Collaborative Care

- Symptoms typically have a sudden onset:
  1. Severe headache
  2. Fever, chills, fatigue, weakness, muscle aches
  3. Sore throat, cough, watery nasal discharge
  4. Influenza type B can lead to nausea, vomiting, and diarrhea.
- Viral infections do not respond to antibiotic therapy. Neuraminidase inhibitor (NAI) antiviral drugs such as oseltamivir, zanamivir, peramivir, and baloxavir have been effective in the prevention and treatment of some strains of influenza.
  1. To be most effective as treatment rather than for prevention, these antiviral drugs must be taken within 24 to 48 hours after symptoms begin.

See Chapter 25 in the main text for more information on influenza.

IRRITABLE BOWEL SYNDROME

- Irritable bowel syndrome (IBS) is a functional GI disorder that causes chronic or recurrent diarrhea, constipation, and/or abdominal *pain* and bloating.
- Increased or decreased bowel transit times result in changes in the normal *bowel elimination* pattern to one of these classifications: diarrhea (IBS-D), constipation (IBS-C), or a mix of diarrhea and constipation (IBS-M).
- The etiology is unclear and a combination of environmental, immunologic, genetic, hormonal, and stress factors has a role in the development and course of IBS.

Interprofessional Collaborative Care
Recognize Cues: Assessment
- Assess for and document:
  1. Fatigue, malaise
  2. Abdominal *pain* or cramps, particularly in the left lower quadrant of the abdomen
  3. Changes in the bowel pattern (diarrhea, constipation, or an alternating pattern of both) or consistency of stools and the passage of mucus
  4. Food intolerance
  5. Serum albumin, CBC, erythrocyte sedimentation rate, and *Helicobacter pylori* testing to detect infection and nutritional deficits
     - Some health care providers request a *hydrogen breath test* or small-bowel bacterial overgrowth breath test. When small-intestinal bacterial overgrowth or malabsorption of nutrients is present, an excess of hydrogen is produced. Some of this hydrogen is absorbed into the bloodstream and travels to the lungs, where it is exhaled. Patients with IBS often exhale increased amounts of hydrogen.
  6. Occult blood or melena

Take Actions: Interventions
- The patient with IBS is usually managed on an ambulatory care basis and learns self-management strategies. Interventions include health teaching, drug therapy, and stress reduction.
- Diet therapy includes:
  1. Suggesting a symptom diary to help identify triggers and bowel habits
  2. Helping the patient identify and eliminate foods associated with exacerbations

3. Consulting with the dietitian to promote intake of fiber and fluid
   - Teaching the patient to ingest 30 to 40 g of fiber daily
   - Teaching the patient to drink 8 to 10 glasses of liquid per day
- Drug therapy includes the following:
  1. Bulk-forming laxatives, such as psyllium hydrophilic mucilloid, may be taken at mealtimes with a glass of water to prevent dry, hard, or liquid stools.
  2. Lubiprostone can be used to increase intestinal fluid and promote bowel elimination in IBS-C.
  3. Linaclotide is the newest drug for IBS-C, which works by simulating receptors in the intestines to increase fluid and promote bowel transit time. The drug also helps relieve *pain* and cramping that are associated with IBS.
  4. Antidiarrheal agents such as loperamide may be used to decrease cramping and frequency of stools.
  5. Alosetron, a serotonin-selective (5-HT$_3$) drug, may be used with caution for women with diarrhea-predominant IBS-D; it has many drug-drug interactions.
  6. Patients with IBS who have bloating and abdominal distention without constipation may be prescribed rifaximin, an antibiotic with little systemic absorption.
  7. For IBS in which pain is the predominant symptom, tricyclic antidepressants, such as amitriptyline, have also been used successfully.
  8. Complementary and integrative health includes:
     - Probiotics to reduce bacteria and alleviate GI symptoms of IBS
     - Peppermint oil capsules to reduce GI symptoms
     - Stress management such as meditation, imagery, and/or yoga to decrease GI symptoms

See Chapter 48 in the main text for more information on irritable bowel syndrome.

KIDNEY DISEASE, CHRONIC: ELIMINATION
✳ CONCEPT EXEMPLAR

Overview
- Chronic kidney disease (CKD) is a progressive, irreversible disorder lasting longer than 3 months (Ferri, 2022).
- CKD is classified in five stages based on the glomerular filtration rate (GFR) category.

Stages of Chronic Kidney Disease

Stage	Estimated Glomerular Filtration Rate	Intervention
Stage 1		
At risk; normal kidney function but urine findings indicate kidney disease	>90 mL/min/ 1.73 m^2	Screen for risk factors and manage care to reduce risk: • Uncontrolled hypertension • Diabetes with poor glycemic control • Congenital or acquired anatomic or urinary tract abnormalities • Family history of genetic kidney diseases • Exposure to nephrotoxic substances
Stage 2		
Slightly reduced kidney function	60–89 mL/min/ 1.73 m^2	Focus on reduction of risk factors.
Stage 3		
Moderately reduced kidney function	30–59 mL/min/ 1.73 m^2	Implement strategies to slow disease progression.
Stage 4		
Severely reduced kidney function; a noticeable jaundice can occur, particularly around the eyes	15–29 mL/min/ 1.73 m^2	Manage complications. Discuss patient preferences and values. Educate about options and prepare for renal replacement therapy.
Stage 5		
End-stage kidney disease (ESKD)	<15 mL/min/ 1.73 m^2	Implement renal replacement therapy or kidney transplantation.

- The risk for progression of CKD, ESKD, and mortality is increased when urine albumin increases.
- Albumin in the urine is a marker of kidney damage, whereas GFR reflects kidney function.
- Three albuminuria stages also are considered in evaluating CKD. These stages are defined by the albumin-to-creatinine ratio in urine.
  1. The first stage (A1) is a none to mildly increased albumin, up to 29 mg/g creatinine (<3 mg/mmol) and is sometimes called *microalbuminuria*.
  2. The second (A2) stage has values of 30 to 300 mg/g creatinine (3 to 30 mg/mmol).
  3. The stage of greatest kidney damage (A3) has values >300mg/g creatinine (>30 mg/mmol).
- The combined values help to identify adults at risk for progression of CKD and its complications, and help to guide interventions.
- CKD with greatly reduced GFR causes many problems, including abnormal urine production, severe disruption of **fluid and electrolyte balance**, and metabolic abnormalities.
  1. Kidney changes
     - Because healthy nephrons become larger and work harder, urine production and water **elimination** are sufficient to maintain essential homeostasis until about three-fourths of kidney function is lost.
     - As the disease progresses, the ability to produce diluted urine is reduced, resulting in urine with a fixed osmolarity (*isosthenuria*).
  2. Metabolic changes
     - Creatinine comes from proteins in skeletal muscle. The rate of creatinine excretion depends on muscle mass, physical activity, and diet. Creatinine is partially excreted by the kidney tubules, and a decrease in kidney function leads to a buildup of serum creatinine.
     - Early in CKD, the patient is at risk for *hyponatremia* (sodium depletion) because there are fewer healthy nephrons to reabsorb sodium and sodium is lost in the urine.
     - In the later stages of CKD, kidney excretion of sodium is reduced as urine production decreases. Then sodium retention and high serum sodium levels (*hypernatremia*) occur.
     - Hyperkalemia results from an increase in potassium load, including ingestion of potassium in drugs, failure to restrict potassium in the diet, blood transfusions, and excess bleeding.
     - Other metabolic changes in CKD include changes in pH (metabolic acidosis), calcium (hypocalcemia) and

K

phosphorus (hyperphosphatemia) imbalances, and vitamin D insufficiency.
- Renal osteodystrophy is skeletal demineralization manifested by bone pain, pseudo fractures, sclerosis of the spine, skull demineralization, osteomalacia, reabsorption of bone, and loss of tooth lamina.
- Hypophosphatemia results in parathyroid dysfunction and accelerates bone loss.

3. Cardiac changes
- Hypertension is common in most patients with CKD. It may be either the cause or the result of CKD. Hyperlipidemia, heart failure, uremic cardiomyopathy, and pericarditis may also occur.
- **Cardiorenal syndrome** refers to disorders of the kidney or heart that cause dysfunction in the other organ. The kidney and the heart have a reciprocal relationship that can make an alteration in one cause an alteration in the other (Ferri, 2022).

4. Hematologic and immunity changes
- Anemia is common in patients in the later stages of CKD and worsens CKD symptoms.
- The causes of anemia include a decreased erythropoietin level with reduced red blood cell (RBC) production, decreased RBC survival time from uremia, and iron and folic acid deficiencies. The patient may have increased bleeding or bruising as a result of impaired platelet function.

5. Gastrointestinal changes
- Uremic stomatitis, anorexia, peptic ulcer disease, nausea, and vomiting
- Altered mouth and GI tract flora (microbiome) affect mucous membrane integrity and immunity.

Interprofessional Collaborative Care
- Because patients with CKD are at risk for so many adverse outcomes (not just ESKD), the interprofessional care team includes many specialists and health care providers (e.g., nephrologists, nephrology nurses, pharmacists, registered dietitian nutritionists [RDNs], mental health therapists, physical therapists, case managers, social workers, and clergy or pastoral care workers).

Recognize Cues: Assessment
- Obtain patient information about:
  1. Age
  2. Height and weight, including recent weight gain or loss

   3. Current and past medical conditions
   4. Drugs, prescription and OTC
   5. Family history of kidney disease
   6. Dietary and nutritional habits, including food preferences
   7. History of GI problems, such as nausea, vomiting, anorexia, diarrhea, or constipation
   8. Recent injuries and abnormal bruising or bleeding
   9. Activity intolerance, weakness, and fatigue
  10. Detailed urinary elimination history

- Assess for and document:
  1. Neurologic symptoms
     - Changes in mentation or new lethargy
     - Changes in sensation or weakness in extremities, indicating uremic neuropathy
  2. Cardiovascular symptoms of CKD, which result from fluid overload, hypertension, or cardiac disease
     - Extra heart sounds (particularly S_3)
     - Peripheral edema
  3. Respiratory symptoms of CKD vary.
     - Breath that smells like urine (uremic fetor or halitosis)
     - Kussmaul pattern or deep sighing or yawning to release carbon dioxide, compensating for metabolic acidosis
     - Tachypnea or shortness of breath
     - Lung sounds congruent with pulmonary edema (crackles) or pleural effusion (rub)
  4. Hematologic symptoms
     - Anemia with fatigue, pallor/ash gray skin, and shortness of breath with exertion
     - Abnormal bleeding (skin, GI, vaginal); bruising, petechiae
  5. GI symptoms
     - Mouth ulceration
     - Abdominal pain or cramping
     - Nausea or vomiting
  6. Urinary symptoms
     - Change in urinary amount, frequency, and appearance of urine
     - Proteinuria or hematuria
  7. Skin symptoms
     - Yellow coloration from pigment deposition; darkening of skin for some Black individuals
     - Severe itching (pruritus)
     - Uremic frost, a layer of uremic crystals from evaporated sweat on the face, eyebrows, axilla, and groin (rare)
     - Bruises or purple patches and rashes

K

8. Psychosocial considerations because CKD affects family relations, social activity, work patterns, body image, and sexual activity
   - Anxiety and depression are common responses to CKD.
   - Self-management is essential to attain optimal health outcomes.
- Diagnostic testing may include:
  1. Serum creatinine, blood urea nitrogen (BUN), sodium, potassium, calcium, phosphorus, bicarbonate, hemoglobin, and hematocrit
  2. Urinalysis
  3. A 24-hour urinalysis for creatinine to calculate GFR
  4. Ultrasound, computed tomography (CT) scan, or x-ray to detect small and fibrotic kidneys

Analyze Cues and Prioritize Hypotheses: Analysis
- The priority problems for patients with CKD include:
  1. Fluid overload due to the inability of diseased kidneys to maintain body fluid balance
  2. Decreased cardiac function due to reduced stroke volume, dysrhythmias, fluid overload, and increased peripheral vascular resistance
  3. Weight loss due to inability to ingest, digest, or absorb food and nutrients as a result of physiologic factors
  4. Potential for injury due to effects of kidney disease on bone density, blood clotting, and drug elimination
  5. Potential for psychosocial compromise due to chronic kidney disease

Generate Solutions and Take Actions: Planning and Implementation
- The overall goal of care is to slow the rate of disease progression and preserve elimination for as long as possible.

Managing Fluid Volume
- Achieve and maintain acceptable fluid balance with drug therapy, nutrition therapy, fluid restriction, and dialysis.
  1. Prevent fluid overload with diuretics and, if needed, fluid restriction.
  2. Monitor weight daily.
  3. Monitor serum electrolytes.
  4. Measure and record intake and output, and report concerning imbalances to provider.
- Pulmonary edema can result from left-sided heart failure related to fluid overload or from blood vessel injury.
  1. Assess for early signs of pulmonary edema, such as restlessness, dyspnea, decreased peripheral oxygenation (Spo_2), and crackles.

2. If the patient is dyspneic, place the patient in a high-Fowler's position and give oxygen to maximize lung expansion and improve gas exchange.
3. Assess the cardiovascular system for fluid overload: S_3 heart sounds, peripheral edema, jugular venous distention, tachycardia, hypotension, or hypertension.
4. Provide drug therapy.
   - Diuretics for stages 1 through 4 CKD; monitor for ototoxicity with loop diuretics
   - Morphine to reduce myocardial oxygen demands; monitor for respiratory depression
   - Vasodilators such as nitroglycerin

Improving Cardiac Function

- Cardiac output alterations are related to hypovolemia or hypervolemia, dysrhythmias, cardiomyopathy, pericarditis, and greater peripheral vascular resistance influenced by CKD.
  1. Determine and assist in attaining BP goals typically around 130/80 mm Hg.
     - Administer calcium channel blockers, angiotensin-converting enzyme (ACE) inhibitors, alpha- and beta-adrenergic blockers, and vasodilators as prescribed.
  2. Teach the family to measure the patient's BP and weight daily and to bring these records when visiting the physician, nurse, or nutritionist.
  3. Monitor the patient for decreased cardiac output, heart failure, and dysrhythmias.
     - Notify the health care provider of increasing peripheral edema or decreasing peripheral pulses.
     - Teach the patient and family about the relationships between diet, drug therapy, and cardiovascular health.

Enhancing Nutrition

- The nutritional needs and diet restrictions for the patient with CKD vary according to the degree of remaining kidney function and the type of renal replacement therapy used.
  1. Common changes include control of protein intake; fluid intake limitation; restriction of potassium, sodium, and phosphorus intake; taking vitamin and mineral supplements; and eating enough calories to meet metabolic demand.
  2. Consult with the registered dietitian nutritionist (RDN) to provide nutritional teaching and planning and to assist the patient in adapting the diet to food preferences, ethnic background, and budget.

K

Preventing Injury
- Potential for injury is related to the effects of kidney disease on bone density, blood clotting, drug elimination, and infection.
  1. Implement falls precaution.
  2. Use skin pressure reduction strategies to reduce risk for pressure injury.
  3. Use interprofessional collaboration with the pharmacist to adjust drug doses to avoid toxicity from reduced renal clearance.
  4. Administer drugs to control hyperphosphatemia to prevent renal osteodystrophy.
  5. Avoid drugs that interfere with clotting, such as aspirin.
  6. Monitor the patient closely for drug-related complications.
  7. Teach the patient to avoid certain drugs that can increase kidney damage, such as nonsteroidal antiinflammatory drugs (NSAIDs), antibiotics, antihypertensives, and diuretics, in the presence of hypovolemia.
  8. Instruct the patient to avoid compounds containing magnesium.
  9. Monitor carefully for indicators of infection. These indicators include:
     - Fever
     - Lymph node enlargement
     - Elevated WBC counts
     - Positive cultures
  10. Administer opioid analgesics in patients with stage 3 or 4 CKD or ESKD with caution as the effects often last longer.

Minimizing Psychosocial Compromise
- Fatigue is related to kidney disease, anemia, and reduced energy production.
  1. Establish patient preferences to conserve energy and preserve the ability to perform self-care, retain interest in surroundings, and sustain mental concentration.
  2. Provide vitamin and mineral supplementation.
  3. The anemic patient with CKD is treated with agents to stimulate red blood cell production. The desired outcome of this therapy is to maintain a hemoglobin level around 10 g/dL (100 g/L).
  4. Monitor dietary intake (improved appetite challenges patients in their attempts to maintain limits on protein and potassium) and fluid restriction.

Kidney Replacement Therapies
- Renal replacement therapy is needed when the symptoms of kidney disease present complications that are potentially life-threatening or that pose continuing discomfort to the patient.

- *Hemodialysis* removes excess fluid and waste products and restores chemical and electrolyte balance. It is based on the principle of diffusion, in which the patient's blood is circulated through a semipermeable membrane that acts as an artificial kidney.
  1. Dialysis settings include the acute care facility, freestanding centers, and the home.
  2. Total dialysis time is usually 12 hours per week, which usually is divided into three 4-hour treatments.
  3. A vascular access route is needed to perform hemodialysis.
     - Long-term vascular access for hemodialysis is accomplished by arteriovenous (AV) fistula or graft.
     - Temporary vascular access for hemodialysis is accomplished by a specially designed catheter inserted into the subclavian, internal jugular, or femoral vein.
     - Complications of vascular access include:
       - Thrombosis or stenosis
       - Infection
       - Ischemia
       - Loss of patency

! NURSING SAFETY PRIORITY

Action Alert

Because repeated compression can result in the loss of the vascular access, avoid taking the blood pressure or performing venipunctures in the arm with the vascular access. Do not use an AV fistula or graft for general delivery of IV fluids or drugs.

- Nurses are specially trained to perform hemodialysis.
- Postdialysis care includes:
  1. Closely monitoring for side effects: hypoglycemia, hypotension, headache, nausea, malaise, vomiting, dizziness, and muscle cramps
  2. Obtaining the patient's weight and vital signs
  3. Avoiding invasive procedures for 4 to 6 hours because of anticoagulation used during dialysis
  4. Monitoring for signs of bleeding
  5. Monitoring laboratory results
- Complications of hemodialysis include:
  1. Dialysis disequilibrium syndrome caused by rapid shifts of electrolytes
  2. Hypotension
  3. Cardiac events
  4. Reactions to dialyzers

K

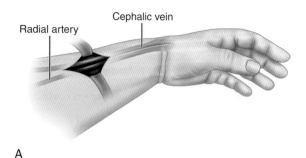

Radial artery

Cephalic vein

A

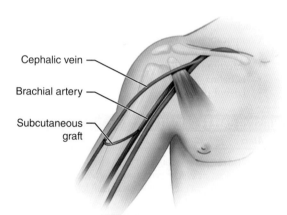

Cephalic vein

Brachial artery

Subcutaneous graft

B

Frequently used means for gaining vascular access for hemodialysis include arteriovenous fistula (A), arteriovenous graft (B), external arteriovenous shunt (C), femoral vein catheterization (D), and subclavian vein catheterization (E). **A** and **B** are options for long-term vascular access for hemodialysis. **C, D,** and **E** are used for short-term access for intermittent hemodialysis or for continuous renal replacement therapy in acute care.

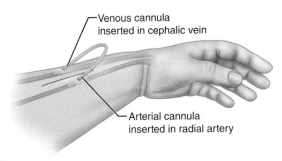

C

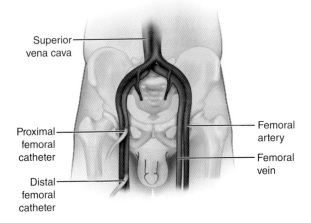

D

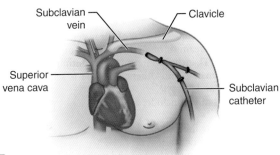

E

Types of Vascular Access for Hemodialysis

Access Type	Description	Location	Time to Initial Use
Permanent			
Arteriovenous (AV) fistula	An internal anastomosis of an artery to a vein	Forearm Upper arm	2–3 months or longer
Arteriovenous (AV) graft	Looped plastic tubing tunneled beneath the skin, connecting an artery and a vein	Forearm Upper arm Inner thigh	1–3 weeks after surgery
Temporary			
Dialysis catheter	A specially designed catheter with separate lumens for blood outflow and inflow	Subclavian vein, internal jugular, or femoral vein	Immediately after insertion and x-ray confirmation of placement
Subcutaneous catheter	An internal device with two access ports and a cuff or dual-lumen catheter inserted into a large central vein	Subclavian vein, internal jugular, or femoral vein	Dedicated use; do not access for blood sampling or drug administration

AV, Arteriovenous.

- *Peritoneal dialysis* (PD), an alternative and slower dialysis method, is accomplished by the surgical insertion of a silicone rubber catheter into the abdominal cavity to instill dialysis solution into the abdominal cavity.
- Candidates for PD include:
  1. Patients who are unable to tolerate anticoagulation
  2. Patients who lack vascular access
  3. Patients without peritoneal adhesions and without extensive abdominal surgery
- The PD process occurs by means of a transfer of fluid and solutes from the bloodstream through the peritoneum.
- The types of PD include intermittent, continuous ambulatory (CAPD), automated, and others; the type is selected based on patient ability and lifestyle.
- Complications of PD include:
  1. Pain
  2. Poor dialysate flow
  3. Leakage of the dialysate
  4. Exit site and tunnel infection and peritonitis

➕ NURSING SAFETY PRIORITY

Critical Rescue

Monitor the patient closely during dialysis to recognize hypotension, which is common. Heat transfer from warm solutions can result in vasodilation and a drop in blood pressure. When this occurs, reduce the temperature of the dialysate to 35°C (95°F). Fluid shifts from the plasma volume related to differences in electrolyte concentrations between HD solutions and blood also reduce blood pressure. Respond to modest declines in blood pressure by adjusting the rate of dialyzer blood flow and placing the patient in a legs-up (Trendelenburg) position. Respond to sustained or symptomatic hypotension by giving a fluid bolus of 100 to 250 mL of normal saline, albumin, or mannitol (if prescribed). A second bolus may be needed. If hypotension persists, new-onset myocardial injury or pericardial disease may be a contributing factor; respond by applying oxygen, reducing the blood flow, and notifying the primary health care provider urgently. Discontinue HD when hypotension continues despite two bolus infusions.

❗ NURSING SAFETY PRIORITY

Action Alert

Monitor the patient to recognize indications of peritonitis (e.g., cloudy dialysate outflow (effluent), fever, abdominal tenderness, abdominal pain, general malaise, nausea, and vomiting). *Cloudy or opaque effluent is the earliest indication of peritonitis.* Examine all effluent for color and clarity to detect peritonitis early. When peritonitis is suspected, respond by sending a specimen of the dialysate outflow for culture and sensitivity study, Gram stain, and cell count to identify the infecting organism.

- Nursing interventions include:
  1. Implementing and monitoring PD therapy and instilling, dwelling, and draining the solution, as ordered
  2. Maintaining PD flow data and monitoring for negative or positive fluid balances
  3. Obtaining baseline and daily weights
  4. Monitoring laboratory results to measure the effectiveness of the treatment
  5. Maintaining accurate intake and output records
  6. Taking vital signs every 15 to 30 minutes during initiation of PD
  7. Performing an ongoing assessment for signs of respiratory distress or pain

- Kidney transplantation is appropriate for selected patients with ESKD.
  1. Discussion about kidney transplant can occur at any time during CKD; it need not wait until stage 5 or dialysis is started. The median wait time for a kidney transplant is 4 years.

Care Coordination and Transition Management
- Case managers can plan, coordinate, and evaluate care.
  1. The physical and occupational therapist collaborates with the patient and family to evaluate the home environment and to obtain needed equipment before discharge.
  2. Refer the patient to home health nursing as needed.

! NURSING SAFETY PRIORITY
Action Alert

Teach patients with mild CKD that carefully managing fluid volume, blood pressure, electrolytes, and other kidney-damaging diseases by following prescribed drug and nutritional therapies can prevent damage and slow the progression to ESKD.

- Provide in-depth health teaching about diet and pathophysiology of kidney disease and drug therapy:
  1. Provide information and emotional support to assist the patient with decisions about treatment course, personal lifestyle, support systems, and coping.
  2. Teach the patient about the hemodialysis treatment.
  3. Teach the patient about care of the vascular access.
  4. Provide patients with home-based renal replacement therapy with extensive teaching, and assist the patient to obtain the needed equipment and supplies. Emphasize the importance of strict sterile technique and of reporting manifestations of infection at any dialysis access site.
  5. Assist the patient and family to identify coping strategies to adjust to the diagnosis and treatment regimen.
  6. Instruct patients and family members in all aspects of diet therapy, drug therapy, and complications. Assist patients to schedule drugs so that drugs will not be unintentionally eliminated by dialysis.
  7. Teach patients and family members to report complications, such as fluid overload, bleeding, and infection.
  8. Stress that although uremic symptoms are reduced as a result of dialysis procedures, patients will not return completely to their previous state of well-being.

9. Instruct the family to monitor the patient for any behaviors that may contribute to nonadherence to the treatment plan and to report such to the health care provider.
10. Refer the patient to a home health nurse and to local and state support groups and agencies such as the National Kidney Foundation.

Evaluate Outcomes: Evaluation

- Evaluate the care of the patient with CKD based on the identified priority problems. The expected outcomes are that, with appropriate management, the patient should:
  1. Achieve and maintain appropriate fluid and electrolyte balance
  2. Maintain an adequate nutritional status
  3. Avoid infection at the vascular access site
  4. Use effective coping strategies
  5. Prevent or slow systemic complications of CKD, including osteodystrophy
  6. Report an absence of physical signs of anxiety or depression

See Chapter 60 in the main text for more information on kidney disease, chronic.

KIDNEY DISEASE, POLYCYSTIC

- Polycystic kidney disease (PKD) is a genetic kidney disorder in which fluid-filled cysts develop in nephrons.
- Growing cysts damage the nephron (i.e., glomerular and tubular membranes), reducing kidney function and causing hypertension.
  1. The cysts do not filter blood; kidney failure will occur over time.
  2. The fluid-filled cysts are at increased risk for infection, rupture, and bleeding; they contribute to kidney stone formation.
  3. Each cystic kidney may enlarge to two to three times its normal size, causing discomfort and abdominal organ displacement.
- Cysts may occur in other tissues, such as the liver or blood vessels.

Interprofessional Collaborative Care
Recognize Cues: Assessment

- Obtain patient information about:
  1. Family history and genetic testing because PKD can be autosomal dominant (most common form of PKD with several different subtypes) or autosomal recessive (more severe, with death typically occurring in early childhood)
  2. Current health status
  3. Changes in urine or pattern of urination
  4. Hypertension

K

- Assess for and document:
  1. Pain (flank or abdominal)
  2. Distended abdomen
  3. Enlarged, tender kidney on palpation
  4. Changes in urine, including hematuria, clarity, odor
  5. Changes in pattern of urination, including nocturia
  6. Dysuria
  7. Vital signs, noting hypertension and fever as needing intervention
  8. Edema
  9. Uremic symptoms: nausea, vomiting, pruritus, and fatigue
  10. Emotional responses such as anger, resentment, futility, sadness, or anxiety related to chronicity or inheritable condition
- Diagnostic studies may include:
  1. Urinalysis with findings of proteinuria and hematuria
  2. Urine culture and sensitivity if infection is suspected
  3. Serum creatinine and BUN to assess kidney function
  4. Renal sonography, CT scan, or MRI to assess the presence and size of cysts

Take Actions: Interventions

- Manage pain.
  1. Provide drug therapy.
     - Administer analgesics for comfort; use NSAIDs cautiously.
     - Administer antibiotics if a cyst infection is causing discomfort.
- Provide hypertension and fluid management.
  1. Administer antihypertensive agents, including ACE inhibitors, vasodilators, beta-blockers, and calcium channel blockers, as prescribed.
  2. Monitor daily weight to detect fluid-related weight gain.
- Implement diet therapy with registered dietitian nutritionist consultation to slow the progression of kidney injury with fluid, sodium, and protein restrictions.
- Provide counseling, support, and teaching about health maintenance to promote self-management.

See Chapter 59 in the main text for more information on kidney disease, polycystic.

KIDNEY INJURY, ACUTE

- Acute kidney injury (AKI) is a rapid decrease in kidney function, resulting in failure to maintain fluid, electrolyte, and **acid-base balance**, along with impaired urinary **elimination** with accumulation of metabolic wastes.
- AKI can result from conditions that reduce **perfusion** to the kidneys (prerenal); damage kidney tissue (glomeruli, interstitial tissue, or tubules [intrarenal or intrinsic]); or obstruct urine outflow (postrenal); or from combinations of these mechanisms of injury.
- The most current definition of AKI is an increase in serum creatinine by 0.3 mg/dL (26.2 mcmol/L) or more within 48 hours; or an increase in serum creatinine to 1.5 times or more from baseline, which is known or presumed to have occurred in the previous 7 days; or a urine volume of less than 0.5 mL/kg/hr for 6 hours.

Interprofessional Collaborative Care
Recognize Cues: Assessment
- Obtain patient information about:
  1. Recent surgery or trauma, transfusions, allergic (hypersensitivity) reactions, or other factors that could lead to decreased kidney perfusion
  2. History of diseases that contribute to impaired kidney function, such as diabetes mellitus, systemic lupus erythematosus, and hypertension

The KDIGO Classification System for Severity of Acute Kidney Injury

Stage	Serum Creatinine	Urine Output
Stage 1	1.5–1.9 times baseline OR ≥0.3 mg/dL (≥26.5 mmol/L) increase over 48 hr	<0.5 mL/kg/hr for 6–12 hr
Stage 2	2.0–2.9 times baseline	<0.5 mL/kg/hr for ≥12 hr
Stage 3	1 times baseline OR Increase in serum creatinine to ≥4.0 mg/dL (≥353.6 mmol/L) OR Initiation of renal replacement therapy OR In patients <18 yr, decrease in eGFR to <35 mL/min/ 1.73 m^2	Anuria lasting for ≥12 hr OR <0.3 mL/kg/hr for >24 hr

eGFR, Estimated glomerular filtration rate; *KDIGO*, Kidney Disease: Improving Global Outcomes (2012). From Kidney Disease Improving Global Outcomes (KDIGO). (2012). Clinical Practice Guideline for Acute Kidney Injury, *Kidney Int Suppl* 2:1–138.

K

3. History of acute infections, including influenza, colds, gastro-enteritis, and sore throat or pharyngitis that contribute to glomerulonephritis
4. Recent dehydration or intravascular volume depletion (from surgery or trauma) or the need for transfusion
5. History of urinary obstructive disease, such as prostatic hypertrophy or kidney stones
- Assess for and document:
  1. Mean arterial pressure <65 mm Hg or symptoms of hypovolemia such as hypotension, tachycardia, decreased mentation, and low urine output

✚ NURSING SAFETY PRIORITY

Critical Rescue

In any acute care setting, preventing volume depletion and providing intervention early when volume depletion occurs are nursing priorities. Reduced **perfusion** from volume depletion is a common cause of AKI. Assess continually to recognize the signs and symptoms of volume depletion (low urine output, decreased systolic blood pressure, decreased pulse pressure, orthostatic hypotension, thirst, rising blood osmolarity). Respond by intervening early with oral fluids or, in the patient who is unable to take or tolerate oral fluid, requesting an increase in IV fluid rate from the primary health care provider to prevent permanent kidney damage.

2. Urine output of less than 0.5 mL/kg for 2 or more hours
3. Abnormal or sharply increasing values for BUN and serum creatinine and electrolytes
4. Reduced, estimated, or measured creatinine clearance (GFR)
5. Protein in urine or signs of a urinary tract or kidney infection (dysuria, urgency, frequency, foul urine odor, flank pain)
6. Symptoms of fluid overload, including pulmonary edema (dyspnea, crackles, reduced Spo_2) and peripheral edema
7. Symptoms of electrolyte derangements, including nausea and vomiting, anorexia, impaired cognition, acute abnormalities in neuromuscular function, and ECG changes
- Diagnostic studies may include:
  1. Serum CBC (WBC for infection) and basic metabolic panel
  2. Urinalysis
  3. Urine and serum electrolytes, creatinine, and BUN
  4. Abdominal or pelvic ultrasound to assess the size of the kidneys and CT without contrast dye to identify obstruction
  5. Renal biopsy if immunologic disease is suspected

Take Actions: Interventions

- Avoid hypotension and maintain fluid balance (*euvolemia*) to prevent AKI and manage *elimination.*
- Monitor fluid and electrolyte status to detect imbalance and abnormal values. The patient may move from an oliguric phase (fluids and electrolytes are retained) to a diuretic phase, in which hypovolemia and electrolyte loss are the main problems during the course of AKI.
- Fluid challenges and diuretics are commonly used to promote fluid balance and kidney perfusion; avoid hypervolemia that can lead to lung or intestinal damage.
- With the interprofessional team, review drugs and drug-drug interactions to reduce nephrotoxicity.
- Communicate with the radiologist to avoid large doses or nephrotoxic contrast (dye) during imaging and ensure adequate hydration to clear contrast before and after imaging.
- Indications for hemodialysis or PD in patients with AKI are symptomatic uremia (pericarditis or encephalopathy), persistent hyperkalemia or other electrolyte abnormalities, uncompensated metabolic acidosis, fluid overload, and uncontrolled inflammation. (See *Kidney Disease, Chronic* for a discussion of dialysis.)
- Continuous kidney replacement therapies (CKRTs), an alternative to dialysis, may be used in the intensive care unit (ICU).

Care Coordination and Transition Management

- The needs of the patient depend on the status of the disease on discharge (see *Care Coordination and Transition Management* under *Kidney Disease, Chronic*).
- Follow-up care may include medical visits, laboratory tests, consultation with a nutritionist, temporary dialysis, home nursing care, and social work assistance.
- Be sure the primary health care provider is aware of occurrence of AKI because it increases risk for CKD and may necessitate more frequent monitoring of kidney function or health status in the immediate posthospitalization care.

See Chapter 60 in the main text for more information on kidney injury, acute.

K

LACERATIONS, EYE

- Lacerations are wounds caused by sharp objects and projectiles.
- The most commonly injured areas involved in eye lacerations are the eyelids and the cornea.

Interprofessional Collaborative Care

- Eyelid lacerations:
  1. Minor lacerations of the eyelid can be sutured in an emergency department, an urgent care center, or an eye-care provider's office.
  2. A microscope is needed in the operating room if the patient has a laceration that involves the eyelid margin, affects the lacrimal system, involves a large area, or has jagged edges.
- Corneal lacerations:
  1. Are an emergency because eye contents may prolapse through the laceration
  2. Symptoms include severe eye pain, photophobia, tearing, decreased vision, and inability to open the eyelid

! NURSING SAFETY PRIORITY
Action Alert

An object protruding from the eye is removed only by an eye-care provider because it may be holding the eye structures in place. Improper removal can cause structures to prolapse out of the eye.

  3. Antibiotics are given to reduce the risk for infection.
  4. If the eye injury is severe, enucleation (surgical removal of the eyeball) may be indicated.

See Chapter 39 in the main text for more information on lacerations of the eye.

LEIOMYOMAS (UTERINE FIBROIDS): SEXUALITY CONCEPT EXEMPLAR

Overview

- Uterine leiomyomas, also called *fibroids* or *myomas,* are benign, slow-growing solid tumors of the uterine myometrium (muscle layer) that can affect *sexuality*.

- These tumors are classified according to their position in the layers of the uterus and anatomic position. The most common types are:
  1. *Intramural leiomyomas,* contained in the uterine wall in the myometrium
  2. *Submucosal leiomyomas,* which protrude into the cavity of the uterus
  3. *Subserosal leiomyomas,* which protrude through the outer uterine surface and may extend into the broad ligament

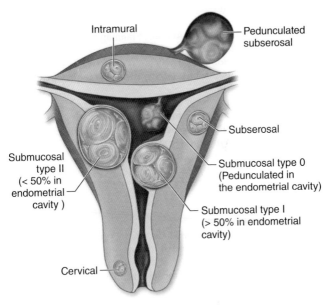

Classifications of uterine leiomyomas.

Interprofessional Collaborative Care
Recognize Cues: Assessment
- Assessment findings include:
  1. Abnormal uterine bleeding or heavy vaginal bleeding with menstruation
  2. Reports of a feeling of pelvic pressure
  3. Constipation
  4. Urinary frequency or retention
  5. Increased abdominal size

L

6. Dyspareunia (painful intercourse)
7. Infertility
8. Abdominal pain occurring with torsion of the fibroid around a connecting stalk
9. Uterine enlargement on abdominal, vaginal, or rectal examination

Analyze Cues and Prioritize Hypotheses: Analysis

- The priority collaborative problem for patients with uterine leiomyoma is:
   1. Potential for prolonged or heavy bleeding due to abnormal uterine growth

Generate Solutions and Take Actions: Planning and Implementation
Managing Bleeding

- Asymptomatic leiomyomas may not require treatment. Leiomyomas in menopausal women usually shrink, so surgery may not be necessary.
- Management depends on the size and location of the tumor, as well as the woman's desire for future pregnancy.
- Women who want to become pregnant may be prescribed drug therapy or have a myomectomy procedure to remove the tumor.
- Uterine artery embolization, endometrial ablation, and hysterectomy are choices for women who no longer desire pregnancy.
- Mild leiomyoma symptoms can be managed with hormonal therapies.

Surgical Management

- Surgical management depends on whether future childbearing is desired, the age of the woman, the size of the fibroid, and the degree of symptoms.
- A *myomectomy* (removal of the leiomyomas with preservation of the uterus) is performed to preserve childbearing capabilities and relieve the symptoms.

✚ NURSING SAFETY PRIORITY
Critical Rescue

Monitor the client who had hysteroscopic myomectomy. The fluid used to distend the uterine cavity during the procedure can be absorbed, resulting in fluid overload (Bradley, 2022). Although this potential complication is rare, assess carefully for signs and symptoms of pulmonary edema or heart failure, such as dyspnea, cough with frothy sputum, subjective report of "suffocating" or "smothering," and palpitations. Report this information to the surgeon immediately.

- *Hysterectomy,* surgical removal of the uterine body, is the usual surgical management in the older woman who has multiple leiomyomas and unacceptable symptoms. One of three approaches may be used: vaginal, abdominal, or laparoscopic.
- Provide preoperative nursing care and:
  1. Listen to the patient's concerns about her sexuality
  2. Identify the patient's support system
- Provide postoperative care.

Postoperative Nursing Care of the Patient After Open Total Abdominal Hysterectomy

Following hysterectomy, assess and monitor:
- Vital signs, including pain level
- Activity tolerance level
- Temperature and color of the skin
- Heart, lung, and bowel sounds
- Incision characteristics
  - Presence or absence of bleeding at the site (a small amount is normal)
  - Intactness of incision
  - Pain at site of incision
- Dressing and drains for color and amount of drainage
- Fluid intake (via IV until peristalsis returns and oral intake is tolerated)
- Urine output
  - Provide catheter care (catheter will be removed in approximately 24 hours).
- Red blood cell, hemoglobin, and hematocrit levels
- Vaginal discharge and/or bleeding
  - Provide perineal care.
  - Assess perineal pads for vaginal bleeding and clots (should be less than one saturated perineal pad in 4 hours).

Care Coordination and Transition Management

 PATIENT AND FAMILY EDUCATION

Care After a Hysterectomy

Expected Physical Changes
- You will no longer have a period, although you may have some vaginal discharge for a few days after you go home.
- It will not be possible for you to become pregnant, and birth control methods are no longer needed. (Condoms should still be used to decrease the chance of getting a sexually transmitted infection [STI].)

Continued

PATIENT AND FAMILY EDUCATION—cont'd

Care After a Hysterectomy

- If your ovaries were removed, you may experience menopausal symptoms, such as hot flushes, night sweats, and vaginal dryness.
- It is normal to tire more easily and require more sleep and rest during the first few weeks after surgery.

Activity (Typically for Vaginal and Traditional Open Surgeries)

- Limit stair climbing, following your surgeon's recommendations if you have stairs in your home.
- Do not lift anything heavier than you can pick up with one hand.
- Gradually increase walking as exercise, but stop before you become fatigued.
- Avoid a sitting position for extended periods. When you sit, do not cross your legs at the knees.
- Avoid strenuous activity and exercise for 2 to 6 weeks, depending on which type of surgical procedure was performed.
- Do not drive until your surgeon has cleared you and opioid medications are discontinued.

Sexual Activity

- Do not engage in sexual intercourse for 6 weeks or as prescribed by your surgeon.
- If you had a vaginal "repair" as part of your surgery, you may experience some tenderness or pain the first time you have intercourse because the vaginal walls are tighter. Careful intercourse and the use of water-based lubricants can help reduce this discomfort.

Complications

- Take your temperature twice each day for the first 3 days after surgery. Report fevers of over 100°F (38°C).
- Check any incisions daily for signs of infection (increasing redness/hyperpigmentation, open areas, drainage that is thick or foul-smelling, incisional **pain**).

Symptoms to Report to Your Surgeon

- Increased vaginal drainage or change in drainage (bloodier, thicker, foul-smelling)
- Signs of infection at an incision site
- Temperature over 100°F (38°C)
- Pain, tenderness, redness/hyperpigmentation, or swelling in the calves
- Pain or burning on urination

Evaluate Outcomes: Evaluation

- Evaluate the care of the patient with leiomyomas on the basis of the identified priority problem. The expected outcome is that the patient:
  1. Has relief of bleeding after effective management

 See Chapter 63 in the main text for more information on leiomyoma.

⁂ LEUKEMIA: IMMUNITY CONCEPT EXEMPLAR

Overview

- Leukemia is cancer with uncontrolled production of immature white blood cells (WBCs) in the bone marrow, altering ***immunity***. The bone marrow is overcrowded with immature, nonfunctional cells ("blast" cells), and the production of normal blood cells is greatly decreased.
- Leukemia may be acute, with a sudden onset, or chronic, with a slow onset and symptoms that persist for years.
- Leukemias are classified as one of two major cell types, and the classification of cell types and subtypes guides treatment:
  1. Lymphocytic (lymphoblastic) leukemias have cells from lymphoid pathways.
  2. Myelogenous (myelocytic) leukemias have abnormal cells originating in myeloid pathways.
- The basic problem causing leukemia involves damage to genes controlling cell growth. This damage then changes cells from a normal to a malignant (cancer) state.

Interprofessional Collaborative Care

- Leukemia affects every aspect of a patient's life and is best managed by an interprofessional team. Like many disorders, leukemia management is most effective when the patient and family are full partners with the health care team.

Recognize Cues: Assessment

- Obtain patient information about:
  1. Age
  2. Exposure to agents or ionizing radiation that increase the risk for leukemia
  3. Recent history of frequent or severe infections (e.g., influenza, pneumonia, bronchitis) or unexplained fevers
  4. A tendency to bruise or bleed easily or for a long period, including hematuria and gastrointestinal (GI) bleeding; platelet function is often decreased with leukemic disorders
  5. Weakness and fatigue or related symptoms of headaches, behavioral changes, increased somnolence, decreased attention span, lethargy, muscle weakness, loss of appetite, or weight loss

L

- Assess for and document the signs and symptoms of leukemia.
- Assess psychosocial issues and concerns, especially anxiety and fear about the diagnosis, treatment, and outcome.
- Laboratory assessment includes:
  1. Decreased hemoglobin and hematocrit levels
  2. Low platelet count and abnormal coagulation values (INF, aPTT)
  3. WBC count (low, normal, or elevated) and differential
- Diagnosis of leukemia is based on findings from a bone marrow biopsy. The leukemia type is diagnosed by cell surface antigens and chromosomal or gene markers.

 KEY FEATURES

Acute Leukemia

Integumentary Signs and Symptoms
- Ecchymoses
- Petechiae
- Open infected lesions
- Pallor of the conjunctivae, the nail beds, the palmar creases, and around the mouth

Gastrointestinal Signs and Symptoms
- Bleeding gums
- Anorexia
- Weight loss
- Enlarged liver and spleen

Renal Signs and Symptoms
- Hematuria

Musculoskeletal Signs and Symptoms
- Bone pain
- Joint swelling and pain

Cardiopulmonary Signs and Symptoms
- Tachycardia at basal activity levels
- Orthostatic hypotension
- Palpitations
- Dyspnea on exertion

Neurologic Signs and Symptoms
- Fatigue
- Headache
- Fever

Analyze Cues and Prioritize Hypotheses: Analysis

- The priority collaborative problems for patients with acute myelogenous leukemia (AML), the most common type of acute leukemia seen in adults, include:
  1. Potential for *infection* due to reduced *immunity*
  2. Potential for injury due to poor *clotting* from thrombocytopenia and chemotherapy
  3. Fatigue due to reduced *gas exchange* and increased energy demands

Generate Solutions and Take Actions: Planning and Implementation
Preventing Infection

- Prevent infection due to decreased *immunity* and chemotherapy. Infection is a major cause of death in the patient with leukemia because the WBCs are immature and cannot function or WBCs are depleted from chemotherapy, leading to sepsis.
  1. Prevent auto- and cross-contamination with best practices in infection control.
  2. Teach and support self-management to avoid situations of increased risk for infection transmission.
  3. Communicate early and urgently to the provider if the patient has signs of infection, particularly if neutropenia is present.

✚ NURSING SAFETY PRIORITY
Critical Rescue

A temperature elevation of even 1°F (or 0.5°C) above baseline is an indication of *infection* for a patient with reduced *immunity*. Monitor patients closely to recognize signs of infection. When any temperature elevation is present in a patient with leukemia, respond by reporting it to the oncology health care provider immediately, and implement standard infection protocols.

Minimizing Injury

- Minimize risk for injury due to thrombocytopenia and chemotherapy.
  1. Poor clotting from decreased platelets and coagulation factors can lead to excessive bleeding.
     - The platelet count is decreased as a side effect of chemotherapy. During the period of greatest bone marrow suppression (the nadir), the platelet count may be less than 10,000/mm^3 (10 × 10^9/L). The patient is at extreme risk for bleeding once the platelet count falls below 50,000/mm^3 (50 × 10^9/L), and spontaneous bleeding may occur when the count is lower than 20,000/mm^3 (20 × 10^9/L).

2. Monitor laboratory values daily, especially CBC, to assess bleeding risk.
3. Implement institutional bleeding precautions for patients to communicate risk.

Conserving Energy
- Conserve energy related to fatigue, decreased gas exchange, and increased energy demands.
  1. Nutritional therapy can help meet caloric intake goals; consult the registered dietitian nutritionist.
  2. Use institutional policy to transfuse red blood cells (RBCs) and other blood products.
  3. Administer drug therapy with colony-stimulating growth factors to reduce the duration of anemia and neutropenia.
  4. Actively manage the periods of rest and activity to meet patient-centered goals of care.

Care Coordination and Transition Management
- Teach the patient and family about:
  1. Measures to prevent infection
  2. The importance of continuing therapy and medical follow-up
  3. The symptoms of infection and when to seek provider advice
  4. The precautions to avoid injury, and to detect and manage problematic bleeding when clotting is impaired
  5. Care of the central catheter if in place at discharge
- Make referrals to resources for psychological and financial support and for role and self-esteem adjustment.
- Assess the patient's need for a home care nurse, aide, or equipment.

Evaluate Outcomes: Evaluation
- Evaluate the care of the patient with leukemia based on the identified priority patient problems. The expected outcomes include that with appropriate interventions and support the patient will:
  1. Remain free of infection and sepsis
  2. Avoid episodes of bleeding
  3. Be able to balance activity and rest
  4. Use energy conservation techniques

 See Chapter 34 in the main text for more information on leukemia.

LYME DISEASE

- Lyme disease is a reportable systemic infection transmitted by deer ticks infected with the spirochete *Borrelia burgdorferi*.
- The disease can be prevented by avoiding heavily wooded areas or areas with thick underbrush; by wearing long-sleeved tops, long pants, and socks; and by using an insect repellent on skin and clothing when in an area where infected ticks are likely to be found.

PATIENT AND FAMILY EDUCATION
Prevention and Early Detection of Lyme Disease

- Avoid heavily wooded areas or areas with thick underbrush, especially in the spring and summer months.
- Walk in the center of the trail, away from brush, trees, and weeds.
- Use an insect repellent (DEET) on your skin and clothes when in an area where ticks are likely to be found.
- Choose to wear lighter-colored clothing to make spotting ticks easier.
- Wear long-sleeved tops and long pants; tuck your shirt into your pants and your pants into your socks or boots.
- Wear closed shoes or boots and a hat or cap.
- Bathe immediately after being in an infested area, and inspect your body for ticks (about the size of a pinhead); pay special attention to your arms, legs, and scalp.
- Check your pets for ticks.
- If a tick is found, gently remove it with tweezers by pulling upward with steady pressure to avoid breaking it.
- Dispose of the tick by putting it in alcohol, placing it into a sealed bag, wrapping it tightly in tape, or flushing it down the toilet.
- Do not attempt to place nail polish, petroleum jelly, or heat onto a tick to make it detach from the skin.
- After removal, clean the tick area with an antiseptic, such as rubbing alcohol, or with soap and water.
- Contact your primary health care provider if you develop a rash or fever within several weeks of experiencing a tick bite.
- Report symptoms such as a rash or influenza-like illness to your primary health care provider immediately.

Data from Centers for Disease Control and Prevention. (2022). *Tick removal and testing.* https://www.cdc.gov/lyme/removal/index.html.

Interprofessional Collaborative Care

- Symptoms appear in three stages:
  1. Stage I symptoms appear in 3 to 30 days after the tick bite and resemble the flu but with a distinctive rash.
     - Low-grade fever
     - Spreading, oval, or "bull's-eye" rash (erythema migrans)
  2. Stage II symptoms appear 3 to 12 weeks after the tick bite (if untreated or if the treatment is unsuccessful).
     - Continued flulike symptoms, with pain in the joints
     - Dysrhythmias, palpitations, dyspnea, and encephalopathy may occur.
  3. Stage III, chronic persistent Lyme disease, occurs weeks to years after the tick bite.
     - The most common symptoms are arthritis in the knee and radicular pain.
     - Cognitive deficits can accompany this stage.
- Management of acute or chronic infection consists of antibiotic therapy with the type or duration of antibiotic varying with the stage of Lyme disease.
- Management of joint inflammation is similar to that for rheumatoid arthritis.

See Chapter 17 in the main text for more information on Lyme disease.

LYMPHOMA, HODGKIN AND NON-HODGKIN

- Lymphomas (also called *malignant lymphomas*) are cancers of the lymphoid tissues with abnormal overgrowth of lymphocytes. Lymphomas are cancers of committed lymphocytes rather than stem cell precursors (as in leukemia). The two major adult forms of lymphoma are Hodgkin lymphoma (HL) and non-Hodgkin lymphoma (NHL).
  1. HL usually starts in a single lymph node or a single chain of nodes and contains a specific cancer cell type, the Reed-Sternberg cell. HL often spreads predictably from one group of lymph nodes to the next.
  2. NHL includes all lymphoid cancers that do not have the Reed-Sternberg cell. There are more than 60 subtypes of NHL, divided into either indolent or aggressive lymphoma.
  3. HL affects any age-group, but it is most common among teens and young adults and among adults over 60. NHL is more common in older adults.

4. Lymph node biopsy provides the basis for an exact diagnosis, classified by subtype and staged to determine the extent of the disease and to individualize therapy.

5. Computerized tomography (CT), MRI, and positron emission tomography (PET) scan also are useful to determine the extent of disease and the patient's response to therapy.

Interprofessional Collaborative Care
Recognize Cues: Assessment

- The most common sign of any lymphoma is lymphadenopathy, or a large but painless lymph node (or nodes).
- Other signs may include fever, night sweats, and unexplained weight loss.

Take Actions: Interventions

- HL is a type of cancer that responds well to aggressive therapy, and long-term survival for decades is now the normal expectation (Xin & Corcoran, 2019). For earlier disease stages, the treatment is external radiation of involved lymph node regions. With more extensive disease, radiation and combination chemotherapy are used to achieve remission.
- Treatment options for patients with NHL vary based the subtype of the tumor, stage of the disease, performance status, and overall tumor burden. Options include combinations of chemotherapy drugs, targeted therapies, localized radiation therapy, radiolabeled antibodies, and investigational agents.
- Nursing management of the patient undergoing radiation therapy for HL or NHL focuses on decreasing the adverse effects of therapy, especially:
  1. Skin problems at the site of radiation
  2. Fatigue and taste changes
  3. Permanent sterility after receiving extensive chemotherapy or radiation to the abdominopelvic region; some cancer centers offer sperm and egg storage for reproductive options
  4. Specific interventions listed under *Cancer*.

See Chapter 34 in the main text for more information on lymphoma.

MACULAR DEGENERATION

- **Macular degeneration,** also known as age-related macular degeneration (AMD), is the deterioration of the macula (the area of central vision) and can be age related or exudative. It is the leading cause of blindness in individuals in the United States who are over the age of 65 years.
- Age-related macular degeneration (AMD) has two types.
  1. Dry AMD is caused by gradual blockage of retinal capillaries, which allows retinal cells in the macula to become ischemic and necrotic. Central vision declines first, but eventually the person loses all central vision.
  2. Wet (exudative) AMD progresses quickly. Patients experience a sudden decrease in vision after a detachment of pigment epithelium in the macula. Newly formed blood vessels, which have very thin walls, invade this injured area and cause fluid and blood to collect under the macula (like a blister), with scar formation and visual distortion. Wet (exudative) AMD can occur at any age, in only one eye or in both eyes. The patient with dry AMD can also develop wet (exudative) macular degeneration.
- The loss of central vision reduces the ability to read, write, recognize safety hazards, and drive.

Interprofessional Collaborative Care

- Dry AMD has no cure. Management in the community setting is focused on slowing the progression of the vision loss and helping the patient maximize remaining vision and quality of life.
  1. The risk for dry AMD can be reduced by increasing long-term dietary intake of the carotenoids *lutein* and *zeaxanthin* (American Optometric Association, 2022).
  2. Suggest alternative strategies (e.g., large-print books, public transportation) and referrals to community organizations that provide a wide range of adaptive equipment.
- See *Visual Impairment (Reduced Vision)* for further discussion of patients' care needs.
- Management of wet macular degeneration focuses on slowing the process and identifying further changes in visual perception.
  1. Laser therapy to seal the leaking blood vessels in or near the macula can limit the extent of the damage.
  2. Vascular endothelial growth factor inhibitors (VEGFIs) injected monthly into the vitreous can also slow disease progression.

See *Chapter 39* in the main text for more information on macular degeneration.

MASTOIDITIS

- Mastoiditis is an ***infection*** of the mastoid air cells caused by progressive otitis media.
- Antibiotic therapy is used to treat the middle ear infection before it progresses to mastoiditis.
- If mastoiditis is not managed appropriately, it can lead to brain abscess, meningitis, and death.

Interprofessional Collaborative Care
Recognize Cues: Assessment
- Signs and symptoms of mastoiditis include:
  1. Swelling behind the ear and ***pain*** when moving the ear or the head.
  2. The pinna usually is edematous, and the auricle is displaced posteriorly or downward.
  3. Patients may have low-grade fever, malaise, and ear drainage.
  4. CT scan should be performed if mastoiditis is suspected.

Take Actions: Interventions
- Interventions focus on halting the ***infection*** before it spreads to other structures.
- Management involves IV antibiotics and surgical removal of the infected tissue if the infection does not respond to antibiotic therapy. A mastoidectomy with myringotomy is the most common treatment.

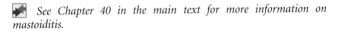 *See Chapter 40 in the main text for more information on mastoiditis.*

MELANOMA

- Melanomas are pigmented cancers arising in the melanin-producing epidermal cells. This most often starts as a benign growth of a nevus (mole).
- Melanoma is highly metastatic, and survival depends on early diagnosis and treatment.
- Risk factors include genetic predisposition, excessive exposure to ultraviolet (UV) light or certain occupational chemical carcinogens, and the presence of one or more precursor lesions that resemble unusual moles.
- It is most common among non-Hispanic white individuals, and risk increases with age.

M

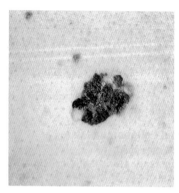

Melanoma.

Interprofessional Collaborative Care
Recognize Cues: Assessment
- Obtain patient information about:
  1. Age and race
  2. Family history of skin cancer
  3. Any past surgery for removal of skin growths
  4. Recent changes in the size, color, or sensation of any mole, birthmark, wart, or scar
  5. Sun exposure
  6. Exposure to arsenic, coal tar, pitch, radioactive waste, or radium
- Assess for and document all lesions for:
  1. Location, size, and color
  2. Surface features (ABCDE)
     - *A*symmetry of shape
     - *B*order irregularity
     - *C*olor variation within one lesion
     - *D*iameter greater than 6 mm
     - *E*xudate presence and quality
- Diagnosis is made based on biopsy findings.

Take Actions: Interventions
- Surgical and nonsurgical interventions are combined for the effective management of skin cancer. Treatment is determined by the size and severity of the malignancy, the location of the lesion, and the age and general health of the patient.
- Melanoma is usually treated by excision using Mohs micrographic surgery.

- Lymph node dissection may be necessary if a node or nodes are found to be abnormally hard or large, or if melanoma is found in a node (American Cancer Society, 2019).
- Immunotherapy and targeted therapy (e.g., BRAF and MEK inhibitors) are often used early in treatment of melanoma.
- Chemotherapy can be used if other treatments have not worked, but it is not as effective in treating melanoma as immunotherapy and targeted therapy agents.
- Radiation is not usually used to treat melanoma unless surgery cannot be done; it is given following lymph node removal, or it is offered as palliative therapy.
- General management issues for the care of patients undergoing radiation therapy are presented under *Cancer*.

 See Chapter 21 in the main text for more information on melanoma.

MÉNIÈRE DISEASE

- Ménière disease is a condition that includes a classic trio of symptoms—episodic vertigo (the sensation of whirling or turning in space), tinnitus, and hearing loss (Moskowitz & Dinces, 2022).
- Episodes, also called "attacks," can last several days, although some patients report ongoing symptoms of varying intensity at all times.
- Patients can be almost to totally incapacitated during an attack, and recovery can take hours to days.
- Although most patients have a window of forewarning when an attack is beginning, others experience Tumarkin otolithic crises, known as *sudden drop attacks,* which happen without warning (Wu et al., 2019).

Interprofessional Collaborative Care
Recognize Cues: Assessment
- Signs and symptoms include:
  1. Vertigo
  2. Hearing loss
  3. Tinnitus
  4. Vertigo is often accompanied by nausea, vomiting, headache, and nystagmus (rapid eye movements).
  5. Blood pressure, pulse, and respirations may be elevated.
  6. Hearing loss occurs first with the low-frequency tones; in some patients, it progresses to include all levels and eventually

M

becomes permanent. Patients may describe the tinnitus as having variable pitch and intensity, which may fluctuate or remain continuous.

Take Actions: Interventions
- Teach patients about attack prevention strategies, including:
  1. Making slow head movements to prevent worsening of the vertigo
  2. Diet modification if foods seem to be a trigger
- Administer drug therapy to reduce symptoms. This may include:
  1. Mild diuretics
  2. Antiemetics to control nausea associated with vertigo
  3. Intratympanic therapy with gentamycin and corticosteroid to control infection or inflammation

Surgical Management
- Surgical procedures such as a labyrinthectomy resect the vestibular nerve or remove the labyrinth. This is reserved for extreme cases in which the patient already has significant hearing loss or continuous disabling vertigo. This surgical procedure results in total hearing loss on the operative side.

See Chapter 40 in the main text for more information on Ménière disease.

MENINGITIS

Meningitis is an ***infection*** of the meninges of the brain and spinal cord, specifically the pia mater and arachnoid.
- Viral meningitis is the most common type, sometimes referred to as *aseptic meningitis* because no organisms are typically isolated from culture of the CSF.
  1. Common viral organisms causing meningitis are enterovirus, herpes simplex virus type 2 (HSV-2), varicella zoster virus (VZV) (also causes chicken pox and shingles), mumps virus, and the human immunodeficiency virus (HIV) (Rogers, 2023).
- The most frequently involved organisms responsible for bacterial meningococcal meningitis are Streptococcus pneumoniae (pneumococcal disease) and Neisseria meningitidis. N. meningitidis meningitis is also known as meningococcal meningitis.
  1. *Meningococcal meningitis is a medical emergency with a fairly high mortality rate, often within 24 hours.*

❗ NURSING SAFETY PRIORITY

Action Alert

People ages 16 through 21 years have the highest rates of infection from life-threatening ***N. meningitidis*** meningococcal infection. The Centers for Disease Control and Prevention (CDC) recommends an initial meningococcal vaccine between ages 11 and 12 years with a booster at age 16 years (www.cdc.gov). Adults are advised to get an initial or a booster vaccine if they are living in a shared residence (e.g., residence hall, military barracks, or group home), traveling or residing in countries in which the disease is common, or if they are immunocompromised as a result of a damaged or surgically removed spleen, or a serum complement deficiency. If the patient's baseline vaccination status is unclear and the immediate risk for exposure to ***N. meningitidis*** infection is high, the CDC recommends vaccination. It is safe to receive a booster as early as 8 weeks after the initial vaccine.

KEY FEATURES

Meningitis

- Decreased level of consciousness
- Disorientation to person, place, and time
- Pupil reaction and eye movements:
  - **Photophobia** (sensitivity to light)
  - **Nystagmus** (involuntary condition in which the eyes make repetitive uncontrolled movements)
- Motor response:
  - Normal early in disease process
  - Hemiparesis (weakness on one side of the body), hemiplegia (paralysis on one side of the body), and decreased muscle tone possible later
  - Cranial nerve dysfunction, especially CN III, IV, VI, VII, VIII
- Memory changes:
  - Attention span (usually short)
  - Personality and behavioral changes
- Severe, unrelenting headaches
- Generalized muscle aches and pain (myalgia)
- Nausea and vomiting
- Fever and chills
- Tachycardia
- Red macular rash (meningococcal meningitis)

M

Interprofessional Collaborative Care
Recognize Cues: Assessment
Perform a complete neurologic and neurovascular assessment to detect signs and symptoms associated with a diagnosis of meningitis or suspected meningitis

- Diagnostic studies may include the following:
  1. The most significant laboratory test used in the diagnosis of meningitis is the analysis of the *cerebrospinal fluid (CSF)*.
  2. Complete blood count (CBC) with WBC differential and basic metabolic panel for kidney function and electrolytes
  3. Computed tomography (CT) scan to detect increased intracranial pressure, abscess (encapsulated pus), or hydrocephalus

---

▶▶ **BEST PRACTICE FOR PATIENT SAFETY AND QUALITY CARE**

Care of the Patient With Meningitis

- Prioritize care to maintain airway, breathing, and circulation.
- Take vital signs and perform neurologic checks every 2 to 4 hours as needed.
- Perform cranial nerve assessment, with particular attention to cranial nerves III, IV, VI, VII, and VIII, and monitor for changes.
- Manage pain with drug and nondrug methods.
- Perform a vascular assessment, and monitor for changes.
- Give drugs and IV fluids as prescribed and document the patient's response.
- Record intake and output carefully to maintain fluid balance and prevent fluid overload.
- Monitor body weight to identify fluid retention early.
- Monitor laboratory values closely; report abnormal findings to the physician or nurse practitioner promptly.
- Position carefully to prevent pressure injuries.
- Perform range-of-motion exercises every 4 hours as needed.
- Decrease environmental stimuli:
  - Provide a quiet environment.
  - Minimize exposure to bright lights from windows and overhead lights.
  - Maintain bed rest with head of bed elevated 30 degrees.
- Maintain Transmission-Based Precautions per hospital policy (for bacterial meningitis).
- Monitor for complications:
  - Increased intracranial pressure
  - Vascular dysfunction
  - Fluid and electrolyte imbalance
  - Seizures
  - Shock

Take Actions: Interventions

- Prevent meningitis by teaching people to obtain vaccination.
  1. The most important nursing interventions for patients with meningitis are accurate monitoring of and documentation of their neurologic status.

> **! NURSING SAFETY PRIORITY**
>
> *Action Alert*
>
> For the patient with meningitis, assess neurologic status and vital signs at least every 4 hours or more often if clinically indicated. *The priority for care is to monitor for early neurologic changes that may indicate increased intracranial pressure (ICP), such as decreased level of consciousness (LOC).* The patient is also at risk for seizure activity.

- Administer drugs such as antimicrobials and analgesics as ordered.
- Monitor for complications, such as vascular compromise from emboli, shock, coagulation disorders, prolonged fever, and septic complications.

> **! NURSING SAFETY PRIORITY**
>
> *Action Alert*
>
> Place the patient with bacterial meningitis that is transmitted by droplets on Droplet Precautions *in addition to* Standard Precautions. When possible, place the patient in a private room. Stay at least 3 feet from the patient unless wearing a mask. Patients who are transported outside of the room should wear a mask. Teach visitors about the need for these precautions and how to follow them.

See Chapter 36 in the main text for more information on meningitis.

METABOLIC SYNDROME

- Metabolic syndrome is the simultaneous presence of metabolic factors known to increase the risk for developing type 2 diabetes and cardiovascular disease.
  1. Features of the syndrome include:
     - Abdominal obesity: waist circumference of 40 inches (100 cm) or more for men and 35 inches (88 cm) or more for women
     - Hyperglycemia: fasting blood glucose level of 100 mg/dL or more or on drug treatment for elevated glucose
     - Hypertension: systolic blood pressure (BP) of 140 mm Hg or more or diastolic BP of 90 mm Hg or more, or on drug treatment for hypertension

- Hyperlipidemia: triglyceride level of 150 mg/dL or more or on drug treatment for elevated triglycerides; high-density lipoprotein (HDL) cholesterol of less than 40 mg/dL for men or less than 50 mg/dL for women
- Management consists of addressing each of the features (e.g., drug therapy for hypertension and hyperlipidemia) and teaching patients about the lifestyle changes that can improve health and reduce obesity.

See Chapter 56 in the main text for more information on metabolic syndrome.

MULTIDRUG-RESISTANT ORGANISMS (MDROs)

- Multidrug-resistant organisms (MDROs) are infectious agents that are no longer responsive to antibiotics.
- The most common MDROs are methicillin-resistant *Staphylococcus aureus* (MRSA), vancomycin-resistant *enterococcus* (VRE), and carbapenem-resistant *enterococcus* (CRE).
  1. MRSA is spread by direct contact and invades hospitalized patients through indwelling urinary catheters, vascular access devices, open wounds, and endotracheal tubes. It is susceptible to only a few antibiotics, such as vancomycin and linezolid. IV ceftaroline is the first cephalosporin antibiotic approved to treat MRSA (Burchum & Rosenthal, 2022).
  2. *Enterococci* are bacteria that live in the intestine and are important for digestion. VRE can live on almost any surface for days or weeks and still be able to cause an infection. Contamination of toilet seats, door handles, and other objects is very likely for a lengthy period. The most common infections caused by VRE include wound infections, urinary tract infections (UTIs), and bloodstream infections.
  3. *Klebsiella* and *Escherichia coli* (*E. coli*) are types of *Enterobacteriaceae* that are located within the intestinal tract; these bacteria have become increasingly resistant to carbapenem antibiotics, which are most often given for abdominal infections.

Interprofessional Collaborative Care

! NURSING SAFETY PRIORITY

Action Alert

To help prevent the transmission of an MDRO, wear scrubs and change clothes before leaving work. Keep work clothes separate from personal clothes. Take a shower when you get home, if possible, to rid your body of any unwanted pathogens.

- Experts suggest several strategies to decrease the incidence of this growing problem.
  1. Perform frequent hand hygiene, including using hand sanitizers.
  2. Use chlorohexidine (2% dilution) when bathing to prevent CRE or decrease colonization and other types of infections from MDROs.
  3. Stop administering multiple antimicrobials when a specific effective drug is identified from culture results.
  4. Use best practices in infection control in hospital and other health care settings, including the use of personal protective equipment (staff and visitors) and cleaning surfaces and equipment.
  5. Teach patients and primary health care providers to avoid the use of antibiotics to treat common viral illnesses such as colds.
  6. Follow guidelines or best practices to ensure selection of the most effective antibiotic, the correct dose for the condition, and the duration of treatment.

See Chapter 19 in the main text for more information on multidrug-resistant organisms.

✳ MULTIPLE SCLEROSIS: IMMUNITY CONCEPT EXEMPLAR

Overview
- Multiple sclerosis (MS) is a chronic disease caused by immune, genetic, and/or infectious factors that affect the myelin and nerve fibers of the brain and spinal cord.
- It is one of the leading causes of neurologic disability in young and middle-aged adults.
- MS is characterized by periods of remission and exacerbation (flare), which is commonly referred to as a relapsing-remitting course.
- Patients progress at different rates and over different lengths of time.
- As the severity and duration of the disease progress, the periods of exacerbation become more frequent.
- MS often mimics other neurologic diseases, which makes the diagnosis difficult and prolonged.
- The four major types of MS are:
  1. Clinically isolated syndrome (CIS), which is an episode of neurologic symptoms often attributed to MS that lasts for at least 24 hours; MRI may or may not show evidence, so a diagnosis is not yet possible.

M

2. Relapsing-remitting MS (RRMS), which is characterized as mild or moderate, depending on the degree of disability; symptoms develop and resolve in a few weeks to months, after which the patient may return to baseline.

3. Primary progressive MS (PPMS), which is characterized by a steady and gradual neurologic deterioration without remission of symptoms; the patient has progressive disability with no acute attacks. Patients with this type of MS tend to be between 40 and 60 years old at onset of the disease.

4. Secondary progressive MS (SPMS) begins with a relapsing-remitting course that later becomes steadily progressive. About half of all people with RRMS develop SPMS within 10 years. The current addition of disease-modifying drugs as part of disease management may decrease the development of SPMS.

👤 PATIENT-CENTERED CARE: GENDER HEALTH
Women and Multiple Sclerosis

MS affects women two to three times more often than men, suggesting a possible hormonal role in disease development. Some studies show that the disease occurs up to four times more often in women than men. However, the exact reason for this difference is not known (National Multiple Sclerosis Society, 2020).

Interprofessional Collaborative Care
Recognize Cues: Assessment
- Assess for and document:
  1. Progression of symptoms
  2. Factors that aggravate symptoms
     - Stress
     - Fatigue
     - Overexertion
     - Temperature extremes such as a hot shower or bath
- No single specific laboratory test is definitively diagnostic for MS. Collective results of a variety of tests are usually conclusive.
- Diagnostic testing may include:
  1. MRI to determine the presence of plaques in the central nervous system (CNS)
  2. Lumbar puncture for analysis of CSF

KEY FEATURES

Multiple Sclerosis

Common Symptoms and Conditions
- Muscle weakness and spasticity
- Fatigue (usually with continuous sensitivity to temperature)
- Flexor muscle spasms
- Numbness or tingling sensations (paresthesia)
- Visual changes such as diplopia, nystagmus, decreased visual acuity, scotomas
- Bowel and bladder dysfunction (flaccid or spastic)
- Alterations in sexual function, such as erectile dysfunction
- Cognitive changes, such as memory loss, impaired judgment, and decreased ability to solve problems or perform calculations
- Depression
- Dysesthesia ("MS hug") squeezing sensation around the torso, often one of the first symptoms of the disease or a relapse
- Difficulty walking (including **dysmetria** (inability to direct or limit movement and ataxia)
- Vertigo (dizziness)
- Pain and itching
- Emotional changes

Less Common Symptoms and Conditions
- **Intention tremors** (tremor when performing an activity)
- **Hypoalgesia** (decreased sensitivity to pain)
- **Dysarthria** (difficulty speaking due to slurred speech)
- **Dysphagia** (difficulty swallowing)
- Decreased hearing acuity
- **Tinnitus** (ringing in the ears)
- Loss of taste
- Seizures

Analyze Cues and Prioritize Hypotheses: Analysis
- The priority collaborative problems for patients with MS include:
  1. Impaired **immunity** due to the disease and drug therapy for disease management
  2. Decreased or impaired **mobility** due to muscle spasticity, intention tremors, and/or fatigue
  3. Decreased visual acuity and **cognition** due to dysfunctional brain neurons

M

Generate Solutions and Take Actions: Planning and Implementation

- The purpose of management is to modify the effect of the disease on the immune system, prevent exacerbations, manage symptoms, improve function, and maintain quality of life.

Managing Impaired Immunity

- Drug therapy:
  1. Current therapies are designed to alter the immune system responses associated with MS.
     - Interferon-beta preparations, immunomodulators that modify the course of the disease and have antiviral effects
     - Glatiramer acetate, a synthetic protein that is similar to myelin-based protein
     - Natalizumab, a monoclonal antibody that binds to WBCs to prevent further damage to the myelin
     - Fingolimod, teriflunomide, or dimethyl fumarate to modulate the immune system
     - Mitoxantrone, an IV antineoplastic antiinflammatory agent used to resolve relapses but with risks for leukemia and cardiotoxicity
     - Medical marijuana (cannabis) has been shown to reduce pain, muscle stiffness, and spasticity for some patients with MS.

💊 NURSING SAFETY PRIORITY

Drug Alert

The interferons and glatiramer acetate are subcutaneous injections that patients can self-administer. Teach patients how to give and rotate the site of interferon-beta and glatiramer acetate injections because local injection site (skin) reactions are common. The first dose of these drugs is given under medical supervision to monitor for allergic response, including anaphylactic shock. Teach patients receiving these drugs to avoid crowds and people with infections because these drugs can cause bone marrow suppression. Remind them to report any sign or symptom associated with infection immediately to their primary health care provider. Instruct patients about flulike reactions that are very common for patients receiving any of the interferons. These symptoms can be minimized by starting at a low drug dose and giving acetaminophen or ibuprofen. Adverse effects of glatiramer are not common (Burchum & Rosenthal, 2022).

Improving Mobility

- The symptoms of MS that affect **mobility** include spasticity, tremor, pain, and fatigue.
  1. Refer to rehabilitative services (physical and occupational therapy).
  2. Adjunctive therapy to treat muscle spasticity and paresthesia
     - For spasticity, the primary health care provider may prescribe baclofen or tizanidine.
  3. Provide sufficient time to complete activities of daily living (ADLs); as a result of weakness and fatigue, the patient requires more time or assistance.

Managing Decreased Visual Acuity and Cognition

- Alterations in visual acuity and cognition can occur at any time during the course of the disease process. Areas affected include attention, memory, problem solving, auditory reasoning, handling distractions, and visual perception.
  1. For diplopia: An eye patch that is alternated from eye to eye every few hours may relieve this condition.
  2. For peripheral vision deficits: Teach scanning techniques to help compensate for the visual deficit.
  3. Complementary and integrative health therapies such as reflexology, massage, and yoga may be successful in decreasing symptoms of MS.

Care Coordination and Transition Management

- Self-management education includes:
  1. Avoiding factors that may exacerbate the symptoms, including overexertion, extremes of temperatures (fever, hot baths, overheating, excessive chilling), humidity, and exposure to infection
  2. Providing drug information
  3. Encouraging the patient to follow the exercise program developed by the physical therapist (PT) and to remain independent in all activities for as long as possible
  4. Encouraging the patient to engage in regular social activities, obtain adequate rest, and manage stress
  5. Teaching the family strategies to cope with personality changes
  6. Reinforcing established bowel and bladder, skin care, and nutritional programs
  7. Identifying community organizations and support groups for education and to promote adaptive psychosocial coping

See Chapter 37 in the main text for more information on multiple sclerosis.

M

NEPHROTIC SYNDROME

- **Nephrotic syndrome (NS)** is an immunologic kidney disorder in which glomerular permeability increases so that larger molecules pass through the membrane into the urine and are then excreted. This process causes massive loss of protein into the urine, edema formation, and decreased plasma albumin levels.
- The main features are severe proteinuria, hypoalbuminemia, hyperlipidemia, lipiduria, facial/periorbital edema, and hypertension.

 KEY FEATURES

Nephrotic Syndrome

Sudden onset of these symptoms:
- Massive proteinuria
- Hypoalbuminemia
- Edema (especially facial and periorbital)
- Lipiduria
- Hyperlipidemia
- Delayed clotting or increased bleeding with higher-than-normal values for serum-activated partial thromboplastin time (aPTT) coagulation or international normalized ratio for prothrombin (INR, PT)
- Reduced kidney function with elevated blood urea nitrogen (BUN) and serum creatinine and decreased glomerular filtration rate (GFR)

Interprofessional Collaborative Care

- Treatment depends on what is causing the disorder (identified by renal biopsy) and may include:
  1. Angiotensin-converting enzyme inhibitors to preserve kidney function in early stages
  2. Cholesterol-lowering drugs/drugs to control hypercholesterolemia
  3. Heparin to reduce clot formation and extension (clots form as part of the inflammatory response)
  4. Diuretics
  5. Diet changes, including fluid and sodium restriction
- Assess the patient's hydration status and monitor for dehydration. If the plasma volume is depleted, kidney problems worsen.
- Assess laboratory values for changes in kidney function, including serum blood urea nitrogen (BUN), creatinine, glomerular filtration rate, electrolytes, and urinalysis.

See Chapter 59 in the main text for more information on nephrotic syndrome.

NEUROMA, ACOUSTIC

- An acoustic neuroma is a benign tumor of the vestibulocochlear nerve (cranial nerve VIII) that often damages other structures as it grows. Damage to hearing, facial movements, and sensation can occur as the tumor grows.
  1. An acoustic neuroma can cause many neurologic signs and symptoms as the tumor enlarges in the brain.

Interprofessional Collaborative Care

- Symptoms begin with tinnitus and progress to gradual sensorineural hearing loss in most patients. Constant mild vertigo occurs later.
- Diagnosis is made by CT or MRI.
- Treatment involves surgery, radiation, or watchful observation.
- Surgical removal is usually achieved by a craniotomy. If surgery is performed, risks include hearing loss, facial weakness, persistent headaches, and/or vestibular disturbances (Park et al., 2023). See *Hearing Loss* for a review of care needs for the patient whose hearing is reduced.

See Chapter 40 in the main text for more information on neuroma, acoustic.

✳ OBESITY: NUTRITION CONCEPT EXEMPLAR

Overview

- The terms *obesity* and *overweight* are often used interchangeably, but they refer to different health problems.
  1. Overweight is reflected by a body mass index (BMI) of 25 to 29.
  2. **Obesity** is reflected by a BMI of 30 or above (CDC, 2022b). Obesity is subdivided into three categories (CDC, 2022b):
     - Class I—BMI of 30 to <35
     - Class II—BMI of 35 to <40
     - Class III—BMI of 40 or higher (sometimes called "extreme" or "severe" obesity

Common Complications of Obesity	
Cardiovascular • Coronary artery disease (CAD) • Hyperlipidemia • Hypertension • Peripheral artery disease (PAD)	**Integumentary** • Delayed wound healing • Susceptibility to infections
Endocrine • Insulin resistance • Metabolic syndrome • Type 2 diabetes	**Musculoskeletal** • Chronic back and/or joint pain • Early onset of osteoarthritis
Gastrointestinal • Cholelithiasis	**Neurologic** • Stroke
Genitourinary/Reproductive • Erectile dysfunction in men • Menstrual irregularities in women • Urinary incontinence	**Psychiatric** • Depression **Respiratory** • Obesity hypoventilation syndrome • Obstructive sleep apnea

  3. Approximately one-third of the U.S. population is overweight or obese. This problem is a leading cause of preventable death.
  4. Bariatrics is a branch of medicine that manages patients with obesity and its related diseases.
  5. Causes of obesity include high-fat and high-cholesterol diets, physical inactivity, drug treatment (corticosteroids, nonsteroidal antiinflammatory drugs [NSAIDs]), dysregulation of

hormones that affect appetite and fat metabolism, and familial or genetic factors.

6. Complications of obesity primarily affect the cardiovascular and respiratory systems. Excess weight can also cause degeneration of the musculoskeletal system, especially weight-bearing joints such as the hips and knees.

Interprofessional Collaborative Care
Recognize Cues: Assessment

- Approach patients with obesity by using the acronym RESPECT, created by The Ohio State University:
  1. Create *R*apport in an *E*nvironment that is *S*afe.
  2. Ensure *P*rivacy.
  3. *E*ncourage realistic goals.
  4. Provide *C*ompassion.
  5. Utilize *T*act in conversation.
- In addition to a complete history regarding present and past health problems, collect this information about the patient in collaboration with the registered dietitian nutritionist (RDN):
  1. Appetite
  2. Attitude toward food
  3. Presence of any chronic diseases
  4. Drugs, including prescriptive, over-the-counter (OTC), and herbal or food additives
  5. Physical activity and functional ability
  6. Accurate height and weight
  7. Family history of obesity
  8. Psychosocial assessment to determine circumstances and emotional factors that might prevent successful weight loss or that might be worsened by intervention

Analyze Cues and Prioritize Hypotheses: Analysis

- The priority collaborative problem for the patient with obesity is:
  1. Weight gain, which stresses all vital organs, due to excessive intake of calories

Generate Solutions and Take Actions: Planning and Implementation
Improving Nutrition

- Weight loss may be accomplished by **nutrition** modification with or without the aid of drugs and in combination with a regular exercise program.

Nonsurgical Management

- Diet programs managed through close interaction among the patient, registered dietitian nutritionist, and primary health care provider

- Exercise programs to include aerobic activity
- Behavioral management
- Drug therapy
    1. Four medications are FDA-approved for overweight and obesity treatment. The health care provider will work with the patient to determine which, if any, of these drugs are appropriate.

Surgical Management
- Certain adults may be considered for weight loss surgery. These include patients who:
    1. Do not respond to traditional interventions
    2. Have a body mass index (BMI) of 40 or greater
    3. Have a BMI of 35 or greater, with other health risk factors
- Surgical procedures include gastric bypass, sleeve gastrectomy, adjustable gastric band, biliopancreatic diversion with duodenal switch (BPD/DS), and single anastomosis duodenal-ileal bypass with sleeve gastrectomy (SADI-S) (American Society for Metabolic and Bariatric Surgery [ASMBS], 2023)
    1. The most common bariatric surgery performed in the United States is the Roux-en-Y gastric bypass (RNYGB), most commonly called a gastric bypass.

Roux-en-Y Gastric Bypass

Pouch (20–30 mL capacity)

Stoma

Duodenum

Jejunum

Roux-en-Y gastric bypass (RNYGB). (From Silvestri, L., & Silvestri, A. [2020]. *Saunders Comprehensive review for the NCLEX-RN examination* [8th ed.]. St. Louis: Elsevier.)

- Provide routine postoperative care after bariatric surgery:
    1. Attend to airway management because a thick neck may lead to a compromised airway.
    2. Monitor vital signs with peripheral oxygen saturation (Spo_2).

3. Focus on patient and staff safety, using bariatric equipment to promote mobility and reduce skin complications.

4. Monitor the patency of the nasogastric tube (NGT), and record the amount of drainage.

! NURSING SAFETY PRIORITY

Action Alert

Some patients who have bariatric surgery have an NGT put in place, especially after open surgical procedures. In gastroplasty procedures, the NGT drains both the proximal pouch and the distal stomach. Closely monitor the tube for patency. ***Never reposition the tube, because its movement can disrupt the suture line!*** The NGT is removed on the second day if the patient is passing flatus.

5. Monitor for symptoms of anastomotic leak if this process was part of the surgical approach. Symptoms of leak are increasing back, shoulder, or abdominal pain; restlessness; unexplained tachycardia; and oliguria (scant urine). Report any of these findings to the surgeon immediately. *Anastomotic leaks are the most common serious complication and cause of death after gastric bypass surgery.*

6. Apply an abdominal binder to prevent wound dehiscence.

7. Place the patient in a semi-Fowler's position to improve breathing and decrease the risk for sleep apnea, pneumonia, or atelectasis.

8. Provide oxygen delivery, or bi-level or continuous positive airway pressure (BiPAP or CPAP) ventilation as prescribed.

9. Implement best practices for maintaining skin integrity, and observe skinfolds for redness/hyperpigmentation, excoriation, or breakdown.

10. Observe for dumping syndrome, manifested by frequent liquid stools after eating.

11. Apply sequential compression stockings and administer prophylactic anticoagulant therapy as prescribed to prevent thromboembolitic complications, including pulmonary embolism (PE).

12. Follow the institutional protocol about starting and advancing oral intake; avoid large volumes of liquid intake to avoid discomfort and stimulation of hyperperistalsis.

Care Coordination and Transition Management

- Discuss community resources, such as Overeaters Anonymous and the American Obesity Association.
- In collaboration with the RDN, provide health teaching regarding the diet and the importance of maintaining a healthy eating pattern.
- Encourage the patient to increase physical activity, decrease fat intake and reliance on drug use, establish a normal eating pattern in response to physiologic hunger, and address medical and psychological problems.

- Emphasize the necessity for follow-up after bariatric surgery to avoid complications and ensure safe weight loss.

 PATIENT AND FAMILY EDUCATION

Discharge Teaching Topics for the Patient After Bariatric Surgery

Nutrition: Diet progression, nutrient (including vitamin and mineral) supplements, hydration guidelines

Drug therapy: Analgesics and antiemetic drugs, if needed; drugs for other health problems

Wound care: Clean procedure for open or laparoscopic wounds; cover during shower or bath

Activity level: Restrictions, such as avoiding lifting; activity progression; return to driving and work

Signs and symptoms to report: Fever; excessive nausea or vomiting; epigastric, back, or shoulder pain; red, hot, and/or draining wound(s); pain, redness/hyperpigmentation, or swelling in legs; chest pain; difficulty breathing

Follow-up care: Health care provider office or clinic visits, support groups and other community resources, counseling for patient (and caregiver, if needed)

Continuing education: Nutrition and exercise classes; follow-up visits with registered dietitian nutritionist (RDN)

Evaluate Outcomes: Evaluation

Evaluate the care of the patient with obesity based on the identified priority patient problem. The primary expected outcome is that the patient consumes appropriate, nutrient-dense foods to meet metabolic demands without overeating.

 See Chapter 52 in the main text for more information on obesity.

OBSTRUCTION, INTESTINAL: ELIMINATION CONCEPT ✳ EXEMPLAR

Overview

- Intestinal obstructions can be partial or complete and are classified as mechanical or nonmechanical. With either condition, *elimination* is compromised by this common and serious disorder.
  1. *Mechanical obstruction* occurs when the bowel is physically obstructed by problems outside the intestine (e.g., adhesions), in the bowel wall (e.g., Crohn's disease), or in intestinal lumens (e.g., tumors).

2. *Nonmechanical obstruction (paralytic ileus or functional obstruction)* occurs when peristalsis is decreased or absent, resulting in a slowing of the movement or a backup of intestinal content.
- Intestinal contents accumulate at and above the area of obstruction, leading to distention.
- With distention, peristalsis and intestinal secretions increase, leading to further distention and bowel edema.
- The changes in the bowel contribute to increased capillary permeability and leakage of fluid and electrolytes into the interstitial space, resulting in reduced circulatory blood volume (hypovolemia) and electrolyte imbalances.
- Edema in the bowel and surrounding issue can lead to increased intra-abdominal pressure and acute abdominal compartment syndrome, a complication that leads to bowel ischemia, injury, and necrosis.
- Vascular circulation to the bowel can become compromised with hypovolemia and with edema pressing on capillaries, leading to peritonitis and sepsis.
- It is a surgical emergency when there is obstruction with compromised blood flow.

Interprofessional Collaborative Care
Recognize Cues: Assessment
- Obtain patient information about:
  1. Medical history, including abdominal surgical procedures, radiation therapy, and bowel diseases such as Crohn's disease, ulcerative colitis, diverticular disease, gallstones, hernia repair, trauma, and peritonitis
  2. Diet history and drug use
  3. Bowel elimination patterns, including the presence of blood in the stool
  4. Familial history of colorectal cancer
  5. Nausea and vomiting, including the characteristics of emesis
- Assess for and document:
  1. The quality of abdominal pain, onset, and aggravating and alleviating factors associated with pain
  2. Vital signs, including symptoms of hypovolemia (tachycardia, hypotension, low urine output) or infection (fever)
  3. Abdominal distention (hallmark sign)
  4. Bowel sounds (borborygmi): high-pitched bowel sounds may be heard early in an obstructive process and absent bowel sounds in later stages
  5. Nausea, vomiting, and characteristics of emesis
     - Obstruction above the ileum causes early and profuse vomiting of partially digested food and chyme, changing to watery contents containing bile and mucus.

- Obstruction in the large intestine produces vomitus with an orange-brown color and a foul odor caused by bacterial overgrowth, which may be fecal contamination.
6. Presence or absence of stool or flatus and characteristics of stool
   - No passage of stool (obstipation) or flatus, a characteristic of total small- and large-bowel mechanical obstruction
   - Diarrhea may be present with a partial obstruction.
7. Hiccups (singultus), which are common with all types of intestinal obstruction
- Diagnostic studies include:
   1. Computerized tomography (CT) scan
   2. A screening abdominal ultrasound may be used to evaluate the type of obstruction.

 KEY FEATURES

Small-Bowel and Large-Bowel Obstructions

Small-Bowel Obstructions	Large-Bowel Obstructions
Abdominal discomfort or pain, possibly accompanied by visible peristaltic waves in upper and middle abdomen	Intermittent lower abdominal cramping
Upper or epigastric abdominal distention	Lower abdominal distention
Nausea and early, profuse vomiting (may contain fecal material)	Minimal or no vomiting
Obstipation	Obstipation or ribbonlike stools
Severe fluid and electrolyte imbalances	No major fluid and electrolyte imbalances
Metabolic alkalosis (not always present)	Metabolic acidosis (not always present)

Analyze Cues and Prioritize Hypotheses: Analysis
- The priority collaborative problem for patients with intestinal obstruction is:
   1. Potential for life-threatening complications due to reduced flow or blocked flow of intestinal contents.

Generate Solutions and Take Actions: Planning and Implementation
Reducing the Risk of Life-Threatening Complications
- Decompress the GI tract by inserting or maintaining a gastric tube, which can be inserted nasally or orally.
   1. Monitor and record quantity and character of nasogastric output every 4 hours.
   2. Assess the patient for nausea, vomiting, increased abdominal distention, and placement of the tube.

3. If the NGT is repositioned or replaced, confirmation of proper placement may be obtained by x-ray.

! NURSING SAFETY PRIORITY
Action Alert

At least every 4 hours, assess the patient with an NGT for proper placement of the tube, tube patency, and output (quality and quantity). Monitor the nasal skin around the tube for irritation. Use an approved device that secures the tube to the nose to prevent accidental removal. Assess for peristalsis by auscultating for bowel sounds with the suction disconnected (suction masks peristaltic sounds).

- If paralytic or partial obstruction, drugs to enhance gastric mobility may be given.
- Obstruction caused by fecal impaction may resolve after disimpaction that can be manual or aided with enema administration.
- Intussusception may respond to hydrostatic pressure changes during a barium enema.
- Administer fluid and electrolyte replacement.
  1. Administer intravenous (IV) fluid because of dehydration from NPO status, lack of normal reabsorption in the intestine, increased intestinal secretions, and NG suction.
  2. Monitor fluid status with vital signs, adequacy of urine output, and daily weight.

Managing Pain
- Report uncontrolled or severe pain to the health care provider, including pain that significantly increases or changes from a colicky, intermittent type to constant discomfort.
- Provide a position of comfort, including the semi-Fowler's position, to relieve the pressure of abdominal distention and facilitate thoracic excursion and normal breathing patterns.
- Broad-spectrum antibiotics are given if surgery is anticipated.

Surgical Management
- Surgical management is required for complete mechanical obstruction and for many cases of incomplete mechanical obstruction.
- An exploratory laparotomy is performed to locate the obstruction and determine the nature of the problem.
- The specific surgical procedure performed depends on the cause and location of the obstruction. Examples of procedures include lysis of adhesions, colon resection with anastomosis for obstruction resulting from tumor or diverticulitis, and embolectomy or thrombectomy for intestinal infarction. A colon resection and colostomy may be necessary.

Care Coordination and Transition Management

- Education for the patient and family depends on the specific cause and treatment of the obstruction.
  1. Report signs that may indicate recurrent obstruction, including abdominal pain or distention, nausea, vomiting, or constipation (for nonmechanical obstruction after surgery or trauma).
  2. Develop a structured bowel regimen, such as a high-fiber diet or fiber supplements and daily exercise with sufficient oral intake of water for prevention of recurrences of fecal impaction.
- Information about incision care (if surgery was performed), drug therapy, and activity restriction is given to the patient and family.

See Chapter 48 in the main text for more information on obstruction, intestinal.

OBSTRUCTION, UPPER AIRWAY

- Upper airway obstruction is an interruption in airflow through the nose, mouth, pharynx, or larynx. When gas exchange is impaired, airway obstruction can be life-threatening.
  1. Causes include:
     - Tongue edema (surgery, trauma, angioedema as an allergic response to a drug)
     - Tongue occlusion (e.g., loss of gag reflex, loss of muscle tone, unconsciousness, coma)
     - Laryngeal edema from any cause (e.g., smoke or toxin inhalation, local or generalized inflammation, allergic reactions, anaphylaxis)
     - Peritonsillar and pharyngeal abscess
     - Head and neck cancer
     - Thick secretions
     - Stroke and cerebral edema
     - Facial, tracheal, or laryngeal trauma
     - Foreign body aspiration
  2. One preventable cause of airway obstruction leading to asphyxiation is thickly crusted oral and nasopharyngeal secretions

Interprofessional Collaborative Care
Recognize Cues: Assessment

- Partial obstruction may have only subtle or general manifestations, such as diaphoresis, tachycardia, and elevated blood pressure.

- Observe for hypoxia and hypercarbia, restlessness, increasing anxiety, sternal retractions, a "seesawing" chest, abdominal movements, or a feeling of impending doom from air hunger.
- Use pulse oximetry or end-tidal carbon dioxide ($ETco_2$ or $PETco_2$) for ongoing monitoring of *gas exchange*. Continually assess for stridor, cyanosis, and changes in level of consciousness.

❗ NURSING SAFETY PRIORITY

Action Alert

Assess the oral care needs of the patient with risk factors for thickly crusted secretions daily. Ensure that whoever provides oral care understands the importance and the correct techniques for preventing secretion buildup and airway obstruction.

Take Actions: Interventions
- Management depends on the cause of the obstruction.
  1. Prevent airway obstruction from thick, hardened oral and nasopharyngeal secretions with regular oral hygiene and adequate hydration.
  2. For tongue occlusion or excessive secretions, slightly extend the patient's head and neck, insert a nasal or oral airway, then suction to remove secretions.
  3. For a foreign body, perform abdominal thrusts.

❗ NURSING SAFETY PRIORITY

Action Alert

Abdominal thrust maneuver is performed on an unconscious patient instead of chest compressions *only* when a known obstruction is present and the patient has a palpable pulse. If no obstruction has been observed in an unconscious person, chest compressions are started instead of abdominal thrusts because many more unconscious adults have cardiac problems rather than airway obstruction.

  4. For complete obstruction from edema, cancer, or abscesses, anticipate the need for direct visualization of the airway (laryngoscopy) by a health care provider or placement of an artificial airway, including:
     - Cricoidectomy
     - Endotracheal intubation
     - Tracheotomy

See Chapter 23 in the main text for more information on obstruction, upper airway.

OBSTRUCTIVE SLEEP APNEA: GAS EXCHANGE CONCEPT ✳ EXEMPLAR

Overview

- Obstructive sleep apnea is a breathing disruption during sleep that lasts at least 10 seconds and happens a minimum of five times in an hour.
- The most common cause of sleep apnea is upper airway obstruction by the soft palate or tongue. Factors that contribute to sleep apnea include obesity, a large uvula, a short neck, smoking, enlarged tonsils or adenoids, and oropharyngeal edema.
- The most accurate test for sleep apnea is an overnight sleep study in which the patient is directly observed while wearing a variety of monitoring equipment to evaluate the depth of sleep, type of sleep, respiratory effort, oxygen saturation, and muscle movement.

Interprofessional Collaborative Care

Recognize Cues: Assessment

- Patients are often unaware that they have sleep apnea. The disorder is suspected for any adult who has persistent daytime sleepiness or reports "waking up tired," particularly if they also snore heavily.
  1. Assess for and document:
     - General appearance, including height and weight
     - Oral cavity, including the size and shape of the pharynx, the uvula, and tongue thickness and position
     - Blood pressure, heart rate and rhythm.
     - Personality changes, irritability, or depression
- An overnight sleep study known as **polysomnography** may be used for diagnosis in which the patient is directly observed during a full sleep time while wearing a variety of monitoring equipment to evaluate depth of sleep, type of sleep, respiratory effort, oxygen saturation, carbon dioxide exhalation, and muscle movement.

Analyze Cues and Prioritize Hypotheses: Analysis

- The primary collaborative problem for the patient with obstructive sleep apnea syndrome is:
  1. Persistent poor gas exchange and hypoxia due to abnormal sleep pattern

Generate Solutions and Take Actions: Planning and Implementation:
Improving the Duration of Restorative Sleep

- Management strategies for OSA vary with the severity of the problem and the patient's willingness to participate in the treatment process. Both nonsurgical and surgical management approaches are available to help correct the problem, depending on the cause and the severity.

1. A common method to prevent airway collapse is the use of noninvasive positive-pressure ventilation (NPPV) to hold open the upper airways.

2. A change in sleeping position, weight loss, or devices to prevent the tongue or neck anatomy from obstructing the airways may correct mild sleep apnea.

3. Surgical intervention is considered when patients are unable to tolerate CPAP or when its use does not improve OSA.

Care Coordination and Transition Management
- An important issue with CPAP therapy for OSA management is appropriate maintenance of the compressor and the mask/tubular system.

Evaluation: Evaluate Outcomes
- Evaluate the care of the patient with obstructive sleep apnea based on the priority patient problem.

See Chapter 23 in the main text for more information on obstructive sleep apnea.

ORGAN TRANSPLANTATION

- Organs are transplanted to improve quantity or quality of life when an organ fails or to replace bone marrow associated with immunity dysregulation.
- Common organ transplants in the United States are kidney, pancreas, liver, heart, lung, and intestine. Sometimes double transplants of kidney/pancreas or heart/lung are performed.
- Vascularized composite allografts (VCAs) are now also possible, including face and hand transplantation.
- Transplant centers specialize in the surgical care and ongoing management of organ recipients.
- The patient for potential transplantation undergoes extensive physiologic and psychological assessment and evaluation by primary health care providers and transplant coordinators.
- Generally, the patient has a chronic disabling condition that must be stabilized before transplant, but rapid progressive organ failure may result in organ transplantation.
- Donor organs are obtained primarily from deceased donors (trauma or other conditions) and living-related donors.

- Organs are distributed through a nationwide program—the United Network of Organ Sharing (UNOS). This system distributes donor organs based on regional considerations and patient acuity.
- Candidates with the highest level of acuity receive the highest priority.
- Most organ recipients require lifelong immune modulation through drug therapy to avoid rejection of the transplanted organ.

Organ transplantation is discussed in the main text in chapters related to the specific organ involved.

✳ OSTEOARTHRITIS: MOBILITY CONCEPT EXEMPLAR

Overview

- Osteoarthritis (OA) is the most common arthritis, with joint pain and loss of function leading to impaired ***mobility.***
- The disease includes progressive deterioration and loss of cartilage in one or more joints (articular or hyaline cartilage), especially the hips and knees, the vertebral column, and the hands.
    1. Enzymes, such as stromelysin, break down the articular matrix.
    2. As cartilage and the bone beneath the cartilage begin to erode, the joint space narrows and *osteophytes* (bone spurs) form.
    3. As the disease progresses, fissures, calcifications, and ulcerations develop and the cartilage thins.
    4. Cartilage disintegrates and pieces of bone and cartilage "float" in the diseased joint, causing *crepitus,* a grating sound caused by the loosened bone and cartilage.
    5. Joints become painful and stiff, and the body's normal repair process cannot overcome the rapid process of degeneration.
- Risk factors for OA include aging, genetics, obesity, joint trauma, metabolic and blood disorders, and smoking.

👤 PATIENT-CENTERED CARE: GENDER HEALTH

Osteoarthritis in Women

More men than women younger than 55 years have OA caused by athletic injuries. After age 55 women have the disease more often than men. Although the cause for this difference is not known, contributing factors may include increased obesity in women after having children and broader hips in women than men (Arthritis Foundation, 2022). Be sure to assess all patients in the hospital or community-based setting, particularly those who are older and obese, for signs and symptoms of OA.

Interprofessional Collaborative Care
Recognize Cues: Assessment
- Obtain patient information about:
  1. Joint pain and function
     - The nature and location of joint pain, stiffness, or swelling
     - What relieves or increases pain or stiffness
     - Any loss of mobility or difficulty in performing ADLs
  2. Trauma or recurrent stress to joints from occupational and recreational activity or sports
  3. Weight history
  4. Family history of arthritis
- Assess for and document:
  1. Chronic joint pain and stiffness
  2. Aggravating and relieving factors, such as activity and rest
  3. Limitations in range of motion (ROM)
  4. Crepitus (a continuous grating sensation felt or heard as the joint goes through its ROM)
  5. Joint enlarged from bony hypertrophy
  6. Joint warmth or inflammation (indicates a secondary synovitis)
  7. Hand changes with Heberden nodes (at the distal interphalangeal [DIP] joints) and Bouchard nodes (at the proximal interphalangeal [PIP] joints)
  8. Joint effusions (excess joint fluid), especially in the knee
  9. Compression of spinal nerve roots that produces radiating pain, stiffness, and muscle spasms in one or both extremities with vertebral involvement
  10. Reduced mobility and function
- Imaging assessment may include x-rays or MRI.

Analyze Cues and Prioritize Hypotheses: Analysis
- The priority collaborative problems for patients with OA include:
  1. Persistent **pain** due to joint swelling, cartilage deterioration, and/or secondary joint **inflammation**
  2. Potential for decreased **mobility** due to joint **pain** and muscle atrophy

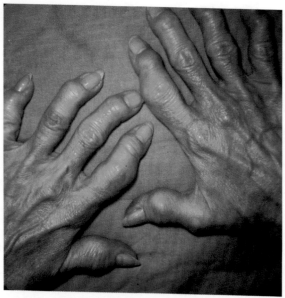

Osteoarthritic hands with Heberden (distal interphalangeal) and Bouchard (proximal interphalangeal) nodes on both index fingers and thumbs. Note angular changes at distal joints as a result of loss of joint cartilage and instability. (Beaty, J.H., Azar, F.M. [2021]. *Campbell's Operative orthopaedics* [14th ed.]. St. Louis: Elsevier.)

Generate Solutions and Take Actions: Planning and Implementation: *Managing Persistent Pain*
Nonsurgical Management
- Drug therapy
  1. Analgesic drugs
     - The American Pain Society, American Geriatrics Society, and OARSI committee recommend regular *acetaminophen* or NSAIDs as the primary drugs of choice (Bannuru et al., 2019)
  2. Topical drug applications
     - Diclofenac 1% topical gel (topical NSAID)

Drug Alert

The standard ceiling dose of acetaminophen is 4000 mg each day. However, patients may be at risk for liver damage if they take more than 3000 mg daily or have alcoholism or liver disease. *Older adults are particularly at risk because of normal changes of aging, such as slowed excretion of drug metabolites.* Remind patients to read the labels of over-the-counter (OTC) or prescription drugs that could contain acetaminophen before taking them. Teach them that their liver enzyme levels may be monitored while taking this drug.

O

3. NSAIDs as oral or topical agents
   • Cyclooxygenase (COX)-2–inhibiting selective agents such as celecoxib
   • Nonselective COX-inhibiting agents such as ibuprofen

Drug Alert

All of the COX-2–inhibiting drugs are thought to cause cardiovascular disease, such as myocardial infarction and hypertension, due to vasoconstriction and increased platelet aggregation (clumping). All NSAIDs can cause GI side effects, bleeding, and acute kidney injury if used long term (Burchum & Rosenthal, 2022). Therefore, they are prescribed at the lowest effective dose. Remind patients to take celecoxib with food to decrease GI distress. Teach your patient about potential adverse effects and the need to report them to the primary health care provider. Examples include having dark, tarry stools; shortness of breath; edema; frequent dyspepsia (indigestion); hematemesis (bloody vomitus); and changes in urinary output.

• Nonpharmacologic measures
   1. Position joint to avoid excessive flexion of involved joint and maintain normal extension.
      • Teach the patient to position joints in their functional position to avoid flexion contracture formation.
      • Supportive shoes or foot insoles can relieve pressure on painful metatarsal joints.
   2. Heat or cold applications (hot showers and baths, hot packs or compresses, moist heating pads)
   3. Weight control or weight loss can lessen stress on weight-bearing joints.

4. Complementary and integrative therapies (topical capsaicin products, acupuncture, acupressure, tai chi, music therapy) reduce pain and pain perception
5. Patients with osteoarthritis pain have reported the effectiveness of cannabinoids, and there is a growing body of scientific evidence that supports these reports.

Surgical Management

- Surgery may be indicated to manage the pain of OA and to improve mobility.
  1. *Total joint arthroplasty* (TJA) (surgical creation of a joint), also known as *total joint replacement* (TJR), is the most common type of surgery for OA. Almost any synovial joint of the body can be replaced with a prosthetic system that consists of at least two parts, one for each joint surface.
  2. *Total hip arthroplasty* (THA) with a replacement prosthesis can be done by a variety of procedures, including open hip incision or minimally invasive surgery (MIS). The replacement joint consists of four parts, the acetabular component (this has two parts) and the femoral component (this has two parts).
- Provide preoperative care.
  1. Assess the patient's level of understanding about the surgery.
  2. Identify a **joint coach** (care partner) who can help the patient through the perioperative period and assist with discharge needs.
  3. *Preoperative rehabilitation,* or "prehab," is essential to prevent functional decline after surgery and provide a quicker functional recovery.
- Provide postoperative care.
- Prevent operative joint dislocation by:
  1. Maintaining correct positioning (supine position with the head slightly elevated)
  2. Placing and supporting the affected leg in neutral rotation
  3. For the patient who had a *posterior surgical approach*, placing an abduction pillow between the legs to prevent adduction beyond the midline of the body, according to agency policy or surgeon preference.
  4. Following agency policy or surgeon preference for postoperative turning
  5. Observing for signs of possible hip dislocation (increased hip pain, shortening of the affected leg, and leg rotation)
- Prevent thromboembolic complications by:
  1. Administering prescribed anticoagulants, such as subcutaneous low-molecular-weight heparin or factor Xa inhibitors as prescribed
  2. Assessing for signs of venous thromboembolism (VTE) (leg swelling, pain)

3. Teaching leg exercises (plantar flexion and dorsiflexion, circles of the feet, gluteal and quadriceps muscle setting, straight-leg raises)
4. Applying prescribed antiembolic stockings or devices
5. Collaborating with the PT to promote early ambulation
- Manage postoperative pain.
  1. A *multimodal pain management* approach is best practice for patients who undergo a major joint arthroplasty.
  2. Immediate pain control may be achieved with short-term PCA or IV opioids.
  3. Nonopioids are also used, such as peripheral nerve block, NSAIDs, NMDA receptor antagonists, and gabapentinoids.
- Promote postoperative mobility.
  1. Collaborate with the PT to teach the patient how to follow weight-bearing restrictions. Most patients will use a walker.

! NURSING SAFETY PRIORITY

Action Alert

Be sure to assist the patient the first time getting out of bed to prevent falls and observe for dizziness. When getting the patient out of bed, put a gait belt on and then stand on the same side of the bed as the affected leg. After the patient sits on the side of the bed, remind the patient to stand on the unaffected leg and pivot to the chair with guidance. *To avoid injury, do not lift the patient!*

- Promote postoperative self-management.
  1. The length of stay in the acute care hospital is typically less than 3 days if there are no complications.
  2. Acute rehabilitation usually takes several weeks, depending on the patient's age and progress.

PATIENT AND FAMILY EDUCATION

Care of Patients With Total Hip Arthroplasty After Hospital Discharge

Hip Precautions
- Do not sit or stand for prolonged periods.
- Do not cross your legs beyond the midline of your body.
- For *posterolateral or direct lateral surgical approach* patients: Do not bend your hips more than 90 degrees.
- For *anterior surgical approach* patients: Do not hyperextend your operative leg behind you.

Continued

PATIENT AND FAMILY EDUCATION—cont'd

Care of Patients With Total Hip Arthroplasty After Hospital Discharge

- Do not twist your body when standing.
- Use the prescribed ambulatory aid, such as a walker, when walking.
- Call 911 if you experience any signs or symptoms of hip dislocation, including sudden difficulty bearing weight on the surgical leg, leg shortening or rotation, or a feeling that the hip has "popped" with immediate intense ***pain***.
- Resume sexual intercourse as usual on the advice of your surgeon.

Pain Management
- Report increased hip or anterior thigh pain to the surgeon immediately.
- Take oral analgesics as prescribed and only as needed.
- Do not overexert yourself; take frequent rests.
- Use ice or cryotherapy as needed on the operative hip to decrease or prevent swelling and minimize pain.

Incisional Care
- Follow the instructions provided regarding dressing changes, if needed. Some surgeons use specialty clear dressings that do not need to be changed. No dressing may be needed if a skin sealant was used.
- Inspect your hip incision every day for redness/hyperpigmentation, heat, or drainage; if any of these are present, call your surgeon immediately.
- Do not bathe the incision or apply anything directly to the incision unless instructed to do so.
- Shower according to the surgeon's instructions.

Other Care
- Continue to walk and to perform leg exercises as you learned them in the hospital. Do not increase the amount of activity unless instructed to do so by the therapist or surgeon.
- To help prevent blood clots, do not cross your legs.
- Report pain, redness/hyperpigmentation, or swelling in your legs to your surgeon immediately.
- Call 911 for acute chest pain or shortness of breath (could indicate pulmonary embolus).
- Follow the bleeding precautions learned in the hospital to prevent bleeding; avoid using a straight razor, avoid injuries, and report bleeding or excessive bruising to your surgeon immediately.
- Be sure to follow up with outpatient physical therapy for your exercise and ambulation program to build strength, ***mobility***, and endurance (if discharged to home).
- Follow up with visits to the surgeon's office as instructed.

- *Total knee arthroplasty* (TKA) can be performed by traditional open surgery or by MIS procedures for some patients.
  1. Provide preoperative care.
     - Care as described for THA
     - Explanation and demonstration of a continuous passive motion (CPM) machine (if prescribed)
  2. Provide postoperative care.
     - Care to prevent complications as described for THA
     - Implement the CPM machine as prescribed for ROM and cycles per minute.
     - Apply cryotherapy to decrease surgical site swelling and hematoma formation.
     - Ensure safe use of peripheral nerve blockade (PNB) for pain control.
     - Maintain the knee in a neutral position, not rotated internally or externally.
     - Ensure that the surgical knee is not hyperextended.
     - Monitor neurovascular status frequently to check for compromise to the distal operative leg every time vital signs are taken.

✚ NURSING SAFETY PRIORITY

Critical Rescue

If the patient has a continuous femoral nerve blockade (CFNB), perform and document neurovascular assessment every 2 to 4 hours, or according to hospital protocol. Be sure that patients can perform dorsiflexion and plantar flexion motions of the affected foot without pain in the lower leg. In addition, monitor these patients for signs and symptoms that indicate absorption of the local anesthetic into the patient's system, including:

- Metallic taste
- Tinnitus
- Nervousness
- Slurred speech
- Bradycardia
- Hypotension
- Decreased respirations
- Seizures

Document and report these new-onset signs and symptoms to the surgeon, anesthesiologist/nurse anesthetist, or Rapid Response Team immediately, and carefully continue to monitor the patient for any changes.

- *Total shoulder arthroplasty* (TSA) can be performed either as a TJR or as a hemiarthroplasty (replacement of part of the joint, typically the humeral component). These surgeries are most commonly performed using traditional open incisions, but minimally invasive shoulder arthroplasty can be used instead for some patients.
  1. Preoperative care and postoperative care are similar to the care provided for other joint replacement surgeries.
  2. A sling is applied to immobilize the joint and prevent dislocation until therapy begins.
  3. This may require an overnight stay or is often performed as a same-day procedure.
  4. Rehabilitation with an OT usually takes 2 to 3 months.

Improving Mobility

- Reinforce the techniques and principles of exercise, ambulation, and promotion of ADLs.
- Collaborate with the physical therapist to implement regular exercise.
- Assist the patient in considering recreational activities such as swimming to maintain muscle strength and joint mobility.
- Collaborate with the occupational therapist (OT) to provide suggestions and devices for assistance for ADLs.
- Use active rather than active-assist or passive exercise independent activity.

Care Coordination and Transition Management

- Teach patients with arthritis what exercises to do, joint protection techniques, and energy conservation guidelines to avoid impaired mobility.
- Teach patients who have OA or are prone to the disease to lose weight (if obese), avoid trauma, and limit strenuous weight-bearing activities.
- Collaborate with the discharge planner and the primary health care provider to determine the best placement for the patient with OA at discharge, particularly after joint replacement surgery.
- Implement interventions for patients having total TJA to prevent venous thromboembolic complications (e.g., anticoagulants, exercises, sequential compression devices); observe patients for bleeding when they are taking anticoagulants.
- Provide health teaching.
  1. Explain the general principles of joint protection.
     - Use large joints instead of small ones; for example, place a purse strap over the shoulder instead of grasping the purse with a hand.

- Turn doorknobs toward the thumb (rather than toward the little finger) to avoid twisting the arm and promoting ulnar deviation.
- Use two hands instead of one to hold objects.
- Sit in a chair that has a high, straight back.
- When getting out of bed, do not push off with the fingers; use the entire palm of both hands.
- Do not bend at the waist; instead, bend the knees while keeping the back straight.
- Use long-handled devices, such as a hairbrush with an extended handle.
- Use assistive-adaptive devices, such as Velcro closures and built-up utensil handles, to protect joints.
- Do not use pillows in bed, except a small one under the head.
- Avoid twisting or wringing the hands.

2. Explain the drug protocol, desired and potential side effects, and adverse or toxic effects.
3. Emphasize the importance of reducing weight and eating a well-balanced diet to promote tissue healing.
4. Refer the patient to the Arthritis Foundation for up-to-date information about new treatments and helpful complementary and alternative practices.
5. Provide written instructions about the required care, regardless of whether the patient goes home or to another inpatient facility.
6. Refer the patient to the nutritionist, counselor, home health nurse, rehabilitation therapist, financial counselor, and local and state support groups as needed.

Evaluating Outcomes: Evaluation

- Evaluate the care of the patient with OA on the basis of the identified priority problems. The expected outcomes are that the patient:
  1. Achieves pain control to a pain intensity level of 2 to 3 on a 0-to-10 scale or at a level that is acceptable to the patient
  2. Does not experience complications associated with total joint arthroplasty (if performed)
  3. Moves and functions in own environment independently with or without assistive devices

See Chapter 43 in the main text for more information on osteoarthritis.

OSTEOMYELITIS

- Osteomyelitis is an infection in bone caused by bacteria, viruses, or fungi.
- Osteomyelitis is difficult to treat and can result in chronic recurrence of infection, loss of function and mobility, amputation, and even death.
- Categories of osteomyelitis include:
  1. *Exogenous osteomyelitis,* in which infectious organisms enter from outside the body, as in an open fracture
  2. *Endogenous osteomyelitis,* also called *hematogenous osteomyelitis,* in which organisms are carried by the bloodstream from other areas of infection in the body
  3. *Contiguous osteomyelitis,* in which bone infection results from skin infection of adjacent tissues, as with surgical site infection or soft tissue infections from penetrating trauma
- Common causes include bacteremia or preexisting conditions that interfere with immune health or wound healing, such as diabetes, trauma, long-term IV therapy, hemodialysis, *Salmonella* infection of the GI tract, sickle cell disease, poor dental hygiene, periodontal infection, and infections with multidrug-resistant organisms (MDROs) like MRSA.

Interprofessional Collaborative Care
Recognize Cues: Assessment
- Assess for and document:
  1. Bone pain described as a constant, localized, pulsating sensation that worsens with movement
  2. Fever, usually greater than 101°F (38°C) during acute presentation
  3. Swelling, tenderness, erythema/hyperpigmentation, and heat around the site of infection
  4. Ulcerations on the feet or hands
  5. Sinus tract formation and drainage with chronic infection
  6. Elevated WBC, neutrophils, and erythrocyte sedimentation rate (ESR)
  7. Positive blood or wound cultures

Take Actions: Interventions
- The specific treatment for osteomyelitis depends on the type and number of microbes present in the infected tissue. If other measures fail to resolve the infectious process, surgical management may be needed.

- Nonsurgical interventions include:
  1. Early, acute diagnosis and appropriate management to avoid the conversion of acute osteomyelitis to chronic status
  2. Administering IV antibiotic therapy for several weeks, followed by oral antibiotic therapy for weeks or months
  3. Irrigating the wound, either continuously or intermittently, with one or more antibiotic solutions
  4. Packing the wound with beads made of bone cement that have been impregnated with an antibiotic
  5. Administering drugs for **pain** control
  6. Covering the wound to prevent infection spread
  7. Administering hyperbaric oxygen (HBO) therapy for patients with chronic, unremitting osteomyelitis to improve oxygenation via perfusion and promote healing

See Chapter 42 in the main text for more information on osteomyelitis.

OSTEOPOROSIS: CELLULAR REGULATION CONCEPT EXEMPLAR

Overview

- Osteoporosis is a chronic disease of **cellular regulation** in which bone loss causes significant decreased density and possible fracture. It is often referred to as a *silent disease* or *silent thief* because the first sign of osteoporosis in most people follows some kind of fracture.
- Osteoporosis occurs when the bone remodeling process (a type of cellular regulation) changes such that osteoclastic (bone resorption) activity is greater than osteoblastic (bone building) activity.
- Altered bone remodeling results in decreased bone mineral density and thin fragile bone tissue that is at risk for fracture, most often at the spine, hip, and wrist.
- Osteoporosis can be classified as generalized or regional.
  1. Generalized osteoporosis involves many structures in the skeleton and is further divided into two categories.
     - *Primary osteoporosis,* which is more common and occurs in postmenopausal women and in men in their sixth or seventh decade of life
     - *Secondary osteoporosis,* which results from other medical conditions, such as hyperparathyroidism, long-term drug

therapy (such as with corticosteroids), or prolonged immobility

2. Regional osteoporosis occurs when a limb is immobilized related to a fracture, injury, or paralysis for longer than 8 to 12 weeks.

- Risk factors for primary osteoporosis are caused by a combination of genetic, lifestyle, and environmental factors.

1. Nonmodifiable factors include older age, parental history of osteoporosis, history of fracture after age 50, and genetics that determine bone turnover or remodeling.

2. Modifiable factors include sedentary lifestyle; chronic low intake of protein, calcium, and vitamin D, or malabsorption syndromes; low body weight or thin build; alcohol and tobacco use; and long-term use of certain drugs, especially corticosteroids.

👤 PATIENT-CENTERED CARE: GENDER HEALTH
Gender Differences in Osteoporosis

Primary osteoporosis most often occurs in women after menopause or removal of both ovaries as a result of decreased estrogen levels. Obese women can store estrogen in their tissues for use as necessary to maintain a normal level of serum calcium better than thinner women, and are therefore less likely to develop osteoporosis and resulting fractures.

Men also develop osteoporosis as they age because their testosterone levels decrease. Testosterone is the major sex hormone that builds bone tissue. Older men are often underdiagnosed.

Interprofessional Collaborative Care
Recognize Cues: Assessment

- Obtain patient information about:
  1. Age, sex, race, body build, weight
  2. Loss of height (indicating loss of vertebrae integrity)
  3. Back pain after bending, lifting, or stooping (worse with activity, relieved with rest)
  4. Mobility or function
  5. Current drugs
- Assess for and document:
  1. Features of the spinal column, particularly presence of classic "dowager's hump," or kyphosis of the dorsal spine

Height

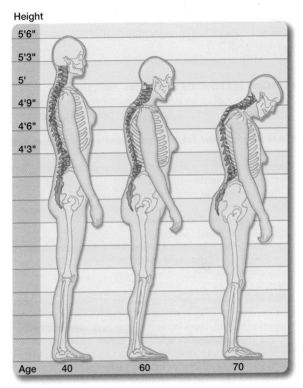

Normal spine at age 40 years and osteoporotic changes at ages 60 and 70 years. These changes can cause a loss of as much as 6 inches in height and can result in the so-called *dowager's hump* (far right) in the upper thoracic vertebrae.

2. Location of all painful areas and signs of fracture, such as swelling and misalignment. Back pain accompanied by tenderness and voluntary restriction of spinal movement suggests one or more compression vertebral fractures—the most common type of osteoporotic or fragility fracture.
3. Constipation, abdominal distention from immobility related to fracture
4. Respiratory compromise
5. Body image disturbance
6. Changes in quality of life and sexuality
- Diagnostic tests may include:
  1. Levels of serum calcium, vitamin D, phosphorus, and protein

2. Imaging to determine bone density:
   - Dual-energy x-ray absorptiometry (DXA)
   - CT-based absorptiometry (qualitative computed tomography [QCT])
   - MRI or magnetic resonance spectroscopy (MRS)

Analyze Cues and Prioritize Hypotheses: Analysis

- The priority problem for patients with osteoporosis or osteopenia is:
  1. Potential for fractures due to weak, porous bone tissue

Generate Solutions and Take Actions: Planning and Implementation

Nutrition Therapy

- Coordinate health teaching and nutrition planning with the registered dietitian nutritionist (RDN).
  1. Teach patients to eat a diet that includes:
     - Calcium and vitamin D; if lactose intolerant, suggest soy and mineral-fortified foods
     - Low-fat protein sources
     - Moderation in alcohol intake (fewer than three drinks daily)
     - A variety of nutrients to maintain bone health

Lifestyle Changes

- Assist with a plan to provide regular weight-bearing exercise.
  1. Coordinate health teaching with the PT for exercises to improve posture, support, and pulmonary capacity; strengthen core and extremity muscles; and improve ROM.
  2. Teach patients to avoid high-impact recreational activities.
- Teach about other lifestyle changes, including:
  1. Smoking cessation and avoiding secondhand tobacco smoke
  2. Preventing falls

Drug Therapy

- Administer drug therapy for prevention and management.
  1. Bisphosphonates to slow bone reabsorption
  2. Estrogen agonist/antagonist
  3. Calcium and vitamin D supplementation; these supplements alone are insufficient to prevent or treat osteoporosis but are important to bone health
  4. Denosumab, a RANK ligand (receptor activator of nuclear factor kappa-B ligand) that prevents osteoclast activation
  5. The newest drug for osteoporosis is a monoclonal antibody called romosozumab, the first drug in a class of sclerostin inhibitors.
  6. Teriparatide and abaloparatide are *parathyroid hormone–related protein drugs* that build bone and may not be used long term

Care Coordination and Transition Management
- Patients with osteoporosis are typically managed in the community and at home.
- Collaborate with members of the interprofessional health team to ensure that the patient's home is safe and hazard-free to help prevent falling.
- Teach patients about diet and lifestyle interventions to slow bone loss.
- Teach patients about drugs used to manage osteoporosis and about the need for ongoing follow-up with their provider.
  1. Remind patients to have follow-up DXA scans as prescribed to determine the effectiveness of drug therapy.

Evaluating Outcomes: Evaluation
- Evaluate the care of the patient with osteoporosis or at risk for osteoporosis based on the identified priority patient problem. Expected outcomes are that the patient:
  1. Continues to follow up with DXA screenings as recommended to assess ongoing bone health
  2. Makes necessary changes in lifestyle to help prevent further bone loss
  3. Does not experience a fragility fracture due to bone loss

 See Chapter 42 in the main text for more information on osteoporosis.

OTITIS MEDIA

- The common forms of otitis media are acute otitis media, chronic otitis media, and serous otitis media. Each type affects the middle ear but has different causes and pathologic changes.
- If otitis media progresses or recurs without treatment, permanent conductive hearing loss may occur.

Interprofessional Collaborative Care
Recognize Cues: Assessment
- Assess for signs of acute or chronic otitis media.
  1. Ear pain with or without movement of the external ear (which is relieved when the eardrum ruptures)
  2. Sensation of fullness in the ear
  3. Reduced or distorted hearing
  4. Tinnitus
  5. Headaches
  6. Dizziness or vertigo
  7. Systemic symptoms of fever, malaise, or nausea and vomiting

8. Otoscopic examination findings
   - Dilated and red eardrum blood vessels
   - Red, thickened, or bulging eardrum
   - Decreased eardrum mobility
   - Eardrum perforation with pus present in the canal

Take Actions: Interventions

- Management begins with a quiet environment and allowing the patient to rest. Bed rest limits head movements that intensify the *pain*.
  1. Systemic antibiotic therapy is needed to address the infection.
  2. Administer analgesics such as ibuprofen and acetaminophen for mild to moderate pain.
  3. Apply low heat to reduce pain.
  4. Administer an antihistamine or decongestant to decrease fluid in middle ear.

Surgical Management

- If pain persists after antibiotic therapy and the eardrum continues to bulge, surgical management with a myringotomy (surgical opening of the eardrum), often combined with tube insertion (to provide ongoing drainage), may be needed to drain fluid.
  1. Postoperatively, teach the patient to keep the external ear and canal free of other substances.
  2. Instruct the patient to avoid washing the hair or showering for 48 hours.

🌣 PATIENT AND FAMILY EDUCATION

Recovery From Ear Surgery

- Avoid straining when you have a bowel movement.
- Avoid drinking through a straw for 2 to 3 weeks.
- Avoid air travel for 2 to 3 weeks.
- Avoid excessive coughing for 2 to 3 weeks.
- Avoid people with respiratory infections.
- When blowing your nose, blow gently, without blocking either nostril and with your mouth open.
- Avoid getting your head wet or washing your hair for several days.
- You may shower; before doing so, place a ball of cotton coated with petroleum jelly in it, or use a waterproof earplug.
- Avoid rapidly moving the head, bouncing, and bending over for 3 weeks.
- If you have a dressing, change it every 24 hours or as directed.
- Report excessive drainage immediately to your health care provider.

 See Chapter 40 in the main text for more information on otitis media.

PAIN

- *Pain* is universal, complex, and a personal experience that everyone has at some point in life. *Pain* is defined as an unpleasant sensory and emotional experience associated with actual or potential tissue damage.

- Self-report is always the most reliable indication of pain.
  1. *Acute pain* results from trauma, surgery, or tissue injury. It is usually temporary, has a sudden onset, and is localized.
  2. *Persistent (chronic) pain* persists for longer than 3 months, is often poorly localized, and is hard to describe. It is often associated with depression, interference with personal relationships, and inability to maintain activities of daily living (ADLs).
- Pain is also categorized as:
  1. Nociceptive, with normal processing of pain signals. This type of pain can be acute or persistent.
  2. **Neuropathic pain** is a descriptive term used to refer to pain that is believed to be sustained by a set of mechanisms driven by damage to or dysfunction of the PNS and/or CNS. In contrast to nociceptive pain, which is sustained by ongoing activation of essentially *normal* neural systems, neuropathic pain is sustained by the *abnormal* processing of stimuli.

Legal/Ethical Considerations
Effective Pain Management

The American Nurses Association (ANA) has a specific position statement regarding the ethical responsibility of nurses to manage pain (ANA, 2018). Although the opioid crisis has presented obstacles to pain management, effective and unbiased pain management remains an ethical responsibility for the nurse. Interprofessional collaboration is required to develop pain management plans that include thorough assessment, goal setting, and ongoing reassessment to determine the efficacy of pain management. Professional nursing implications include recognition of personal bias and deliberate work to relieve inequities that may prevent the relief of pain and suffering (ANA, 2018).

Interprofessional Collaborative Care
Recognize Cues: Assessment

- The primary role of the nurse in *pain* management is to advocate for patients by *accepting* their reports of pain and acting promptly to relieve it while respecting their preferences and values. It is important for the nurse to recognize any potential personal bias or prejudice that could influence the management of patient's pain (ANA, 2018).

- Conduct a comprehensive pain assessment, including:
  1. Location of pain
     - *Localized* pain is confined to the site of origin.
     - *Projected* pain is diffuse around the site of origin and is not well localized.
     - *Referred* pain is felt in an area distant from the site of painful stimuli.
     - *Radiating* pain is felt along a specific nerve or nerves.
  2. Intensity of pain: Ask the patient to rate the severity of the pain using a reliable and valid assessment tool.
     - Numeric Rating Scale
     - Wong-Baker FACES Pain Rating Scale
     - Faces Pain Scale
     - Verbal Descriptor Scale

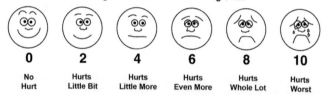

Wong-Baker FACES® Pain Rating Scale

0	2	4	6	8	10
No Hurt	Hurts Little Bit	Hurts Little More	Hurts Even More	Hurts Whole Lot	Hurts Worst

©1983 Wong-Baker FACES® Foundation. Visit us at www.wongbakerFACES.org.
Used with permission. Originally published in Whaley & Wong's Nursing Care of Infants and Children. ©Elsevier Inc.

Wong-Baker FACES® pain rating scale. (From Wong-Baker FACES Foundation [2016]. Wong-Baker FACES® Pain Rating Scale. Retrieved March 12, 2017, with permission from http://www.WongBakerFACES.org.)

  3. Quality: Ask the patient to describe how the **pain** and discomfort feel.
  4. Onset and duration: Ask the patient when the pain started and whether it is constant or intermittent.
  5. Aggravating and relieving factors: Ask the patient what makes the pain worse and what makes it better.
  6. Effect of pain on function and quality of life: The effect of pain on the ability to perform recovery activities should be evaluated regularly.
  7. Comfort-function (pain intensity) outcomes: For patients with *acute pain,* identify expected short-term functional outcomes. Reinforce to the patient that adequate pain control will lead to more successful achievement of those outcomes.

8. Other information: Consider the patient's culture, past pain experiences, and pertinent medical history, such as comorbidities.

👤 PATIENT-CENTERED CARE: OLDER ADULT HEALTH

Effective Pain Assessment

Pain is not a result of aging; however, the incidence is higher in older adults. Sensitivity to pain does not diminish with age. Many older adults, even those with mild to moderate dementia, are able to use a self-report assessment tool if nurses and other caregivers take the time to administer it. Many older adults are reluctant to report pain for a variety of reasons, including the belief that it is normal and that they are bothering the nurse. It is essential that attempts be made to obtain the patient's self-report and that pain be assessed frequently with a focus on functional and quality-of-life indicators in this vulnerable population (Rebar & Heimgartner, 2020).

Take Actions: Interventions
Nonsurgical Management
Drug Therapy

- Multimodal analgesia: Multimodal treatment involves the use of two or more classes of analgesics or interventions to target different pain mechanisms in the PNS or CNS.
  1. A multimodal approach may allow lower doses of each of the drugs in the treatment plan (Czarnecki & Turner, 2018).
  2. Lower doses have the potential to produce fewer side effects.
  3. Multimodal analgesia can result in comparable or greater relief than can be achieved with any single analgesic.
- Preemptive analgesia: Involves the administration of local anesthetics, opioids, and other drugs (multimodal analgesia) in anticipation of pain along the continuum of care during the preoperative, intraoperative, and postoperative periods.
  1. This continuous approach is designed to decrease pain severity in the postoperative period, reduce analgesic dose requirements, prevent morbidity, shorten hospital stay, and avoid complications after discharge.
- Routes of administration: The oral route is the *preferred* route of analgesic administration.
  1. Other routes of administration are used when the oral route is not possible, such as in patients who are NPO, nauseated, or unable to swallow.
- Around-the-clock (ATC) dosing: Controlling pain may require ATC dosing rather than PRN ("as needed") to maintain stable analgesic levels.

1. Patient-controlled analgesia (PCA) is an interactive method of management that allows patients to treat their **pain** by self-administering doses of analgesics.
2. Patients who use PCA must be able to understand the relationships among pain, pressing the PCA button and taking the analgesic, and pain relief.
3. They must also be cognitively and physically able to use any equipment that is used to administer the therapy.

- The three analgesic groups:

1. Nonopioid analgesics
   - Acetaminophen and nonsteroidal antiinflammatory drugs (NSAIDs)
   - Acetaminophen and an NSAID may be given together, and there is no need for staggered doses.
   - Unless contraindicated, all surgical patients should routinely be given acetaminophen and an NSAID in scheduled doses as the foundation of the pain treatment plan throughout the postoperative course, preferably initiated before surgery.
   - The most serious complication of acetaminophen is hepatotoxicity (liver damage) as a result of overdose.
   - NSAIDs have more adverse effects than acetaminophen, with gastric toxicity and ulceration being the most common.

⬧ NURSING SAFETY PRIORITY
Drug Alert

NSAIDs can cause GI disturbances and decrease platelet aggregation (clotting), which can result in bleeding. Therefore, observe the patient for gastric discomfort or vomiting and for bleeding or bruising. Tell the patient and family to stop taking these drugs and report these effects to the primary health care provider immediately if any of these problems occur. Celecoxib has no effect on bleeding time and produces less GI toxicity compared with other NSAIDs.

---

2. Opioid analgesics
   - Opioid analgesics are the mainstay in the management of moderate to severe nociceptive types of pain, such as postoperative, surgical, trauma, and burn pain.
   - Examples are morphine, fentanyl, hydromorphone, oxycodone, oxymorphone, and hydrocodone.
   - Collaborate with the health care provider and patient to provide safe, effective care when opioids are used.

- Monitor and prevent complications from side effects. Side effects can include respiratory depression, sedation, constipation, nausea and vomiting, urinary retention, and pruritus (itching).
- Monitor RR and depth, especially when the patient is sleeping.
- Sedation occurs before opioid-induced respiratory depression, so nurse-monitored sedation levels are recommended by use of a sedation scale for opioid-naive (not currently on an opioid) patients or those receiving opioids intravenously (IV) or epidurally. The key to assessing sedation is determining how easily the patient is aroused.
- Prevent constipation with concurrent administration of a stool softener or bowel stimulant.
- When opioids are prescribed for longer than 3 to 7 days, consider risk for dependence, tolerance, or addiction.
- *Addiction* is a chronic neurobiologic disease with one or more of the following: impaired control over drug use, compulsive use, continued use despite harm, and craving.
- *Tolerance* is a state of adaptation in which exposure to a drug induces changes that result in a decrease in one or more of the drug's effects over time.
- *Physical dependence response* occurs with repeated administration of an opioid for several days. It is manifested by the occurrence of withdrawal symptoms when the opioid is stopped suddenly or rapidly reduced or an antagonist such as naloxone is given. Withdrawal symptoms may be suppressed by the natural, gradual reduction of the opioid as pain decreases or by gradual, systematic reduction, referred to as *tapering. Physical dependence is not the same as addiction.*

PATIENT-CENTERED CARE: OLDER ADULT HEALTH

Opioid Dosing

Although the patient's weight is not a good indicator of analgesic requirement, *age is considered an important factor to consider when selecting an opioid dose.* For older adults the guideline is to "start low and go slow" with all drug dosing. For example, the starting opioid dose may need to be reduced by 25% to 50% in older adults because they are more sensitive to opioid side effects than are younger adults. The subsequent doses are based on patient response, which should be evaluated frequently. Monitor sedation level and respiratory status and promptly reduce the drug dose if sedation occurs or the respiratory rate is markedly decreased, depending on agency policy. Many older adults are admitted to the ED with fractures of the hip, pelvis, and spine, which are very painful and require prompt and adequate *pain* management to promote patient *comfort.*

3. Adjuvant analgesic drugs may be used to relieve pain alone or in combination with other analgesics by potentiating or enhancing the effectiveness of the analgesic.
   - Antiepileptic drugs (AEDs or anticonvulsants)
     - Gabapentin
     - Pregabalin
   - Tricyclic antidepressants
     - Amitriptyline
     - Nortriptyline
   - Other antidepressants
     - Duloxetine
     - Venlafaxine

👤 PATIENT-CENTERED CARE: OLDER ADULT HEALTH

Adjuvant Analgesic Safety

Older adults are often sensitive to the effects of adjuvant analgesics, such as anticonvulsants and antidepressants, which produce sedation and other CNS effects. Therapy should be initiated with low doses, and titration should proceed slowly, with systematic assessment of patient response. Caregivers in the home setting must be taught to take preventive measures to reduce the likelihood of falls and other accidents. A home safety assessment is highly recommended and can be arranged by social services before discharge.

- Local anesthetics relieve *pain* by blocking the generation and conduction of the nerve impulses necessary to transmit pain. The local anesthetic effect is dose related.
- Medical marijuana (Cannabis): Cannabis is a schedule I controlled substance and has been since 1970. However, the use of cannabis and cannabinoids for various medical reasons, including persistent and neuropathic *pain,* is increasing. Currently, 37 jurisdictions have legalized the use of medical cannabis, creating a conflict between state and federal law in the United States (National Conference of State Legislatures, 2022). Medical use of cannibis is legal in Canada.
- Nonpharmacologic interventions include:
  1. Physical modalities
     - Physical therapy
     - Occupational therapy
     - Aquatherapy
     - Functional restoration (also has cognitive-behavioral components)
     - Acupuncture
     - Low-impact exercise programs such as slow walking and yoga

2. Cutaneous (skin stimulation) strategies:
   - Application of heat, cold, or pressure
   - Therapeutic massage
   - Vibration
   - Transcutaneous electrical nerve stimulation (TENS)
3. Cognitive-behavioral modalities
   - Distraction
   - Guided imagery
   - Relaxation (may be combined with music therapy)
   - Hypnosis
   - Mindfulness
   - Biofeedback

Care Coordination and Transition Management

- Pain can be managed in any setting, including the home. Some patients require parenteral pain medications at home; therefore, provide health teaching to ensure continuity of care.
- Refer patients whose pain is difficult to manage to pain specialists and/or pain centers.
- Make appropriate referrals for physical therapy, a clinical nurse specialist in pain management, a social worker, and hospice or palliative care.
- Plan a home care nurse referral for patients who will require assistance or supervision with the patient's pain relief regimen at home.

 See Chapter 6 in the main text for more information on pain.

PAIN, LOW BACK (LUMBOSACRAL)

- The areas of the back most commonly affected by back pain are the cervical and lumbar vertebrae.
- *Acute low back pain* (LBP) occurs along the lumbosacral area of the vertebral column.
  1. Acute pain is caused by muscle strain or spasm, ligament sprain, disk degeneration, or herniation of the center of the disk (herniated nucleus pulposus).
  2. Acute back pain usually results from injury or trauma such as during a fall, vehicular crash, or lifting a heavy object.
- Persistent *(chronic)* LBP persists for 3 or more months.
  1. Acute or repeated back injury can contribute to spinal stenosis, a narrowing of the spinal canal, damage to nerve root canals, or intervertebral foramina malformation.

2. Trauma, arthritis, infection, disk degeneration from aging, and inherited (e.g., ankylosing spondylitis) or congenital conditions such as scoliosis can also contribute to chronic LBP.
3. Back pain may also be caused by *spondylolysis,* a defect in one of the vertebrae, usually in the lumbar spine. Spondylolisthesis occurs when one vertebra slips forward on the one below it, often as a result of vertebral bony defect.

👤 PATIENT-CENTERED CARE: OLDER ADULT HEALTH

Low Back Pain

Older adults are at high risk for acute and chronic LBP. Vertebral fracture from osteoporosis contributes to LBP. Petite, older White women are at high risk for both bone loss and subsequent vertebral fractures. Specific factors that can cause LBP in the older adult include (Touhy & Jett, 2022):

- Spinal stenosis
- Hypertrophy of the intraspinal ligaments
- Osteoarthritis
- Osteoporosis
- Changes in vertebral support structures and malalignment with deformity
- Scoliosis
- Lordosis (an inward abnormal curvature of the lumbar spinal area)
- Vascular changes
- Diminished blood supply to the spinal cord or cauda equina caused by arteriosclerosis
- Blood dyscrasias
- Intervertebral disk degeneration
- Vertebral compression fractures

Interprofessional Collaborative Care
Recognize Cues: Assessment

- Assess and document:
  1. A complete pain assessment, including pain location, quality, radiation, severity, and alleviating and aggravating factors
  2. Posture and gait
  3. Vertebral alignment
  4. Muscle tone and strength; limitations or presence of spasm
  5. Tenderness or swelling of the spinal column
  6. Sensory changes: paresthesia, numbness, or tingling
  7. Vertebral changes seen on an x-ray, computed tomography (CT) scan, or magnetic resonance imaging (MRI) scan
  8. Abnormal electromyography and nerve conduction studies

Take Actions: Interventions

Nonsurgical Management

- To treat acute LBP:
  1. Use the Williams position when in bed (semi-Fowler's bed position with the knees flexed) if a herniated disk is present. In a side-lying position, a pillow between the knees may be helpful.
  2. Collaborate with the physical therapist (PT) to develop an individualized exercise and rehabilitation program to strengthen core and leg muscles after acute pain resolves.
  3. Drug therapy includes NSAIDs (oral and topical) and other drugs to manage acute pain.
- Approaches for treating persistent back pain:
  1. Collaborate with the dietitian to implement a weight-loss program if appropriate.
  2. Collaborate with the occupational therapist (OT) for ergonomic and adaptive furniture and aids.
  3. If complementary and integrative therapy measures along with NSAIDs are ineffective in relieving persistent LBP, ziconotide may be used as a potent analgesic (sometimes used for patients who have severe chronic pain).
  4. Opioids have a very limited role in the treatment of back pain; they are used sparingly and for a very short time
  5. Nonpharmacologic therapy, such as spinal manipulative therapy, distraction, imagery, and music therapy, can reduce the effects associated with persistent pain.

Surgical Management

- Conventional open operative procedures include:
  1. *Discectomy,* in which a portion of the disk is removed
  2. *Laminectomy,* which is the removal of one or more vertebral laminae, plus osteophytes, and the herniated nucleus pulposus through a 3-inch (7.5-cm) incision
  3. *Spinal fusion* to stabilize the affected area. Chips of bone are grafted between the vertebrae for support and to strengthen the back. Metal implants (usually titanium pins, screws, plates, or rods) may be required to ensure the fusion of the spine.
  4. Artificial disk replacement may also be part of this type of surgery.
- Minimally invasive operative procedures include *microdiskectomy* or *percutaneous endoscopic discectomy* (PED), a procedure that may be used with *laser thermodiscectomy* to shrink the herniated disk before removal.

- Provide routine postoperative care.
  1. Postoperative care depends on the type of surgery that was performed.
  2. In the postanesthesia care unit (PACU), vital signs and level of consciousness are monitored frequently, the same as for any surgery.
  3. Patients who have a *minimally invasive spinal surgical procedure* go home the same day or the day after surgery with one or more wound closure tapes over the small incision.
  4. Perform neurologic assessment with vital signs every 4 hours during the first 24 hours.
  5. Check the patient's ability to void. An inability to void may indicate damage to sacral spinal nerves. Opioid analgesics have been associated with difficulty voiding and constipation.
  6. Maintain vertebral alignment with frequent log roll repositioning.

✚ NURSING SAFETY PRIORITY

Critical Rescue

For the patient after back surgery, inspect the surgical dressing for blood or any other type of drainage. Clear drainage may mean cerebrospinal fluid (CSF) leakage. Blood and CSF may be mixed on the dressing, with the CSF being visible as a "halo" around the outer edges of the dressing. The loss of a large amount of CSF may cause the patient to report having a sudden headache. *If a CSF leak is suspected, keep the patient on bed rest, and lower the head of the bed immediately to slow the loss of fluid! Report signs of any drainage on the dressing to the surgeon or Rapid Response Team. Bulging at the incision site may be due to a CSF leak or a hematoma, both of which should also be reported immediately.*

Care Coordination and Transition Management

- After *conventional open back surgery,* the patient may have activity restrictions for the first 4 to 6 weeks, such as:
  1. Limit daily stair climbing.
  2. Restrict or limit driving.
  3. Do not lift objects heavier than 5 lb.
  4. Restrict pushing and pulling activities (e.g., dog walking).
  5. Avoid bending and twisting at the waist.
- In a few patients, back surgery is unsuccessful. This situation (failed back surgery syndrome [FBSS]), is a complex combination of organic, psychological, and socioeconomic factors.
  1. Nerve blocks, implantable spinal cord stimulators (neurostimulators), and other chronic pain management modalities may be needed on a long-term basis to help with comfort.

 See Chapter 37 in the main text for more information on pain, back.

PAIN, CERVICAL NECK

- Cervical neck pain most often results from a bulging or herniation of the nucleus pulposus (HNP) in a cervical intervertebral disk.
- Cervical back pain also may result from muscle strain or ligament sprain, bony spur (from osteoarthritis), arthritis, tumor, infection, poor posture, or history of trauma.

Interprofessional Collaborative Care

- Conservative treatment for acute neck *pain* is the same as described for low back pain except prescribed exercises focus on the shoulders and neck.
- A cervical collar may be prescribed for no more than 10 days; prolonged use can lead to increased pain and decreased muscle strength and range of motion (ROM).

Surgical Management

- Depending on the causative factors, an anterior or a posterior approach may be used to provide a discectomy and spinal fusion.
- Provide routine preoperative and postoperative care.

+ NURSING SAFETY PRIORITY

Critical Rescue

The priority for care in the immediate postoperative period after an anterior cervical discectomy and fusion (ACDF) is to maintain an airway and ensure that the patient has no problem with breathing. Swelling from the surgery can narrow the trachea, causing a partial obstruction. Surgery can also interfere with cranial innervation for swallowing, resulting in a compromised airway or aspiration. If these changes occur, open the patient's airway, sit the patient upright, suction if needed, and provide supplemental oxygen. Promptly notify the surgeon or Rapid Response Team using SBAR, and document your assessment and interventions.

---

1. Monitor for complications:
   - CSF leak from the surgical site
   - Hoarseness or dysphagia resulting from laryngeal injury
   - Esophageal, tracheal, or vertebral artery injury
   - Graft extrusion and screw loosening if a fusion was performed

BEST PRACTICE FOR PATIENT SAFETY AND QUALITY CARE

Care of the Patient After an Anterior Cervical Diskectomy and Fusion

Postoperative Interventions
- Assess **a**irway, **b**reathing, and **c**irculation (first priority!).
- Check for bleeding and drainage at the incision site.
- Monitor vital signs and neurologic status frequently.
- Check for swallowing ability.
- Monitor intake and output.
- Assess the patient's ability to void (may be a problem secondary to opiates or anesthesia).
- Manage *pain* adequately.
- Assist the patient with ambulation within a few hours of surgery, if he or she is able.

Discharge Teaching
- Be sure that someone stays with the patient for the first few days after surgery.
- Review drug therapy.
- Teach care of the incision.
- Review activity restrictions:
  - No lifting
  - No driving until surgeon permission
  - No strenuous activities
- Walk every day.
- Call the primary health care provider if symptoms of pain, numbness, and tingling worsen or if swallowing becomes difficult.
- Wear brace or collar per the primary health care provider's prescription.

 See Chapter 37 in the main text for more information on pain, cervical neck.

PANCREATITIS, ACUTE: INFLAMMATION CONCEPT EXEMPLAR

Overview
- Acute pancreatitis is a serious and, at times, life-threatening *inflammation* of the pancreas caused by premature activation of pancreatic enzymes that destroy ductal tissue and pancreatic cells; it results in autodigestion and fibrosis of the pancreas.
- Pancreatitis can range from mild involvement evidenced by edema and inflammation to *necrotizing hemorrhagic pancreatitis (NHP)*. NHP is diffuse bleeding pancreatic tissue with fibrosis and tissue death (Rogers, 2023).

Interprofessional Collaborative Care
Recognize Cues: Assessment
- Obtain patient information about:
  1. History of abdominal *pain*, especially if related to alcohol ingestion or high intake of fat
  2. Individual and family history of alcoholism, pancreatitis, or biliary tract disease
  3. Previous abdominal surgeries or diagnostic procedures
  4. Medical history, including kidney disease, abdominal surgery or procedures, biliary tract diseases, trauma, hyperparathyroidism, and hyperlipidemia
  5. Recent viral infection
  6. Use of prescription and OTC drugs
- Assess for and document:
  1. Abdominal *pain* (the most frequent symptom), particularly sudden-onset pain in a midepigastric or left upper quadrant location with radiation to the back, left flank, or left shoulder, aggravated by a fatty meal, ingestion of a large amount of alcohol, or lying in the recumbent position
  2. Weight loss, with nausea and vomiting
  3. Jaundice
  4. Gray-blue discoloration of the abdomen and periumbilical area (Cullen's sign)
  5. Gray-blue discoloration of the flanks (Turner's sign)
  6. Absent or decreased bowel sounds
  7. Abdominal tenderness, rigidity, and guarding
  8. Dull sound on abdominal percussion, indicating ascites
  9. Elevated temperature with tachycardia and decreased blood pressure
  10. Adventitious breath sounds, dyspnea, or orthopnea
  11. Elevated serum amylase and lipase levels

✚ NURSING SAFETY PRIORITY
Critical Rescue

For the patient with acute pancreatitis, monitor for significant changes in vital signs that may indicate the life-threatening complication of shock. Hypotension and tachycardia may result from pancreatic hemorrhage, excessive fluid volume shifting, or the toxic effects of abdominal sepsis from enzyme damage. Observe for changes in behavior and level of consciousness (LOC) that may be related to alcohol withdrawal, hypoxia, or impending sepsis with shock.

- Diagnostic studies may include:
  1. Serum lipase, amylase, alkaline phosphatase, alanine amino-transferase (ALT), bilirubin, white blood cell (WBC), hemo-globin, hematocrit, coagulation factors, basic metabolic panel (electrolytes and kidney function), calcium, magnesium, tri-glycerides, and albumin
  2. Imaging of the pancreas and gallbladder with ultrasound or CT scan

Analyze Cues and Prioritize Hypotheses: Analysis
- The priority collaborative problems for patients with acute pancreatitis include:
  1. Severe acute *pain* due to pancreatic *inflammation* and enzyme leakage
  2. Weight loss and inadequate *nutrition* due to inability to ingest food and absorb nutrients

Generate Solutions and Take Actions: Planning and Implementation
Managing Acute Pain
- The priorities for patient care are supportive care by relieving pain and other symptoms, decreasing *inflammation*, and anticipating or treating complications. As for any patient, continually assess for and support the ABCs (airway, breathing, and circulation).
- Decrease *pain* with interventions that reduce GI activity (decrease pancreatic synthesis of enzymes).
  1. Initiate NPO status for 24 to 48 hours.
  2. Consider nasogastric drainage and suction to manage vomiting or biliary obstruction.

❗ NURSING SAFETY PRIORITY
Action Alert

Because paralytic (adynamic) ileus is a common complication of acute pancreatitis, prolonged nasogastric intubation may be necessary. Assess frequently for the return of peristalsis by asking patients whether they have passed flatus or had a stool. The return of bowel sounds is unreliable as an indicator of peristalsis return; passage of flatus or a bowel movement is the most reliable indicator.

- Manage *pain* with nonopioid and opioid analgesics.
  1. Comfort measures include helping the patient assume a side-lying position to decrease abdominal pain and providing antinausea drugs and antiemetics as needed.

2. Histamine receptor antagonists (e.g., famotidine) and proton pump inhibitors (e.g., pantoprazole) help decrease gastric acid secretion. Antibiotics may be prescribed, but they are indicated primarily for patients with acute necrotizing pancreatitis or pancreatic abscess.

! NURSING SAFETY PRIORITY

Action Alert

For the patient with acute pancreatitis, monitor respiratory status every 4 to 8 hours or more often as needed, and provide oxygen to promote comfort in breathing. Respiratory complications such as pleural effusions increase patient discomfort. Fluid overload can be detected by assessing for weight gain, listening for crackles, and observing for dyspnea. Carefully monitor for signs of respiratory failure.

Promoting Nutrition
- Maintain hydration and electrolyte balance with IV fluids.
- Provide jejunal, enteral, or parenteral nutrition unless paralytic ileus is present.
- When food is tolerated, provide small-volume, high-carbohydrate, and high-protein feedings with limited fats.

Care Coordination and Transition Management
- Patient and family health teaching is aimed at preventing both future episodes and disease progression to chronic pancreatitis.
  1. Encourage alcohol abstinence to prevent *pain* and extension of the inflammatory damage.
  2. Teach the patient to notify the primary health care provider of experiences with acute abdominal pain or symptoms of biliary tract disease, such as jaundice, clay-colored stools, and dark urine.
  3. Emphasize the importance of follow-up visits with the primary health care provider.

Evaluate Outcomes: Evaluation
- Evaluate the care of the patient with acute pancreatitis based on the identified priority patient problems. The expected outcomes include that the patient will:
  1. Have control of abdominal *pain*, as indicated by self-report and pain scale measurement
  2. Have adequate *nutrition* available to meet metabolic needs

See Chapter 51 in the main text for more information on pancreatitis, acute.

PANCREATITIS, CHRONIC

- Chronic pancreatitis is a progressive, destructive disease with remissions and exacerbations.
- *Inflammation* and fibrosis of the tissue contribute to pancreatic insufficiency and diminished function of the organ.
  1. Pancreatic insufficiency is characterized by the loss of exocrine function, resulting in a decreased output of enzymes and bicarbonate and altered digestion.
  2. Diabetes results from loss of endocrine function.

Interprofessional Collaborative Care
Recognize Cues: Assessment
- Assess for and document key features of chronic pancreatitis.

 KEY FEATURES

Chronic Pancreatitis

- Intense abdominal *pain*, a major symptom, that is continuous and burning or gnawing
- Abdominal tenderness
- Ascites
- Possible left upper quadrant mass (if pancreatic pseudocyst or abscess is present)
- Respiratory compromise manifesting with adventitious or diminished breath sounds, dyspnea, or orthopnea
- **Steatorrhea**; clay-colored stools
- Weight loss
- Jaundice
- Dark urine
- Polyuria, polydipsia, polyphagia (diabetes mellitus)

Take Actions: Interventions
- The focus of caring for the patient with chronic pancreatitis is to manage acute or persistent *pain*, maintain adequate *nutrition*, and prevent disease recurrence.

Nonsurgical Management
- Drug therapy includes:
  1. Opioid analgesia (the patient may become dependent on opioids with long-term use)
  2. Nonopioid analgesics

3. Pancreatic-enzyme replacement therapy (PERT) is the standard of care to prevent malnutrition, malabsorption, and excessive weight loss.
4. Insulin to control diabetes
5. H_2-blocker or proton pump inhibitor to decrease gastric acid

---

! NURSING SAFETY PRIORITY

Action Alert

P

If the patient has diabetes, insulin or oral antidiabetic agents for glucose control are prescribed. Patients maintained on total parenteral nutrition (TPN) are particularly susceptible to elevated glucose levels and require regular insulin additives to the solution. Monitor blood glucose to control hyperglycemia. Check fingerstick blood glucose (FSBG) or sugar (FSBS) levels every 2 to 4 hours.

- Record daily weight and the number and consistency of stools per day to monitor the effectiveness of drug therapy.
- Diet therapy includes:
  1. Providing total parenteral nutrition (TPN) or total enteral nutrition (TEN)
  2. Consult with the registered dietitian nutritionist (RDN) to provide sufficient calories and protein to maintain health.

Surgical Management
- Surgery is not a primary intervention for the treatment of chronic pancreatitis. However, it may be indicated for ongoing abdominal *pain,* incapacitating relapses of pain, or complications such as a **pancreatic abscess** or **pancreatic pseudocyst** (Bartel, 2020).

Care Coordination and Transition Management
- Health teaching is aimed at preventing further exacerbations.
  1. Avoid known precipitating factors, such as alcohol and foods with a high-fat content.
  2. Comply with diet instructions: high protein, high carbohydrate, and low or no fat.
  3. Follow written instructions and prescriptions for pancreatic enzyme therapy regarding:
     - How and when to take enzymes
     - The importance of maintaining therapy
     - The importance of notifying the health care provider of increased steatorrhea, abdominal distention, cramping, and skin breakdown

4. Comply with elevated glucose management, including oral hypoglycemic drugs or insulin injections and monitoring of blood glucose levels.
5. Keep follow-up visits with the health care provider.
- Refer the patient to case management, financial counseling, social services, vocational rehabilitation, home health services, and Alcoholics Anonymous, as needed.

See Chapter 51 in the main text for more information on pancreatitis, chronic.

✳ PARKINSON'S DISEASE: MOBILITY CONCEPT EXEMPLAR

Overview
- Parkinson's disease (PD) is a progressive neurodegenerative disorder involving the basal ganglia and substantia nigra, leading to a decrease of dopamine in the brain. Loss of dopamine results in difficulty with voluntary movement. Loss of dopamine reduces the sympathetic nervous system influence in the cardiovascular system, contributing to autonomic dysfunction and neuropsychiatric symptoms such as mood disorders.
- The disease is characterized by tremor, muscle rigidity, bradykinesia or akinesia (slow movements), and postural instability.
- The disease involves five stages.
    1. *Stage 1:* mild disease with unilateral limb involvement
    2. *Stage 2:* bilateral limb involvement
    3. *Stage 3:* significant gait disturbances and moderate generalized disability
    4. *Stage 4:* severe disability, akinesia, and muscle rigidity
    5. *Stage 5:* complete dependency in all aspects of ADLs

Interprofessional Collaborative Care
Recognize Cues: Assessment
- Obtain patient information about:
    1. Time and the progression of symptoms, such as tremors, and slowed voluntary and automatic movements, such as a change in handwriting
    2. Family history related to neurologic disorders
- Assess for and document:
    1. Rigidity, which is present early in the disease process and progresses over time
    2. Posture and appearance
        - Stooped posture, flexed trunk

3. Gait
   - Slow and shuffling with short, hesitant steps
   - Propulsive gait
   - Difficulty stopping quickly
4. Speech
   - Change in voice volume, phonation, or articulation
5. Motor dysfunction
   - Bradykinesia or akinesia
   - Tremors, especially at rest
   - "Pill-rolling" movement
   - Masklike face
   - Difficulty chewing and swallowing
   - Difficulty getting into and out of bed
6. Autonomic dysfunction
   - Orthostatic hypotension
   - Excessive perspiration and oily skin
   - Uncontrolled drooling, especially at night
   - Bowel and bladder dysfunction
7. Psychosocial effects
   - Emotional lability, easily upset, rapid mood swings
   - Depression
   - Cognitive impairments
   - Delayed reaction time
   - Sleep disturbances

Analyze Cues and Prioritize Hypotheses: Analysis
- The priority collaborative problems for patients with PD include:
  1. Decreased *mobility* (and possible self-care deficit) due to muscle rigidity, resting tremors, and postural/gait changes
  2. Impaired *cognition* due to neurotransmitter and neuronal changes in the brain

Generate Solutions and Take Actions: Planning and Implementation
Promoting Mobility
Nonsurgical Interventions
- Provide drug therapy.
  1. Administer drug therapy on time to maintain continuous therapeutic drug levels.
     - Dopamine agonists such as apomorphine, pramipexole, and ropinirole
     - Levodopa combinations are less expensive than the dopamine agonists and are better at improving motor function, but long-term use leads to dyskinesia.

- Catechol-*O*-methyltransferase (COMT) inhibitors to interfere with the breakdown of dopamine in the CNS
- Monoamine oxidase type B (MAO-B) inhibitors
- Variety of other drugs and drug combinations

NURSING SAFETY PRIORITY

Drug Alert

Dopamine agonists are associated with adverse effects such as orthostatic (postural) hypotension, hallucinations, sleepiness, and drowsiness, and can be mistaken for signs and symptoms of PD. Remind patients to avoid operating heavy machinery or driving if they have any of these symptoms. Teach them to change from a lying or sitting position to standing by moving slowly. The primary health care provider should not prescribe drugs in this class to older adults because of their severe adverse drug effects.

NURSING SAFETY PRIORITY

Drug Alert

Teach patients taking monamine oxidase inhibitors (MAOIs) about the need to avoid foods, beverages, and drugs that contain tyramine, including cheese and aged, smoked, or cured foods and sausage. Remind them to also avoid red wine and beer to prevent severe headache and life-threatening hypertension (Burchum & Rosenthal, 2022). Patients should continue these restrictions for 14 days after the drug is discontinued.

2. Monitor the patient for drug toxicity, decreased effectiveness of the drug, and adverse effects such as delirium.
   - Drug toxicity can be treated with a decrease in drug dose or frequency or a drug holiday of about 10 days.
- Manage *mobility* impairment:
  1. Nontraditional exercise such as yoga and tai chi
  2. Collaborate with PT and OT to maintain patient flexibility, prevent falling, and promote out-of-bed activity.
  3. If the patient is hospitalized for any reason, be sure to place on Fall Precautions according to agency policy.
  4. Encourage the patient to participate as much as possible in self-management, including ADLs.
  5. Make the environment conducive to independence, including the use of adaptive or assistive devices.
  6. Collaborate with the registered dietitian nutritionist (RDN) and speech-language pathologist to ensure sufficient oral intake and avoid injury from swallowing difficulties.
  7. Together with the interprofessional team, develop a communication plan if the patient has speech difficulties.

Surgical Interventions

- Several options are available if surgery for the patient with PD is needed. Surgery is a last resort, when drugs are ineffective in symptom management. The most common surgeries are stereo-tactic pallidotomy and deep brain stimulation, although newer surgical procedures are being tried.

Managing Cognitive Dysfunction

- About 50% of patients with PD have cognitive dysfunction. Pimavanserin is a new drug that is used only for Parkinson's disease–related hallucinations and delusions (psychoses).

Care Coordination and Transition Management

- The long-term management of PD presents a special challenge in the home care setting.
- A case manager may be required to coordinate interprofessional care and provide support for the patient and family.
- Teach patients and their families about the need to follow instructions regarding the safe administration of drug therapy.
- Remind them to immediately report adverse effects of medication, such as dizziness, falls, acute confusion (delirium), and hallucinations.
- Collaborate with the social worker or case manager to help the family with financial and health insurance issues, as well as respite care or permanent placement if needed.
- Refer the patient and family to social and state agencies, as well as support groups.

Evaluate Outcomes: Evaluation

- Evaluate the care of the patient with PD based on the identified priority patient problems. The expected outcomes include that the patient and/or family will:
  1. Improve **mobility** to provide self-care and not experience complications of impaired mobility
  2. Maintain safety and an acceptable quality of life

See Chapter 36 in the main text for more information on Parkinson's disease.

PELVIC INFLAMMATORY DISEASE: INFECTION CONCEPT EXEMPLAR

Overview

- Pelvic inflammatory disease (PID) is an acute syndrome resulting in tenderness in the tubes and ovaries (adnexa) and, typically, dull pelvic **pain**.

- PID occurs when organisms from the lower genital tract migrate from the endocervix upward through the uterine cavity into the fallopian tubes.
  1. Sexually transmitted organisms are most often responsible, especially *C. trachomatis* and *N. gonorrhoeae* (Ross & Chacko, 2022).
  2. Bacterial vaginosis is also a common causative agent (Ross & Chacko, 2022).
- The infection may spread to other organs and tissues. This may involve one or more of the pelvic structures, including the uterus, fallopian tubes, and adjacent pelvic structures.
- Sepsis and death can occur, especially if treatment is delayed or inadequate.
  1. Complications of PID include chronic pelvic pain, infertility, risk for ectopic pregnancy, and tubo-ovarian abscess (TOA), a serious short-term condition requiring hospitalization in which an inflammatory mass arises on the fallopian tube, ovary, and/or other pelvic organs, and (rarely) fatal intraabdominal sepsis (Ross & Chacko, 2022).
- Although common signs and symptoms include tenderness in the tubes and ovaries (adnexa) and low, dull abdominal pain, some patients have only mild discomfort or menstrual irregularity, and others experience no symptoms at all. These variations can make the diagnosis of PID challenging.

Interprofessional Collaborative Care
Recognize Cues: Assessment
- Obtain patient information about:
  1. Menstrual, obstetric, sexual, and family history
  2. History of previous episodes of PID or other sexually transmitted infection (STI)
  3. Results of cultures or serum analysis congruent with infection or infecting organism
  4. Results of pelvic examination, particularly the presence of purulent cervical discharge or friable cervical tissue
  5. Previous reproductive surgery
  6. Abnormal vaginal bleeding
  7. Dysuria (painful urination)
  8. Increase or change in vaginal discharge
  9. Dyspareunia (painful sexual intercourse)
  10. Risk factors, including:
      - Multiple sexual partners
      - Practicing inconsistent use of condoms
      - Previous episodes of sexually transmitted infection or PID
- Assess for and document:
  1. ***Pain***, especially lower abdominal pain
  2. Fever, chills, generalized aches

3. Hunched-over gait
4. Abdominal tenderness, rigidity, or rebound tenderness
- Assess for psychosocial issues, such as:
  1. Anxiety and fear
  2. Need for reassurance and support during the physical examination
  3. Embarrassment
  4. Discomfort when discussing symptoms or sexual history
- Diagnosis is made based on history, physical symptoms and signs, cervical or vaginal mucopurulent discharge, presence of WBCs on saline microscopy of vaginal secretions, and positive culture or nucleic acid test (e.g., laboratory identification of *N. gonorrhoeae* or *Chlamydia* in urine or genital secretions/discharge). Other tests that may be helpful include ultrasonography, MRI, and endometrial biopsy.

Analyze Cues and Prioritize Hypotheses: Analysis
- The priority collaborative problem for patients with PID is:
  1. ***Infection*** due to invasion of pelvic organs by sexually transmitted pathogens
  2. Pain due to the infectious process

Generating Solutions and Take Actions: Planning and Implementation
Managing Infection and Pain
- Uncomplicated PID is usually treated with oral antibiotics.
- Hospitalization for PID for treatment with intravenous antibiotics is recommended if the patient has a complicated history or presentation (such as pregnancy or tubo-ovarian abscess), does not respond to oral antibiotic therapy, or has severe illness.
- Drug therapy includes oral and/or parenteral antibiotics for 14 days.
- In a small number of patients, a laparotomy may be needed to remove a pelvic abscess.
- Provide nonjudgmental emotional support, and allow time for patients to discuss their feelings.

> **! NURSING SAFETY PRIORITY**
>
> *Action Alert*
>
> Instruct women who are being treated for PID on an ambulatory care basis to avoid sexual intercourse for the full course of antibiotic treatment and until their symptoms have resolved and their partner(s) have been treated for any STIs (Workowski et al., 2021). Teach them to check their temperature twice daily and to report an increase in temperature to their health care provider. Remind them to be seen by the health care provider within 72 hours from starting antibiotic treatment and then 1 and 2 weeks from the time of the initial diagnosis.

Care Coordination and Transition Management

- Counsel the patient to contact sexual partner(s) for examination and treatment.
- Teach the patient about the need to:
  1. Abstain from sexual intercourse during treatment
- Discuss contraception and the patient's need or desire for it. This discussion includes the use of condoms, which can decrease the risk for future episodes of PID.
- Provide referral for follow-up related to serious psychosocial reactions. A patient who has PID may exhibit a variety of feelings (guilt, disgust, anger) about having a condition that may have been transmitted sexually. These feelings may affect relationships with significant others and future sexual partners.

Evaluate Outcomes: Evaluation

- Evaluate the care of the patient with PID based on the identified priority patient problem(s). The expected outcomes include that the patient should:
  1. Show evidence that the **infection** has resolved
  2. Report or demonstrate that **pain** is relieved or reduced and that she feels more comfortable
  3. Articulate a plan for ensuring treatment of her partner, obtaining antibiotics, and returning for follow-up care

See Chapter 65 in the main text for more information on pelvic inflammatory disease (PID).

PERICARDITIS

- Pericarditis is an inflammation or alteration of the pericardium, the membranous sac enclosing the heart. Alterations include fibrotic, serous, hemorrhagic, purulent, and neoplastic changes to the sac or fluid in the pericardial space.
- There are two types of pericarditis.
  1. *Acute pericarditis* is most commonly associated with infective organisms (bacteria, viruses, fungi), postmyocardial infarction syndrome, postpericardiotomy syndrome, and acute exacerbations of systemic connective tissue disease.
  2. *Chronic constrictive pericarditis* is caused by tuberculosis, radiation therapy, trauma, renal failure, and metastatic cancer, with the pericardium becoming rigid, preventing adequate ventricular filling, and resulting in cardiac failure.

Interprofessional Collaborative Care

Recognize Cues: Assessment

- Assess for and document:
  1. The nature of chest discomfort; pericardial **pain** is typically substernal, worse on inspiration and lessens when the patient leans forward
  2. Pericardial friction rub (may be heard with the diaphragm of the stethoscope positioned at the left lower sternal border). This scratchy, high-pitched sound is produced when the inflamed, roughened pericardial layers create friction as their surfaces rub together.
  3. Acute pericarditis diagnostic criteria include two of the following:
     - Pericardial chest pain
     - Presence of pericardial rub
     - New ST elevation in all ECG leads or PR-segment depression
     - New or worsening pericardial effusion
  4. Chronic constrictive pericarditis (lasting longer than 3 months) often exhibits:
     - Right-sided heart failure, including dyspnea, exertional fatigue, and orthopnea
     - Elevated systemic venous pressure with jugular distention
     - Hepatic engorgement
     - Dependent edema

Take Actions: Interventions

- Treatment depends on the type of pericarditis.
- Acute pericarditis is treated by:
  1. Administering NSAIDs, corticosteroids, and antibiotics
  2. Encouraging rest
  3. Colchicine twice a day, orally, for 3 months has been shown to prevent pericarditis recurrence (Imazio, 2023).
- Chronic pericarditis is treated by:
  1. Radiation or chemotherapy if it is associated with malignant disease
  2. Hemodialysis if it is associated with uremia from kidney disease
  3. Surgical excision of the pericardium if the chronic pericarditis is constrictive (e.g., *pericardial window* or *pericardectomy*)
- Complications of pericarditis include pericardial effusion and cardiac tamponade, resulting in decreased cardiac output similar to heart failure.

 See Chapter 29 in the main text for more information on pericarditis.

PERIOPERATIVE CARE

- Patient care before (**preoperative**), during (**intraoperative**), and after (**postoperative**) surgery is the **perioperative** experience.
- Patient *safety* throughout the perioperative period is the number one priority and requires teamwork and interprofessional collaboration.

PERIOPERATIVE CARE: PREOPERATIVE PHASE

- The preoperative period begins when the patient is scheduled for surgery and ends at the time of transfer to the surgical suite.
- The nurse prepares the patient for surgery and ensures patient safety.

Interprofessional Collaborative Care
Recognize Cues: Assessment

Taking a Preoperative History

- Age
- General status of health
- Review of systems
- Medical history
  - Current medical problems and their treatment
  - Allergies, including sensitivity to latex products
  - History of any type of prostheses
- Surgical history
  - Prior surgical procedures and how these were tolerated
  - Prior experience with anesthesia (e.g., difficulty being aroused after surgery, ongoing nausea and vomiting)
  - Prior experience with postsurgical *pain* control
- Social history
  - Use of tobacco, alcohol, or illicit substances, including marijuana (which may be legalized in certain states)
  - Current drugs taken (prescribed and over-the-counter)
  - Use of complementary or alternative therapies or practices such as vitamins, minerals, herbal preparations, folk remedies, or acupuncture
- Family history
  - Relevant information about similar familial surgeries and outcomes
  - History of malignant hyperthermia, cancer, or a bleeding disorder
  - History of reactions or complications associated with anesthesia
- Psychosocial status
  - Knowledge about and understanding of events during the perioperative period

Taking a Preoperative History—cont'd

- Comfort level with understanding the type of surgery planned and the anticipated outcomes
- Adequacy of the patient's support system
- Cultural or spiritual needs
  - Desire for (or against) autologous or directed blood (or blood product) donations
  - Requests for postsurgical cultural needs or spiritual support

P

! NURSING SAFETY PRIORITY

Action Alert

Ask about a history of joint replacement, and document the exact location of any prostheses. Communicate this information to operative personnel to ensure that electrocautery pads, which could cause an electrical burn, are not placed on or near the area of the prosthesis. Other areas to avoid when placing electrocautery pads include on or near bony prominences, pacemakers, scar tissue, hair, tattoos, weight-bearing surfaces, pressure points, and metal piercings.

- A *review of systems* involves the collection of information about body symptoms to understand what signs or symptoms the patient has experienced or may be currently experiencing (Centers for Medicare and Medicaid Services [CMS], 2021).

Review of Systems

General (Constitutional)
- Fevers and/or chills
- Generalized weakness

Eyes
- Dryness or infection of conjunctiva and/or lids
- Blurring or changes in vision

Ears, Nose, Mouth, Throat
- Ear drainage or pain
- Difficulty or changes in hearing

Genitourinary
- Pain or burning on urination
- Frequency, urgency, or incontinence
- Bladder changes or difficulty

Respiratory
- Cough with sputum or blood
- Pain or shortness of breath when breathing
- Obstructive sleep apnea

Continued

Review of Systems—cont'd

Musculoskeletal
- Clubbing or cyanosis in digits or nails
- Pain in joints
- Symmetry of extremities
- Loss of or change in range of motion
- Difficulty or changes in breathing through the nose
- Sinus tenderness
- Oral lesions
- Changes in dentition (e.g., cavities, dentures)
- Difficulty in swallowing

Cardiovascular
- Edema
- Exercise intolerance
- Pain
- Palpitations
- Venous thromboembolism
- History of ischemic heart disease

Gastrointestinal
- New or unusual masses or tenderness
- Bowel changes or difficulty

Integumentary (Includes Skin and Breast)
- Dryness, rashes, lesions, or ulcerations

Neurologic
- Changes in memory or usual state of orientation
- One-sided weakness
- Numbness or tingling
- Loss of balance
- History of cerebrovascular disease

Psychiatric
- General mood
- Depression over diagnosis
- Anxiety about surgery

Endocrine
- Increased thirst or urination
- Unexplained weight loss or gain

Hematologic and Lymphatic
- Swollen nodes
- New or unusual bleeding
- Nonhealing wounds

Allergic and Immunologic
- Seasonal, food, chemical allergies
- Changes in immune system

Analyze Cues and Prioritize Hypotheses: Analysis
- The priority collaborative problems for preoperative patients are:
  1. Need for health teaching due to unfamiliarity with surgical procedures and preparation
  2. Anxiety due to fear of a new or unknown experience, ***pain***, and/or surgical outcomes

PATIENT-CENTERED CARE: OLDER ADULT HEALTH

Preoperative Care

When planning care for older adults in the preoperative phase, recognize that these patients may have:

- Greater incidence of chronic illness (hypertension, diabetes)
- Greater incidence of malnutrition and dehydration
- More allergies
- An increased number of abnormal laboratory values (anemia, low albumin level)
- Increased incidence of impaired self-care abilities
- Inadequate or absent support systems
- Decreased ability to withstand the stress of surgery and anesthesia
- Increased risk for cardiopulmonary complications after surgery
- Risk for a change in mental status when admitted (e.g., related to unfamiliar surroundings, change in routine, drugs)
- Increased risk for a fall and resultant injury
- Mobility changes that affect recovery efforts

P

Generate Solutions and Take Actions: Planning and Implementation

Need for Health Teaching: Providing Information

- Explore the patient's level of knowledge and understanding of the planned surgery. Have patients explain in their own words the purpose of the surgery and expected results.
- As required by The Joint Commission, ensure that the correct site is selected and the wrong site is avoided. A licensed independent practitioner (who will perform the surgery) marks the site and, whenever possible, involves the patient.
- Ensure proper patient identification, including placement of identification bands. Use at least two appropriate identifiers.
- Ensure that informed consent is obtained from the patient (or legal designee) by the surgeon before sedation is given and before surgery is performed. Consent implies that the patient has sufficient information to understand:
  1. The nature of and reason for surgery
  2. Who will perform the surgery and whether others will be present during the procedure
  3. All available options and the risks associated with each option
  4. The risks associated with the surgical procedure and its potential outcomes
  5. The risks associated with the use of anesthesia
  6. The risks, benefits, and alternatives to the use of blood products

> ! **NURSING SAFETY PRIORITY**
>
> *Action Alert*
>
> Before surgery, be certain to provide the patient with information about informed consent (which the surgeon will obtain), dietary restrictions, specific preparation for surgery (e.g., bowel and skin preparations), exercises that will be required after surgery, and plans for pain management following the procedure. This helps to promote the patient's participation in self-care, which will help the patient better achieve the expected outcome.

- Preoperative care includes:
  1. Determining the existence and nature of the patient's advance directives
  2. Implementing and evaluating adherence to oral or dietary restrictions
     - Recommendations include NPO status (no eating or drinking), typically for 6 or more hours for easily digested solid food and 2 hours for clear liquids.
     - Failure to adhere to NPO status can result in cancellation of surgery or increase the risk for aspiration during or after surgery.
  3. Ensuring intestinal preparation
     - Before abdominal, bowel, or intestinal surgery, a simple enema, "enemas until clear," or mild or potent laxatives may be prescribed to empty the large intestine to reduce the potential for contamination of the surgical field.
     - Antibiotics may be administered immediately before orthopedic and abdominal surgery to reduce bacterial load.
  4. Performing skin preparation
     - Skin preparation before surgery is the first step to reduce the risk for *surgical site infection* (SSI) (AORN, 2021).
     - Confirm or assist the patient in the use of an antiseptic solution while showering and removal of oil and skin debris. This intervention reduces the number of organisms on the skin and the potential for a site infection.
     - Remove hair at the surgical site with clippers.
  5. Teaching the patient about the potential use of tubes, drains, and vascular access
     - Reassure the patient that these are temporary and that efforts will be made to reduce discomfort.
     - Common devices include:
       - Foley catheter
       - Nasogastric tube (NGT)
       - Drains (e.g., Penrose, Jackson-Pratt, Hemovac)
       - Vascular access

6. Teaching about postoperative interventions to prevent respiratory complications
   - Deep diaphragmatic and expansion breathing, splinting during cough, and position changes
   - Incentive spirometry
   - Turning and positioning
7. Teaching about identification and prevention of cardiovascular complications
   - Teach that deep venous thrombosis, or DVT (a type of venous thromboembolism [VTE]), is swelling in one leg, the presence of calf pain that worsens with ambulation, or worsening shortness of breath.
   - Use compression stockings or pneumatic compression devices to prevent superficial venous stasis and VTE.
   - Use leg exercises and early ambulation to prevent VTE and promote venous return.
8. Reviewing the plans for pain management postoperatively
   - If the patient is receiving sedation or general anesthesia, stress the importance of having another adult drive the patient home after the procedure.
9. Communicating during hand-off to the operating room (OR) personnel all of the care that has been provided and what care may still be needed
10. Ensuring appropriate clothing removal and storage of valuables
    - Removal and safekeeping of dentures, dental prostheses (e.g., bridges, retainers), jewelry (including body piercing), eyeglasses, contact lenses, hearing aids, wigs, and other prostheses
11. Correctly administer prescribed preoperative drugs, including cardiovascular drugs and antibiotics.

Minimizing Anxiety
- Assess the patient's knowledge about the surgical experience.
- Allow ample time for questions.
- Respond to questions accurately or facilitate communication with the knowledgeable care provider.
- Incorporate family or supportive adults in communications.
- Provide opportunity for distraction, rest, or relaxation.
- Communicate to the perioperative team any of the patient's concerns, fears, or preferences.

Evaluate Outcomes: Evaluation
- Evaluate the care of the preoperative patient based on the identified patient problems. The expected outcomes include that the patient:
  1. States understanding of the informed consent and preoperative procedures

   2. Demonstrates postoperative exercises and techniques for prevention of complications

   3. Verbalizes reduced anxiety

PERIOPERATIVE CARE: POSTOPERATIVE PHASE

- The **postoperative period** starts with completion of the surgical procedure and transfer of the patient to a specialized area for monitoring, such as the PACU or an ICU. This period may extend beyond discharge from the hospital, until activity restrictions have been lifted.

- Postoperative and postanesthesia care is divided into three phases based on the level of care needed, not the physical setting. Not every patient will need all three phases.

   1. Phase 1 includes close monitoring of airway, vital signs (VS), and indicators of recovery every 5 to 15 minutes. The length of time the patient remains at a phase I level of care depends on health status, the surgical procedure, anesthesia type, and rate of progression to regain alertness and hemodynamic stability.

   2. Phase 2 focuses on preparing the patient for care in another setting, such as an acute care unit, ICU, skilled nursing facility (SNF), or home.

   3. Phase 3 occurs in the extended care environment (e.g., hospital, residence) with assisted and self-management.

▶▶ BEST PRACTICE FOR PATIENT SAFETY AND QUALITY CARE

Postoperative Hand-off Report

- Type and extent of the surgical procedure
- Type of anesthesia used; length of time the patient was under anesthesia
- Allergies (especially to latex or drugs)
- Primary language, any sensory impairments, any communication difficulties
- Special requests that were verbalized by the patient before surgery, including communications with caregiver
- Preoperative and intraoperative respiratory function and dysfunction
- Any health problems or pathophysiologic conditions
- Any relevant events or complications during anesthesia or surgery, such as a traumatic intubation
- If intraoperative complications occurred, how were they managed and what were the patient responses (e.g., laboratory values, excessive blood loss, injuries)
- Intake and output, including current IV fluid administration and estimated blood loss

BEST PRACTICE FOR PATIENT SAFETY AND QUALITY CARE—cont'd

Postoperative Hand-off Report

- Type and amount of IV fluids or blood products administered
- Medications administered and when last dose of pain medication given
- When the next dose of antibiotics, cardiac drugs, or other medications is due
- Location and type of incisions, dressings, catheters, tubes, drains, or packing
- Prosthetic devices (existing or applied)
- Joint or limb immobility while in the operating room, especially in the older patient
- Other intraoperative positioning that may be relevant in the postoperative phase
- Status of current vital signs, including temperature and oxygen saturation

Interprofessional Collaborative Care
Recognize Cues: Assessment

- The initial assessment of the patient immediately after surgery includes the respiratory status (including peripheral oxygenation [Spo_2]), level of consciousness, temperature, pulse, and blood pressure.

 NURSING SAFETY PRIORITY

Critical Rescue

During the postoperative period, recognize that all patients remain at risk for pneumonia, shock, cardiac arrest, respiratory arrest, VTE, and gastrointestinal (GI) bleeding. These serious complications can be prevented, or the consequences reduced, by using prudent clinical judgment. If any signs or symptoms of these conditions are noted, respond by immediately notifying the surgeon.

- Examine the surgical area for bleeding and drainage.
- Assess VS on admission and then follow agency protocol for frequency. Changes in heart rate, blood pressure, respiratory rate, or peripheral oxygenation (oximetry, Spo_2) that are concerning need to be communicated urgently to the provider or Rapid Response Team.
- Increase the frequency of VS assessment whenever VS increase or decrease, particularly when there is clinical concern around

maintaining a narrow range of values. High or low values in VS can be early indicators of adverse reaction to operative drugs, blood or volume loss, and postoperative complications, including myocardial infarction or stroke.

> **! NURSING SAFETY PRIORITY**
>
> **Action Alert**
>
> Perform an initial assessment and continue to monitor respiratory assessment for any patient who has undergone general anesthesia or moderate sedation or has received sedative or opioid drugs.

- Routine postoperative monitoring and assessment include:
  1. Respiratory status
     - Evaluate airway patency and adequacy of gas exchange by oxygen saturation, end-tidal carbon dioxide levels, respiratory rate, pattern, and effort.
     - Ensure security and placement (e.g., depth) of an artificial airway (endotracheal tube, nasal trumpet, oral airway).
     - Maintain type of oxygen delivery device and the concentration of oxygen delivered.
     - Auscultate lung fields for breath sounds.
     - Examine the degree of symmetry of breath sounds and chest movement.
     - Determine the presence of snoring and stridor.

> **➕ NURSING SAFETY PRIORITY**
>
> **Critical Rescue**
>
> If you recognize that the patient's oxygen saturation drops below 95% (or below the patient's presurgery baseline), immediately respond by notifying the surgeon or anesthesia provider. If the patient's condition continues to deteriorate or other symptoms arise, an emergency response is imperative.

  2. Cardiovascular status
     - Evaluate the heart rate, quality, and rhythm.
     - Carefully monitor blood pressure values.
     - Monitor electrocardiography for dysrhythmias.
     - Compare distal pulses, color, temperature, and capillary refill on extremities.
     - Examine feet and legs for manifestations of DVT (e.g., redness/hyperpigmentation, pain, warmth, swelling).

- Maintain any prescribed compression devices or antiembolic stockings applied in the preoperative or operative suite.
3. Neurologic status
    - Trending level of consciousness or awareness
    - Presence of lethargy, restlessness, or irritability
    - Patient responses to stimuli (calling the patient's name, touching the patient, and giving simple commands such as "Open your eyes" and "Take a deep breath")
    - Degree of orientation to person, place, and time by asking the conscious patient "What is your name?" (person), "Where are you?" (place), and "What day is it?" (time)
    - Compare the patient's baseline preoperative neurologic status with postoperative findings.

PATIENT-CENTERED CARE: OLDER ADULT HEALTH

Regaining Orientation

An older adult may take longer than a younger adult to return to the level of presurgical orientation. Preoperative drugs and anesthetics can slow the process. Prevention of delirium involves being mindful of sensory needs (glasses, hearing aids), early ambulation (if possible), bedside presence of a family member or caregiver (if possible), effective pain management, mindfulness of sleep and nutritional status, maintenance of a calm environment, and cognitive stimulation (Touhy & Jett, 2023).

4. Motor and sensory function status
    - Ask the patient to move each extremity.
    - Assess the strength of each limb, comparing the results on both sides.
    - Gradually elevate the patient's head and monitor for hypotension.
5. Fluid, electrolyte, and acid-base balance
    - Measure intake and output (including IV fluid intake, emesis, urine, wound drainage, NGT drainage).
    - Check hydration status (e.g., inspecting the color and moisture of mucous membranes; the turgor, texture, and tenting of the skin; the amount of drainage on dressings; and the presence of axillary sweat).
6. Kidney and urinary status
    - Measure intake and output.
    - Assess for urine retention by inspection, palpation, percussion of the lower abdomen for bladder distention, or use of a bladder scanner.

- Perform prescribed intermittent catheterization.
- Assess urine for color, clarity, and amount.

7. GI status
   - Listen for bowel sounds in all four abdominal quadrants and at the umbilicus.
   - Assess for nausea and vomiting; postoperative nausea and vomiting are common with general anesthesia.
   - Administer prescribed antiemetic drugs.
   - Assess for symptoms of paralytic ileus (few or absent bowel sounds, distended abdomen, abdominal discomfort, vomiting, and no passage of flatus or stool).
   - Assess and record the color, consistency, and amount of the NGT drainage.
   - Check NGT placement.

> ! **NURSING SAFETY PRIORITY**
>
> *Action Alert*
>
> After gastric surgery, do not move or irrigate the NG tube unless ordered.

8. Integumentary status
   - Assess the incision (if visible) for redness/hyperpigmentation, increased warmth, swelling, tenderness or pain, and the type and amount of drainage; be sure to look under the patient for pooling, collection, or drainage and blood.
   - Condition of the sutures or staples.
   - Presence of open areas.

9. Dressings and drains
   - Document color, amount, consistency, and odor of drainage.
   - Examine for leakage around or under the patient.
   - Determine patency of drains.
   - Perform neurovascular checks to identify any restriction of circulation or sensation.

10. *Pain* assessment
    - Pain assessment is continuous during recovery.
    - Pain is a subjective experience and must be assessed based on individual conditions.
    - Follow best practices for surgical pain management.

11. Consider the psychological, social, cultural, and spiritual issues of the patient as postoperative care is provided. The patient's age and health history; surgical procedure; and impact of surgery on recovery, body image, roles, and lifestyle are all considerations to consider.

Analyze Cues and Prioritize Hypotheses: Analysis

- The priority collaborative problems for patients in the immediate postoperative period are:
  1. Potential for decreased *gas exchange* due to the effects of anesthesia, *pain*, opioid analgesics, and immobility
  2. Potential for *infection* and delayed healing due to wound location, decreased mobility, drains and drainage, and tubes
  3. Acute *pain* due to the surgical incision and procedure, and surgical positioning
  4. Potential for decreased peristalsis due to surgical manipulation, opioid use, and fluid and electrolyte imbalances

Generate Solutions and Take Actions: Planning and Implementation
Improving Gas Exchange

- Support a patent airway.
  1. Monitor the patient's oxygen saturation.
  2. Position the patient in a semi-Fowler's position unless contraindicated.
  3. Suction the mouth, nose, and throat to keep the airway clear of mucus or vomitus as needed.
- Apply prescribed oxygen by face tent, nasal cannula, or mask.
- Assist the patient to breathe deeply (with the incision splinted) and use the incentive spirometer.
- Assist the patient to reposition every 2 hours and to ambulate as soon as possible.

Preventing Wound Infection and Delayed Healing

- Reinforce the dressing, change the dressing, assess the wound for healing and infection, and care for drains, including emptying drainage containers/reservoirs, measuring drainage, and documenting drainage features.
  1. The surgeon usually performs the first dressing change to assess the wound, remove any packing, and advance (pull partially out) or remove drains. Follow agency policy regarding the timing of the first dressing changes and incision care.
  2. An unchanged wet or damp dressing is a source of infection. Change dressings using aseptic technique until the sutures or staples are removed.
  3. Skin sutures or staples are usually removed 5 to 10 days after surgery, although this varies up to 30 days, depending on the type of surgery and the patient's health.
  4. Generally, administer antibiotics for no longer than 24 hours after surgery unless the patient has a documented infection.

5. *Dehiscence* is a wound opening or rupture along the surgical incision. An *evisceration* is a wound opening with protrusion of internal organs and a surgical emergency.
   • Dehiscence or evisceration may follow forceful coughing, vomiting, or straining and when not splinting the surgical site during movement. The patient may state, "Something popped" or "I feel as if I just split open."
   • Have the patient lie flat (supine) with knees bent to reduce intraabdominal pressure; apply sterile nonadherent dressing materials to the wound and notify the surgeon or Rapid Response Team.

✚ NURSING SAFETY PRIORITY

Critical Rescue

Monitor surgical incisions at least every 8 hours to recognize an impending evisceration. Recognize when a surgical wound evisceration occurs, and respond by staying with the patient while calling for another nurse to immediately notify the surgeon or Rapid Response Team (RRT).

Managing Pain
• Drug therapy is commonly used to manage surgical pain, but drugs may mask or increase the severity of symptoms of anesthesia.
   1. Administer opioids as prescribed, and closely monitor patient responses with the first dose.
   2. Assess the type, location, and intensity of the pain before and after giving pain medication. Monitor the patient's VS for hypotension and hypoventilation after giving opioid drugs.
   3. Use around-the-clock scheduling or use patient-controlled analgesia (PCA) systems for consistent blood levels and more effective surgical pain management.
   4. Monitor epidural analgesia effects when administered intermittently by the anesthesia provider or by continuous infusion through an epidural catheter left in place after surgery. Common drugs given by epidural catheter include the opioids fentanyl, preservative-free morphine, and bupivacaine.
   5. Offer prescribed pain medication 30 to 45 minutes before the patient gets out of bed.
   6. Use nonopioid drugs to augment pain management; typically, acetaminophen or NSAIDs are used.

- Use adjuvant therapy such as distraction, positioning, relaxation techniques, and anxiety-reducing interventions to manage pain.

Promoting Peristalsis
- Monitor bowel sounds, rectal output, and abdominal status (distention) with VS.
  1. Auscultate for bowel sounds in all four abdominal quadrants for up to 1 minute in each quadrant.
  2. Gently palpate the abdomen to determine degree of softness or whether any rigidity is present.
- Ensure adequate hydration with intravenous fluids, oral fluids, and evaluation of intake and output to achieve hydration or fluid balance goals.
- Promote early and progressive out-of-bed mobility.
- Provide drug therapy to maintain or restore intestinal peristalsis.
  1. Alvimopan has been approved to accelerate the time to GI recovery following certain GI surgeries.
  2. Metoclopramide promotes peristalsis by directly stimulating GI motility.

! NURSING SAFETY PRIORITY
Action Alert

Provide written discharge instructions (including medication education sheets) to follow at home. Request that the patient and caregiver explain the regimen in their own words to assess understanding.

Care Coordination and Transition Management
- If the patient is discharged directly to home, assess information about the home environment for safety and the availability of caregivers.
- Reinforce to the patient and family after surgery the specific interventions to use to prevent complications (e.g., hand hygiene, incision splinting, deep-breathing exercises, range-of-motion exercises).
- Collaborate with the social worker or discharge planner to identify needs related to care after surgery, including meal preparation, dressing changes, drain management, drug administration, physical therapy, and personal hygiene.
- If dressing changes and drain or catheter care are needed, instruct the patient and family members on the importance of proper

handwashing to prevent infection. Explain and demonstrate wound care to the patient and family, who then perform a return demonstration.

- Perform a drug reconciliation with the patient before discharge. Ensure that drugs for other health problems are resumed, as needed.
- A diet high in protein, calories, and vitamins promotes wound healing; vitamin supplementation may be temporarily added to home drugs.
- Teach the patient to increase activity level slowly, rest often, and avoid straining the wound or the surrounding area; healing requires both time and avoidance of stress.

Evaluate Outcomes: Evaluation
- Evaluate the care of the patient after surgery based on the identified priority patient problems. The expected outcomes include that the patient:
  1. Attains and maintains adequate lung expansion and respiratory function
  2. Has appropriate wound healing without complications
  3. Has acceptable *pain* management
  4. Has return of peristalsis

See Chapter 9 in the main text for more information on perioperative care.

PERIPHERAL ARTERIAL DISEASE

- Peripheral arterial disease (PAD) is a result of atherosclerosis, a chronic condition in which partial or total arterial blockage decreases perfusion to the extremities, most commonly the legs.
- Inflow PAD obstructions involve the distal end of the aorta and the common, internal, and external iliac arteries, manifested by discomfort in the lower back, buttocks, or thighs.
- Outflow PAD obstructions involve the femoral, popliteal, and tibial arteries and typically cause significant tissue damage.

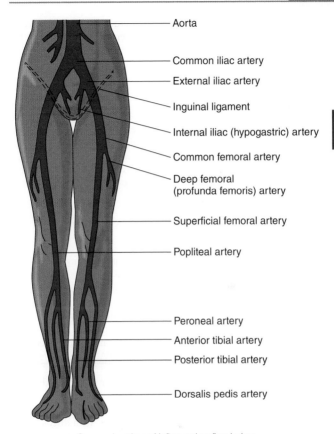

- Aorta
- Common iliac artery
- External iliac artery
- Inguinal ligament
- Internal iliac (hypogastric) artery
- Common femoral artery
- Deep femoral (profunda femoris) artery
- Superficial femoral artery
- Popliteal artery
- Peroneal artery
- Anterior tibial artery
- Posterior tibial artery
- Dorsalis pedis artery

Common locations of inflow and outflow lesions.

- *Chronic* PD can be divided into four stages:
  1. Asymptomatic
  2. Presence of *claudication,* described as pain, cramping, or burning with exercise that is relieved by rest (*intermittent claudication*)
  3. Pain while resting; pain that awakens the patient during sleep; relief of pain when extremity is in a dependent position
  4. Occurrence of ulcers, blackened tissue on toes, forefoot, and heel; gangrene infection of tissues

- *Acute* arterial occlusion occurs when there is an acute obstruction by a thrombus or embolus, causing severe, acute pain below the level of the obstruction.

Interprofessional Collaborative Care
Recognize Cues: Assessment
- Assessment findings include:
    1. Abnormal ankle-brachial index (ABI): The value can be derived by dividing the ankle blood pressure by the brachial blood pressure. *An ABI of less than 0.90 in either leg is diagnostic of PAD. Patients with diabetes are known to have a falsely elevated ABI.*
    2. Leg pain (burning, cramping in calves, ankles, feet, and toes with exercise or rest) or discomfort in the lower back, buttocks, or thighs
    3. Ischemic changes of the extremity
        - Loss of hair on the lower calf, ankle, and foot
        - Dry, scaly skin
        - Thickened toenails
        - Color changes (elevation pallor or dependent rubor)
        - Mottled and cool or cold extremity
    4. Decreased or absent leg pulses: The most sensitive and specific indicator of arterial function is the quality of the posterior tibial pulse because the pedal pulse is not palpable in a small percentage of people.
    5. Painful arterial ulcers that develop on the toes, between the toes, or on the upper aspect of the foot; PAD ulcers differ from diabetic and venous ulcers.
        - Diabetic ulcers develop on the plantar surface of the foot, over metatarsal heads, on the heel, or on pressure areas; they may not be painful.
        - Venous stasis ulcers occur at the ankles, with discoloration of the lower extremity at the ulcer; they cause minimal pain.
- Diagnostic assessment includes:
    1. Blood pressure and ABI measurement
    2. MRI and Doppler/ultrasound to assess blood flow in peripheral arteries

Take Actions: Interventions
Nonsurgical Management
- Teach the following methods of increasing arterial blood flow in chronic arterial disease:
    1. Exercising to promote collateral circulation
    2. Positioning to promote circulation and decrease swelling
        - Elevate legs at rest but not above the level of the heart.
        - Avoid crossing legs and wearing restrictive clothing.

3. Promoting vasodilation
   - Avoid cold exposure to the affected extremity with warm socks and room temperature modulation.
   - Avoid nicotine, caffeine, and emotional stress.
   - Comply with drug therapy, including vasodilator and antiplatelet therapy.
   - Control blood pressure to avoid hypertension.
- Endovascular intervention may be used to dilate the occluded artery, provide atherectomy, or place an endovascular stent or graft to restore arterial circulation. After endovascular intervention, care of the patient includes:
   1. Observing the puncture site for bleeding
   2. Closely monitoring vital signs for hypotension and hypertension
   3. Checking the neurovascular status of limbs (color, warmth, pulses, sensation, and voluntary movement)
   4. Administering antiplatelet or anticoagulation therapy as prescribed, which may continue for 3 to 6 months after the procedure

➕ NURSING SAFETY PRIORITY

Critical Rescue

The priority for nursing care following a percutaneous vascular intervention or atherectomy is to observe for bleeding at the arterial puncture site, which is sealed with a special collagen plug. Monitor for symptoms of impending hypovolemic shock, including a decrease in blood pressure, increased pulse rate, and decreased urinary output. Related complications can include hematoma, retroperitoneal bleeding, pseudoaneurysm, arteriovenous fistula, nerve compression, and atheroembolism. Perform frequent checks of the arterial puncture site and distal pulses in both legs to ensure adequate **perfusion.**

Surgical Management
- Arterial revascularization surgery is used to increase arterial blood flow in an affected limb and includes inflow procedures such as aortoiliac bypass, aortofemoral bypass, and axillofemoral bypass and outflow procedures, including femoropopliteal bypass and femorotibial bypass.
- Grafting materials for bypass surgeries include the autogenous saphenous vein and synthetic graft material.
- Provide postoperative care.
   1. Monitor for the patency of the graft by checking for changes in the extremity:
      - Color
      - Temperature

- Pulse quality; mark the site of pulses for consistent evaluation
- Sensation and pain intensity (typical pain is described as throbbing pain, which occurs from increased blood flow to the affected limb)

2. Monitor the patient's blood pressure, notifying the health care provider about increases and decreases beyond desired ranges.
3. Avoid bending the knee and hip of the affected limb for 6 to 8 hours.
4. Monitor for signs and symptoms of vessel reocclusion at or around the graft and incision sites, such as hardness, tenderness, redness/hyperpigmentation, or coolness or warmth.

- Thrombectomy (removal of the clot) is the most common treatment for acute graft occlusion; thrombolytic therapy may be used.

✚ **NURSING SAFETY PRIORITY**

Critical Rescue

Graft occlusion (blockage) is a postoperative emergency that can occur within the first 24 hours after arterial revascularization. Monitor the patient for and report severe continuous and aching pain, which may be the first indicator of postoperative graft occlusion and ischemia. Many people experience a throbbing pain caused by the increased blood flow to the extremity. Because this alteration in comfort is different from that of ischemic pain, be sure to assess the type of pain that is experienced. Pain from occlusion may be masked by patient-controlled analgesia (PCA). Some patients have ischemic pain that is not relieved by PCA.

Monitor the patency of the graft by checking the extremity every 15 minutes for the first hour and then hourly for changes in color, temperature, and pulse intensity. Compare the operative leg with the unaffected one. *If the operative leg feels cold; becomes pale, ashen, or cyanotic; or has a decreased or absent pulse, contact the surgeon immediately!*

Care Coordination and Transition Management

- Patient and family education includes:
  1. Teaching the patient to monitor tissue perfusion to the affected extremity
     - Distal circulation, sensation, and motion
     - Presence of pain, pallor/ash gray skin, paresthesias, pulselessness, paralysis, and coolness
  2. Reinforcing the need for individualized positioning and an exercise plan

3. Providing written and oral foot care instructions, per agency policy
4. Providing dressing change and incision care instructions, if necessary
5. Providing instructions concerning discharge medications, particularly to improve safety when using antiplatelet and anticoagulant drugs
6. Encouraging healthy diet choices to reduce atherosclerotic plaque formation and growth

P

See Chapter 30 in the main text for more information on peripheral arterial disease (PAD).

PERIPHERAL VENOUS DISEASE

- Peripheral venous disease (PVD) is a condition that alters the natural flow of blood through the veins of the peripheral circulation. Three health problems result in PVD:
  1. Thrombus (thrombosis) formation (see *Venous Thromboembolism [VTE]*) and thrombophlebitis or clot with associated inflammation
  2. Defective valves leading to venous insufficiency and varicose veins
  3. Reduced skeletal muscle activity when weight bearing is limited or muscle tone decreases
     - Skeletal muscles help pump blood in veins.
     - When weight bearing is limited or muscle tone decreases, PVD can develop.

See Chapter 30 in the main text for more information on peripheral venous disease.

✳ PERITONITIS: INFECTION CONCEPT EXEMPLAR

Overview

- **Peritonitis** is a life-threatening, acute *inflammation* and *infection* of the visceral/parietal peritoneum and endothelial lining of the abdominal cavity.
- Peritonitis is most often caused by contamination of the peritoneal cavity by bacteria or chemicals. Bacteria gain entry into the peritoneum by perforation (from appendicitis, diverticulitis, peptic ulcer disease) or from an external penetrating wound, a gangrenous gallbladder or bowel segment, bowel obstruction, or ascending infection through the genital tract.
- Peritonitis is associated with sepsis, hypovolemic and septic shock, respiratory problems, and paralytic ileus or bowel obstruction.

Interprofessional Collaborative Care

Recognize Cues: Assessment

- Obtain patient information about:
  1. History of abdominal trauma or surgery
  2. Character of abdominal pain, onset, duration, location, quality, aggravating and alleviating factors; the cardinal signs of peritonitis are abdominal pain, tenderness, and distention; often, pain is aggravated by coughing or movement and relieved by knee flexion
  3. Assess for key features of peritonitis.

KEY FEATURES

Peritonitis

- Rigid, boardlike abdomen (classic)
- Abdominal *pain* (localized, poorly localized, or referred to the shoulder or chest)
- Distended abdomen
- Nausea, anorexia, vomiting
- Diminishing bowel sounds
- Inability to pass flatus or feces
- Rebound tenderness in the abdomen
- High fever
- Tachycardia
- Dehydration from high fever (poor skin turgor)
- Decreased urine output
- Hiccups
- Possible compromise in respiratory status

- Diagnostic tests may include:
  1. CBC; anticipate an elevated WBC count and neutrophilia
  2. Blood cultures to determine whether septicemia has occurred; can identify the causative organism
  3. Serum electrolytes, blood urea nitrogen (BUN), and creatinine
  4. Abdominal CT scan, x-ray, or ultrasound to determine the presence of dilation, edema, and inflammation of the intestines

Analyze Cues and Prioritize Hypotheses: Analysis

- The priority collaborative problems for patients with peritonitis include:
  1. Acute *pain* due to abdominal *inflammation* and *infection*
  2. Potential for fluid volume shift due to fluid moving into interstitial or peritoneal space

Generate Solutions and Take Actions: Planning and Implementation
Managing Pain
Nonsurgical management
- Monitor vital signs, noting any change that may indicate septic shock, such as unresolved or progressive hypotension, decreased pulse pressure, tachycardia, fever, skin changes, and/or tachypnea.
- Provide and evaluate pain management with analgesics.
- Administer oxygen to maintain Spo₂ greater than 92%.

Surgical management
- Surgical management may be necessary to identify and repair the underlying cause of the peritonitis.
- Surgery is focused on controlling the contamination, removing foreign material from the peritoneal cavity, and draining fluid collections.
- During surgery, the peritoneum is irrigated with antibiotic solution, and drainage catheters are inserted.

! NURSING SAFETY PRIORITY
Action Alert

> Monitor the patient's level of consciousness, vital signs, respiratory status (respiratory rate and breath sounds), and intake and output at least hourly immediately after abdominal surgery. Maintain the patient in a semi-Fowler's position to promote drainage of peritoneal contents into the lower region of the abdominal cavity. This position also helps increase lung expansion.

Restoring Fluid Volume Balance
- Administer hypertonic IV fluids and broad-spectrum antibiotics as prescribed.
- Record intake, output, and daily weight.
- Monitor and record drainage from the nasogastric tube (NGT) used for gastric and intestinal decompression.

Care Coordination and Transition Management
- The patient may be discharged home or to a transitional care unit to complete antibiotic therapy and recovery.
- If the patient is discharged home, collaborate with the case manager to determine the need for assistance.
- Provide written and oral postoperative instructions, including:
  1. The necessity to report any redness/hyperpigmentation, swelling, tenderness, or unusual or foul-smelling drainage from the wound
  2. Care of the incision and dressing; ensuring that the patient has the necessary equipment to perform wound care (dressings,

solutions, catheter-tipped syringe); and stressing the importance of handwashing
3. The need to report fever (typically 101°F [38°C]) or abdominal pain to the primary health care provider
4. Administration and monitoring of drugs for *pain*

Evaluate Outcomes: Evaluation
- Evaluate the care of the patient with peritonitis based on the identified priority patient problems. The expected outcomes are that the patient:
  1. Verbalizes relief or control of pain as *infection* resolves
  2. Experiences restoration of fluid balance

 See Chapter 49 in the main text for more information on pneumonia.

✳ PNEUMONIA: GAS EXCHANGE CONCEPT EXEMPLAR

Overview
- Pneumonia is a common disorder with many causes that reduces *gas exchange*.
- It can be caused by many infectious organisms or by inhalation of irritating agents.
  1. Infectious pneumonias are categorized as community-acquired pneumonia (CAP) or hospital-acquired pneumonia (HAP), and ventilator-associated pneumonia (VAP).
- Inflammation and infection in the lungs result in local capillary leak, edema, and exudate that interfere with gas exchange, leading to hypoxemia that has the potential to cause death.

Interprofessional Collaborative Care
Recognize Cues: Assessment
- Obtain patient information about:
  1. Age
  2. Living, work, and school environments, including exposure to droplet-based infection
  3. Diet, exercise, and sleep routines
  4. Swallowing problems or presence of a nasogastric tube
  5. Tobacco and alcohol use
  6. Past and current use of drugs, including drug addiction or injection drug use
  7. Acute or chronic respiratory problems
  8. Recent skin rashes, insect bites, or exposure to animals
  9. Home respiratory equipment use and cleaning
  10. Date of last influenza, COVID-19, and pneumococcal vaccine

Risk Factors for Pneumonia

Community-Acquired Pneumonia
- Is an older adult
- Has never received the pneumococcal vaccination or received it more than 5 years ago
- Did not receive the influenza vaccine in the previous year
- Did not receive the COVID-19 vaccine series and boosters as recommended
- Has a chronic health problem or other coexisting condition that reduces *immunity*
- Has recently been exposed to respiratory viral or influenza *infection*
- Uses tobacco or alcohol or is exposed to high amounts of secondhand smoke

Nosocomial Pneumonia
(Includes Hospital-Acquired Pneumonia and Ventilator-Associated Pneumonia)
- Is an older adult
- Has a chronic lung disease
- Has presence of Gram-negative colonization of the mouth, throat, and stomach
- Has an altered level of consciousness
- Has had a recent aspiration event
- Has presence of endotracheal, tracheostomy, or nasogastric tube
- Has poor nutritional status
- Has reduced *immunity* (from disease or drug therapy)
- Uses drugs that increase gastric pH (histamine [H_2] blockers, antacids) or alkaline tube feedings
- Is currently receiving mechanical ventilation (ventilator-associated pneumonia [VAP])

👤 PATIENT-CENTERED CARE: OLDER ADULT HEALTH

Pneumonia

The older adult with pneumonia has weakness, fatigue (which can lead to falls), lethargy, confusion, and poor appetite. Fever and cough may be absent, but hypoxemia is often present. The most common symptom of pneumonia in the older adult patient is acute confusion from hypoxia. The WBC count may not be elevated until the infection is severe. Waiting to treat the disease until more typical symptoms appear greatly increases the risk for sepsis and death.

- Assess for and document:
  1. General appearance for signs of flushing and hypoxia-related anxiety
  2. Oxygen saturation, evaluating for hypoxemia
  3. Abnormal lung sounds, particularly crackles, rhonchi, and wheezing
  4. Respiratory rate and dyspnea or increased effort of breathing, such as use of accessory muscles
  5. Cough
  6. Sputum amount and appearance, especially if purulent, blood-tinged, or rust-colored
  7. Chest or pleuritic pain or discomfort
  8. Fever, diaphoresis, chills, and fatigue or weakness
  9. Tachycardia, hypotension
  10. Mental status changes (especially in an older adult)
  11. Laboratory and imaging results, such as elevated WBC, sputum or blood culture results, or consolidation on chest x-ray (CXR)

❗ NURSING SAFETY PRIORITY

Action Alert

Because pneumonia is a frequent cause of sepsis, use a sepsis screening tool to monitor patients who have pneumonia. For patients with pneumonia, always check oxygen saturation with vital signs.

Analyze Cues and Prioritize Hypotheses: Analysis

- The priority interprofessional collaborative problems for patients with pneumonia include:
  1. Decreased *gas exchange* due to decreased diffusion at the alveolar-capillary membrane
  2. Potential for airway obstruction due to *inflammation,* with excessive pulmonary secretions, fatigue, and muscle weakness
  3. Potential for sepsis due to the presence of microorganisms in a very vascular area and reduced *immunity*

Generating Solutions and Take Actions: Planning and Implementation
Improving Gas Exchange

- Interventions to improve *gas exchange* are similar to those for the patient with asthma or chronic obstructive pulmonary disease.
- Nursing priorities include delivery of oxygen therapy and assisting the patient with bronchial hygiene.
  1. Assess lung sounds and pulse oximetry, and administer oxygen by nasal cannula or mask to maintain Spo_2 >95% prescribed.

2. Instruct the patient on cough and deep-breathing technique or the correct use of incentive spirometry (sustained maximal inspiration), and encourage the patient to perform 5 to 10 breaths per session every hour while awake.

Preventing Airway Obstruction

- Because of fatigue, muscle weakness, chest discomfort, and excessive secretions, the patient often has difficulty clearing secretions.
  1. Assist patient to cough and deep breathe at least every 2 hours.
  2. Encourage the alert patient to use the incentive spirometer.
  3. Encourage the alert patient to drink at least 2 L of fluid daily.
  4. Monitor intake and output, oral mucous membranes, and skin turgor for hydration status.
  5. Bronchodilators may be used when bronchospasm is present.

Preventing Sepsis

- Administer prescribed antiinfective therapy based on organism sensitivity.
- For pneumonia resulting from aspiration of food or stomach contents, interventions focus on preventing lung damage and treating the infection.

Care Coordination and Transition Management

- Teach the patient about:
  1. The importance of completing the full course of antibiotic therapy
  2. Notifying the primary health care provider if chills, fever, persistent cough, dyspnea, wheezing, hemoptysis, increased sputum production, chest discomfort, or increasing fatigue recurs or if symptoms fail to resolve
  3. The importance of getting plenty of rest and gradually increasing exercise
  4. Preventing upper respiratory tract infections and viruses by:
     - Using handwashing
     - Avoiding crowds and people who have a cold or flu
     - Avoiding exposure to irritants such as smoke
     - Obtaining vaccinations for influenza, COVID-19, and pneumonia
- Encourage the patient to quit smoking and provide information on smoking cessation because smoking is a risk factor for both onset and severity of pneumonia.

See Chapter 25 in the main text for more information on pneumonia.

PNEUMOTHORAX

- Pneumothorax is air in the pleural space and a reduction in vital capacity that can lead to lung collapse. A common cause of pneumothorax is blunt trauma to the chest. It can also occur as a complication of medical procedures (e.g., central line placement) or spontaneously.
  1. Open pneumothorax: pleural cavity is exposed to outside air such as through an open wound
  2. Closed pneumothorax: spontaneous pneumothorax
  3. **Tension pneumothorax** is a life-threatening complication of pneumothorax in which air continues to enter the pleural space during inspiration and does not exit during expiration. If not promptly detected and treated, tension pneumothorax is quickly fatal.

Interprofessional Collaborative Care
Recognize Cues: Assessment

- Assessment findings for any type of pneumothorax commonly include:
  1. Chest pain and shortness of breath
  2. Reduced (or absent) breath sounds of the affected side on auscultation
  3. Hyperresonance on percussion
  4. Prominence of the involved side of the chest, which moves poorly with respirations
  5. When severe, deviation of the trachea *away* from the midline and side of injury toward the *unaffected* side (indicating pushing of tissues to the unaffected side [a *mediastinal shift*] from increasing pressure within the injured side)
- For tension pneumothorax, additional assessment findings also may include:
  1. Extreme respiratory distress and cyanosis
  2. Distended neck veins
  3. Hemodynamic instability

Take Actions: Interventions

- Initial management of a tension pneumothorax is an immediate needle thoracostomy, with a large-bore needle inserted by the primary health care provider into the second intercostal space in the midclavicular line of the affected side.
  1. This intervention changes a tension pneumothorax to a simple pneumothorax and is only a temporary measure. More definitive treatment is mandatory; chest tube placement until the lung reinflates is generally required.

- An open thoracotomy is needed when there is initial blood loss of 1000 mL from the chest or persistent bleeding at the rate of 150 to 200 mL/hr over 3 to 4 hours.

🔖 *See Chapter 26 in the main text for more information on pneumothorax.*

PRESSURE INJURY: TISSUE INTEGRITY CONCEPT ❋ EXEMPLAR

Overview

- A pressure injury is a loss of ***tissue integrity*** caused when the skin and underlying tissue are compressed between a bony prominence and external surface for an extended period.
- They form most commonly over the sacrum, hips, and ankles but can occur on any body surface.
- Tissue compression from pressure restricts blood flow to the skin, resulting in reduced tissue perfusion and gas exchange, leading to cell death.
- Once formed, pressure injuries lead to complications, increased cost for care, and greater risk for mortality.
- Complications include infection, osteomyelitis, and pain.

Interprofessional Collaborative Care
Recognize Cues: Assessment

Assessing the Patient at Risk for Pressure Injuries
• Perfusion
• Presence or absence of peripheral edema
• Reduced capillary refill
• Cognition
• Impaired level of consciousness
• Lack of orientation to time, place, and person
• Nutrition
• Decreased muscle mass
• Lackluster nails, sparse hair
• Recent weight loss of more than 5% of usual weight
• Impaired oral intake
• Difficulty swallowing

- Obtain patient information about contributing factors and causes of pressure injuries, including:
  1. Prolonged bed rest
  2. Immobility

3. Incontinence
4. Diabetes mellitus and/or peripheral vascular disease
5. Undernutrition
6. Cognitive problems or decreased sensory perception

- Assess for and document:
  1. Inspection of the entire body for areas of skin injury or pressure
  2. General appearance for body weight and the proportion of weight to height (obesity and underweight contribute to skin problems)
  3. Overall cleanliness of the skin, hair, and nails
  4. Any loss of mobility or range of joint motion

- Assess existing wounds on admission, with each dressing change, and in accordance with the facility policy on ongoing assessment.
  1. Location, size (length, width, and depth), color, and extent of tissue involvement, and document this information along with:
     - Presence of blanching if skin is intact
     - Exudate
     - Condition of surrounding tissue, including wound margin
     - Presence of foreign bodies
     - Presence or absence of necrotic tissue (eschar)
     - Presence of undermining and tunneling
     - Comparison of existing wound features with those documented previously to determine the current state of healing or deterioration
     - Inflammation or cellulitis (inflammation of skin and surrounding tissue)
     - Fever or mental status changes associated with acute infection
     - Peripheral edema that can interfere with healing
     - Vascular imaging result indicating poor perfusion to pressure injury, such as ultrasound/Doppler or angiography results

- Assess for psychosocial issues, including:
  1. Altered body image
  2. Coping patterns
  3. Changes in lifestyle and ADLs
  4. Financial resources

- Assess laboratory data:
  1. Wound culturing is not routinely performed, as open pressure injuries are often colonized by bacteria (Grada & Phillips, 2022).
  2. Clinical indicators of infection (e.g., cellulitis, exudate changes, increase in injury size or depth) and systemic signs of bacteremia (e.g., fever, elevated white blood cell [WBC] count) are used to diagnose an infection.

3. Elevated WBC, indicating infection
4. Laboratory reports to determine nutritional deficiencies including prealbumin, albumin, and total protein

Analyze Cues and Prioritize Hypotheses: Analysis
- The priority collaborative problems for patients with pressure injuries include:
  1. Compromised *tissue integrity* due to vascular insufficiency and trauma
  2. Potential for *infection* due to insufficient wound management

Generate Solutions and Take Actions: Planning and Implementation
Improving Tissue Integrity
Nonsurgical Management
- Wound care and dressing techniques are the basis for pressure injury management. A well-designed dressing removes surface debris, protects exposed healthy tissues, and creates a barrier until the ulcer is closed. The frequency of dressing changes is dependent on the nature of the pressure injury and the facility's policies or procedures.

Common Dressing Techniques for Wound Débridement

Technique	Mechanism of Action
Wet-to-damp saline-moistened gauze	Necrotic debris is mechanically removed with less trauma to healing tissue than experienced when the wet-to-dry technique is used.
Continuous wet gauze	The wound surface is continually bathed with a wetting agent of choice, promoting dilution of viscous exudate and softening of dry eschar.
Moisture-retentive dressing	Spontaneous separation of necrotic tissue is promoted by autolysis.

- Nutritional therapy provides adequate nutritional intake of calories, protein, vitamins, minerals, and water.
  1. Coordinate with the registered dietitian nutritionist to encourage the patient to eat a well-balanced diet, emphasizing proteins, vegetables, fruits, whole-grain breads and cereals, and vitamins.
- New technologies may be useful for chronic ulcers that remain open for months.
  1. *Electrical stimulation* is the application of a low-voltage current to a wound area to increase blood vessel growth and promote granulation.

2. *Negative-pressure wound therapy* uses a suction tube covered by a special sponge ("foam"). Closely monitor patients for bleeding for the first 2 hours after placement, and stop suction if bleeding occurs. Suction removes exudate and infectious materials. The foam needs to be changed three times weekly.

> ## ! NURSING SAFETY PRIORITY
> ### Action Alert
>
> Recognize that continuous negative-pressure wound therapy (NPWT) must be closely monitored in patients taking anticoagulants or platelet aggregation inhibitors (U.S. Food and Drug Administration, 2018). Respond by consulting with members of the interprofessional team, such as the primary health care provider and wound nurse, to ascertain that careful monitoring takes place while patients on these types of drug therapies are using NPWT.

3. *Hyperbaric oxygen* therapy (HBOT) is the administration of oxygen under high pressure, which raises the tissue oxygen concentration.
4. *Topical growth factors* are biologically active substances that stimulate cell movement and growth and are applied to the wound.
5. *Skin substitutes* are engineered products that aid in the temporary or permanent closure of various types of wounds.

Surgical Management

- Surgical management includes removal of necrotic tissue (surgical débridement) and skin grafting or use of muscle flaps to close wounds that cannot heal by epithelialization and contraction.

Preventing Infection

- Priority nursing interventions focus on preventing wound infections and promoting progression to complete wound healing.
  1. Monitor the wound appearance using objective criteria.
  2. Reevaluate the treatment plan if wound worsens or shows no progress toward healing within 7 to 10 days.
  3. Check signs and symptoms of wound infection:
     - *Pain*, tenderness, and redness/hyperpigmentation at the wound margins
     - Purulent and malodorous drainage

- Increased size or depth of the wound
- Changes in the color or texture of the granulation tissue

Care Coordination and Transition Management

- Have the patient or family member demonstrate a dressing change successfully before discharge from acute or home health care.
- Explain the signs of wound infection, and remind the patient and family to report these to the primary health care provider or wound care clinic.
- Work with the social worker or case manager to obtain special beds or mattress overlays for the home and assistance for complex care.
- Ensure an accurate hand-off to home care services regarding the wound description and plan for management.
- Encourage the patient to eat a balanced diet with frequent high-protein snacks.
- Emphasize the need to keep the skin of a patient who is incontinent clean and dry; adult absorbent underwear can wick away moisture.
- Make referrals for home care nursing visits, if needed, to monitor wound progress or provide assistance with activity or rehabilitation.

See Chapter 21 in the main text for more information on pressure injury.

PROLAPSE, PELVIC ORGAN

- The pelvic organs are supported by a sling of muscles and tendons, which sometimes become weak and are no longer able to hold an organ in place.
- *Uterine prolapse* is the downward displacement of the uterus. It can be caused by neuromuscular damage of childbirth; increased intraabdominal pressure related to pregnancy, obesity, or physical exertion; or weakening of pelvic support due to decreased estrogen.
- A *cystocele* is a protrusion of the bladder through the vaginal wall (urinary bladder prolapse), which can lead to stress urinary incontinence (SUI) and urinary tract infections (UTIs). (See *Cystocele.*)
- A *rectocele* is a protrusion of the rectum through a weakened vaginal wall (rectal prolapse).

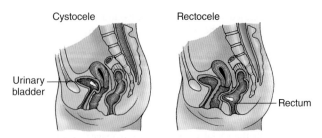

In cystocele, the urinary bladder is displaced downward, causing bulging of the anterior vaginal wall. In rectocele, the rectum is displaced, causing bulging of the posterior vaginal wall.

Interprofessional Collaborative Care

Recognize Cues: Assessment

- Assessment findings include:
  1. Patient's report of feeling as if "something is falling out"
  2. Dyspareunia (painful intercourse)
  3. Backache
  4. Feeling of heaviness or pressure in the pelvis
  5. Protrusion of the cervix when the woman is asked to bear down
  6. Bowel or bladder problems, such as urinary incontinence, constipation, hemorrhoids, or fecal impaction

Take Actions: Interventions

- Interventions are based on the degree of prolapse.
  1. Nonsurgical management may include:
     - Teaching to improve pelvic support and tone by pelvic floor muscle exercises (*Kegel exercises*)
     - Using space-filling devices such as a pessary or sphere worn intravaginally to elevate the uterine prolapse
     - Promoting bladder training and attention to complete emptying
     - Promoting bowel elimination with high-fiber diet and a stool softener or laxative
  2. Surgical management may be recommended for severe symptoms.
     - Most women are treated with a reconstructive procedure, which may or may not include hysterectomy (Jelovsek, 2023). Synthetic mesh is often used in transabdominal pelvic organ prolapse (POP) repair; mesh intended for transvaginal surgical repair was discontinued in the United States in 2019 due to complications associated with this procedure (U.S. Food & Drug Administration, 2021).

- Anterior colporrhaphy (anterior repair) tightens the pelvic muscles for better bladder support.
- Posterior colporrhaphy (posterior repair) reduces rectal bulging.

3. Nursing care is similar to that for a woman undergoing a vaginal hysterectomy.
   - Teach the patient to avoid lifting anything heavier than 5 pounds, strenuous exercises, and sexual intercourse for up to 6 weeks.
   - Instruct her to notify her surgeon if she has signs of infection, such as fever, persistent pain, or purulent, foul-smelling discharge.

See Chapter 63 in the main text for more information on pelvic organ prolapse.

PROSTATIC HYPERPLASIA, BENIGN: ELIMINATION CONCEPT EXEMPLAR

Overview

- When the prostate gland enlarges, it extends upward into the bladder and inward, causing bladder outlet obstruction, impairing urinary *elimination*.
  1. The patient has an increased residual urine (stasis) or acute or chronic urinary retention.
  2. Increased residual urine causes overflow urinary incontinence in which the urine "leaks" around the enlarged prostate, causing dribbling.
  3. Urinary stasis can result in urinary tract infections, hydroureter, hydronephrosis, bladder calculi (stones), and contribute to chronic kidney disease.
- With aging and increased dihydrotestosterone (DHT) levels, the glandular units in the prostate undergo nodular tissue hyperplasia (an increase in the number of cells).
  1. Testosterone and DHT are the major androgens (male hormones) in the adult male.
  2. Testosterone is produced by the testis and circulates in the blood. DHT is a testosterone derivative produced in the prostate gland.

Interprofessional Collaborative Care
Recognize Cues: Assessment

- Evaluate for the presence of risk factors.
- Use a standardized tool such as the International Prostate Symptom Score (I-PSS) to determine the severity of lower urinary tract symptoms.

- Assess for and document:
  1. Current urinary patterns such as frequency, straining to begin urination, number of voids overnight (nocturia), hesitancy, force and size of urinary stream, sensation of bladder fullness after voiding, and postvoid dribbling or leaking
  2. Bladder distention (by palpation or bedside ultrasound)
  3. History or finding by the provider of an enlarged prostate
  4. Psychosocial responses to symptoms or diagnosis, including anxiety, depression, or changes in sexual function
  5. Laboratory diagnostics
     - Urinalysis or urine culture
     - Serum prostate-specific antigen (PSA) and a serum acid phosphatase level to rule out prostate cancer
     - Basic metabolic panel to examine kidney function (BUN and creatinine)
  6. Imaging
     - Transabdominal ultrasound and/or transrectal ultrasound (TRUS)
     - MRI

Analyze Cues and Prioritize Hypotheses: Analysis
- The priority collaborative problem for the patient with benign prostatic hyperplasia (BPH) is:
  1. Urinary retention due to bladder outlet obstruction

Generate Solutions and Take Actions: Planning and Implementation
Improving Urinary Elimination
Nonsurgical Management
- Treatment ranges from careful monitoring with yearly examination to surgery, depending on the degree of impairment the patient is experiencing.
- Drug therapy is usually a combination of agents:
  1. A drug to lower DHT; 5-alpha reductase inhibitors (5-ARI)
     - Finasteride
     - Dutasteride
  2. A drug to improve urine outflow: *alpha*$_1$-adrenergic antagonist
     - Tamsulosin
     - Alfuzosin
     - Doxazosin
     - Silodosin
  3. A drug used to improve lower urinary tract symptoms (also used for ED): alpha$_{1a}$-blocker/5-alpha-reductaste inhibitor
     - Tadalafil

NURSING SAFETY PRIORITY

Drug Alert

Remind patients taking a 5-ARI for BPH that they may need to take it for as long as 6 months before improvement is noticed. Teach about possible side effects, including erectile dysfunction (ED), decreased libido, and dizziness due to orthostatic hypotension. *Remind them to change positions carefully and slowly!*

P

 NURSING SAFETY PRIORITY

Drug Alert

If giving alpha blockers in an inpatient setting, assess for orthostatic (postural) hypotension, tachycardia, and syncope, especially after the first dose is given to older men. If the patient is taking the drug at home, teach about being careful when changing position and to report any weakness, light-headedness, or dizziness to the primary health care provider immediately. Bedtime dosing may decrease the risk for problems related to hypotension.

- Prostatic fluid can be released and obstructive symptoms reduced with frequent sexual intercourse.
- Teach the patient about ways to prevent bladder distention, such as:
  1. Avoiding drinking large amounts of fluid in a short period
  2. Avoiding alcohol, diuretics, and caffeine
  3. Voiding as soon as the urge is felt
  4. Avoiding drugs that can cause urinary retention, especially anticholinergics, antihistamines, antipsychotics, and muscle relaxants
- Minimally invasive techniques to reduce prostate tissue and relieve urinary symptoms include:
  1. *Transurethral needle ablation* (TUNA), in which low-radio-frequency energy shrinks the prostate
  2. *Transurethral microwave therapy* (TUMT), in which high temperatures heat and destroy excess tissue
  3. Aquablation, a waterjet, is used in combination with a cystoscope with ultrasound to remove the prostate tissue
  4. Photoselective vaporization (PVP), in which laser energy is used to vaporize the prostate tissue
  5. Transurethral electro-vaporization of the prostate (TUVP), in which a heated ball or wire loop is inserted through the urethra to heat the prostate tissue, reducing it to vapor

Surgical Management

- Historically, the most common surgery for BPH was a *transurethral resection of the prostate* (TURP), in which the enlarged portion of the prostate is cut into pieces and removed through the urethra by an endoscopic instrument. A similar procedure is the *transurethral incision of the prostate* (TUIP), in which small cuts are made into the prostate to relieve pressure on the urethra.
- Currently, the most common procedure and gold standard is the *holmium laser enucleation of the prostate* (HoLEP).
- Provide preoperative care and:
  1. Correct any misconceptions about the surgery such as concerns about the automatic loss of sexual functioning or permanent incontinence.
  2. Inform the patient if he will have an indwelling bladder catheter for at least 24 hours and may have traction on the catheter.
  3. Explain that the patient will feel the urge to void while the catheter is in place.
  4. Reassure the patient that it is normal for the urine to be blood-tinged after surgery.
- Provide postoperative care and:
  1. Monitor the patient's urine output every 2 to 4 hours with vital signs.
  2. Provide aseptic continuous or intermittent urinary bladder irrigation to maintain patency as prescribed. This is typically associated with a TURP procedure.

✚ NURSING SAFETY PRIORITY

Critical Rescue

> Monitor the patient for the rare, yet critical, complication of TURP syndrome characterized by dilutional hyponatremia related to excessive absorption of hyperosmolar fluids (McVary, 2021). This degree of absorption places stress on the heart. Signs and symptoms include headache, dizziness, hypoxemia, hypertension, bradycardia, and an altered level of consciousness. Notify the surgeon immediately, as the patient will likely need intensive care during diuresis.

---

  3. Monitor for severe bleeding, including serum hemoglobin and hematocrit levels, presence of hematuria, and signs of hypovolemia from blood loss in the first 24 postoperative hours.
  4. Administer antispasmodic drugs as prescribed.
  5. Keep the catheter free of obstruction and kinks; monitor for clots and sudden cessation of urine output.
  6. Instruct the patient to maintain fluid intake to keep the urine clear.

✚ NURSING SAFETY PRIORITY

Critical Rescue

After a TURP, monitor the patient's urine output every 2 to 4 hours and vital signs (including pain assessment) every 4 hours for the first postoperative day or according to agency or surgeon protocol. Assess for postoperative bleeding. *Patients who undergo a TURP are at risk for severe bleeding or hemorrhage after surgery. Although rare, bleeding is most likely within the first 24 hours.* Bladder spasms or movement may trigger fresh bleeding from previously controlled vessels. This bleeding may be arterial or venous, but venous bleeding is more common.

Care Coordination and Transition Management

- Following TURP, patients are typically discharged with a urinary catheter in place for about a week or longer; a catheter at discharge is not common with minimally invasive techniques.
- Teach patients not to take a bath or swim to prevent a urinary tract infection while the catheter is in place.
- When the urinary catheter is removed, the patient may experience burning on urination and some urinary frequency, dribbling, and leakage. Reassure the patient that these symptoms are normal and will decrease.
- Instruct the patient to take in 2000 to 2500 mL of fluid daily to decrease dysuria and keep the urine clear, unless contraindicated by another health condition.
- Instruct the patient to contract and relax his sphincter frequently to reestablish urinary elimination control (pelvic floor or *Kegel* exercises).

Evaluate Outcomes: Evaluation

- Evaluate the care of the patient with BPH based on the identified priority patient problem. The primary expected outcome is that the patient will:
  1. Have improved urinary ***elimination*** as a result of appropriate and effective interprofessional management

🔖 *See Chapter 64 in the main text for more information on prostatic hyperplasia, benign.*

PSORIASIS

- Psoriasis is a chronic, autoimmune scaling skin disorder that has exacerbations and remissions characterized by inflammation.
- Psoriasis lesions are scaled with underlying dermal inflammation from an abnormality in the growth of epidermal cells. Normally basal cells take about 28 days to reach the outermost layer, where they are shed. In a person with psoriasis, the rate of cell division is speeded up so that cells are shed every 4 days (National Psoriasis Foundation, 2022a).

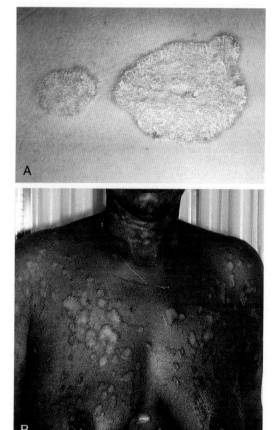

(A) Psoriasis in a patient with white skin. (B) Psoriasis in a patient with dark skin.

- Environmental factors can trigger outbreaks, yet these are very subjective to the individual person. Stress, skin injuries, certain medications (lithium, propranolol, indomethacin, quinidine, and antimalarials), and infection are known triggers (National Psoriasis Foundation, 2022b). Smoking, alcohol use, and obesity have been shown to exacerbate symptoms (Feldman, 2022).
- Some patients can develop a debilitating psoriatic arthritis (PsA) or joint deterioration.

P

Types of Psoriasis

Type	Description
Plaque psoriasis (most common type)	• Raised, red patches covered with silvery white scales • Usually found on scalp, knees, elbows, lower back • May be itchy, painful, or bleeding
Guttate psoriasis	• Small, dotlike lesions • Usually starts after a strep infection
Inverse psoriasis	• Very red lesions in folds of the body (e.g., groin, behind knees, under arms) • Smooth and shiny • Most people have another type of psoriasis in addition to inverse psoriasis
Pustular psoriasis	• White pustules surrounded by reddened skin • Not infectious, nor contagious; the pustules contain white blood cells • Usually occurs on hands and feet
Erythrodermic psoriasis	• Severe form of psoriasis with widespread, fiery redness/hyperpigmentation over most of the body • Causes severe itching and pain • Skin may come off in sheets • Rare; usually seen in people who also have unstable plaque psoriasis
Nail psoriasis	• Nail pits (dents in the nails) • White, brown, or yellow nail discoloration • Crumbling nails or nails that separate from fingers or toes • Buildup or blood that accumulates under the nail

Data from American Academy of Dermatology. (2023). *What is nail psoriasis, and how can I treat it?* https://www.aad.org/public/diseases/psoriasis/treatment/genitals/nails; and National Psoriasis Foundation. (2022). *About psoriasis.* https://www.psoriasis.org/about-psoriasis.

Interprofessional Collaborative Care

Recognize Cues: Assessment

- Obtain patient information about:
  1. Any family history of psoriasis
  2. Current status
     - Age at onset
     - Description of the disease progression
     - Pattern of recurrences
     - Whether fever and itching are present
     - Exposure to precipitating factors, including skin trauma or surgery
- Assess for and document the appearance of psoriasis and its course.

Take Actions: Interventions

- Teach the patient about the disease and its treatment, and provide emotional support for the changes in body image often experienced with psoriasis.
- Three therapeutic approaches are used to manage psoriasis.
  1. Topical therapy includes:
     - Corticosteroid creams or gels with warm, moist dressings or occlusive wraps to enhance absorption
     - Tar preparations applied to the skin lesions as solutions, ointments, lotions, gels, and shampoos
     - Anthralin application alone or in combination with coal tar baths and ultraviolet (UV) light
     - Calcipotriene, a synthetic form of vitamin D that regulates skin cell division
     - Tazarotene, a topical retinoid that can be combined with topical corticosteroid therapy; teratogenic substance

---

🩺 NURSING SAFETY PRIORITY

Drug Alert

Tazarotene and other vitamin A derivatives are *teratogenic* (can cause birth defects) even when used topically. Teach women of childbearing age who are using any of these drugs to adhere to strict contraceptive measures.

2. Phototherapy (also known as light therapy) uses ultraviolet (UV) irradiation therapy to decrease dermal growth rates.
   - Ultraviolet B (UV-B) light therapy
   - Psoralen and UV-A (PUVA) treatments involve the ingestion of a photosensitizing agent (psoralen) before exposure to UVA light
3. Systemic therapy
   - Methotrexate, folic acid, and systemic retinoids (vitamin A derivatives) are examples of systemic therapy.
   - Several biologic and biosimilar agents are also used for psoriasis. Etanercept, certolizumab, and infliximab are common tumor necrosis factor (TNF)-alpha inhibitors. Secukinumab and ustekinumab are monoclonal antibodies.
- Encourage the patient and family members to express their feelings about having an incurable skin problem that can alter appearance and to seek additional support through community-based groups.
- Use touch to communicate acceptance; avoid the use of gloves during an introductory handshake or other social interaction.

 See Chapter 21 in the main text for more information on psoriasis.

PULMONARY ARTERIAL HYPERTENSION

- Primary pulmonary arterial hypertension (PAH) is a problem of the pulmonary blood vessel constriction in the absence of lung disease.
- Primary PAH is considered idiopathic because the causes of this life-threatening disorder are unclear, although exposure to some drugs increases the risk.
- Secondary PAH can occur as a complication of other lung disorders.
- As PAH increases, blood flow decreases, leading to poor lung perfusion and gas exchange. Eventually, the right side of the heart fails *(cor pulmonale)* because of the continuous workload of pumping against the high pulmonary pressures.

Interprofessional Collaborative Care
Recognize Cues: Assessment
- Assess for and document:
  1. Dyspnea and fatigue in an otherwise healthy adult
  2. Angina-like chest pain
- Diagnosis is made from the results of right-sided heart catheterization showing elevated pulmonary pressures.

Take Actions: Interventions
- Drug therapy can reduce pulmonary pressures and slow the development of *cor pulmonale* by dilating pulmonary vessels and preventing clot formation.
  1. Endothelin-receptor antagonists (e.g., bosentan) induce blood vessel relaxation.
  2. Natural and synthetic prostacyclin agents dilate pulmonary blood vessels (e.g., epoprostenol, treprostinil).
  3. *Phosphodiesterase type 5 inhibitors* decrease pressure in the pulmonary artery and have been shown to improve the patient's ability to exercise.
- Surgical management of PAH involves single-lung or whole-lung transplantation.
- If *cor pulmonale* also is present, the patient may need combined heart-lung transplantation.

See Chapter 24 in the main text for more information on pulmonary arterial hypertension.

PULMONARY CONTUSION

- Pulmonary contusion, a potentially lethal injury, most often follows injuries caused by rapid deceleration during vehicular accidents. Hemorrhage and edema occur in and between the alveoli, decreasing lung movement and reducing the area for gas exchange.
- Respiratory failure often develops over time rather than immediately after the trauma.

Interprofessional Collaborative Care
Recognize Cues: Assessment
- Signs and symptoms include:
  1. Dyspnea
  2. Decreased breath sounds
  3. Crackles and wheezes
  4. Tachypnea
  5. Dullness to percussion

Take Actions: Interventions
- Management is aimed at maintenance of ventilation and oxygenation.
  1. Provide oxygen, give IV fluids as ordered, and place the patient in a moderate-Fowler's position.

2. The patient in respiratory distress may need noninvasive positive-pressure ventilation (NIPPV) or mechanical ventilation with positive end-expiratory pressure (PEEP) to maintain open alveoli.

See Chapter 26 in the main text for more information on pulmonary contusion.

PULMONARY EMBOLISM: GAS EXCHANGE CONCEPT ✳ EXEMPLAR

Overview
- Pulmonary embolism (PE) is a collection of particulate matter (solids, liquids, or air) that enters venous circulation and lodges in pulmonary vessels, leading to reduced *gas exchange*.
- Large emboli obstruct pulmonary blood flow, leading to reduced oxygenation, pulmonary tissue hypoxia, decreased perfusion, and potential death.
- Most often a PE occurs because of a deep vein thrombosis (DVT).
- The local response includes blood vessel constriction and pulmonary hypertension, which impair *gas exchange* and tissue perfusion.
- Major risk factors for VTE leading to PE are:
  1. Prolonged immobility
  2. Central venous catheters
  3. Surgery within the last 3 months
  4. Obesity
  5. Advancing age
  6. Conditions that increase blood clotting
  7. History of thromboembolism
  8. Smoking
  9. Pregnancy, and within 3 months postpartum
  10. Heart failure
  12. Cancer
  13. Trauma/traumatic injury

Interprofessional Collaborative Care
The patient who has a pulmonary embolism (PE) is critically ill and at risk for life-threatening complications.

Recognize Cues: Assessment
- Obtain patient information about risk factors for VTE and PE.
- Assess for key features of pulmonary embolism.

KEY FEATURES

Pulmonary Embolism

- Sudden onset of dyspnea
- Sharp, stabbing chest pain
- Apprehension, restlessness
- Feeling of impending doom
- Cough
- Hemoptysis
- Diaphoresis
- Tachypnea

- Crackles
- Pleural friction rub
- Tachycardia
- S_3 or S_4 heart sound
- Fever, low-grade
- Petechiae over chest and axillae
- Hypoxemia

- Signs and symptoms range from vague, nonspecific discomforts to hemodynamic collapse and death. It is important to remember that many patients with PE do not exhibit the ailment's classic signs and symptoms, which means that a diagnosis of PE is often overlooked.

 NURSING SAFETY PRIORITY

Critical Rescue

Monitor patients at risk to recognize signs and symptoms of PE (e.g., shortness of breath, chest pain, hypotension without an obvious cause). If symptoms are present, respond by notifying the Rapid Response Team. If PE is strongly suspected, prompt categorization and management are started before diagnostic studies have been completed.

- Computed tomography pulmonary angiography (CTPA) is the standard for diagnosing a PE.
- Laboratory studies can include a metabolic panel, troponin, B-natriuretic peptide (BNP), and D-dimer (fibrin split product).

Analyze Cues and Prioritize Hypotheses: Analysis

- The priority interprofessional collaborative problems for patients with PE include:
    1. Hypoxemia due to mismatch of lung **perfusion** and alveolar **gas exchange** with oxygenation
    2. Hypotension due to right ventricular failure
    3. Potential for bleeding due to anticoagulation or fibrinolytic therapy

Generate Solutions and Take Actions: Planning and Implementation
Managing Hypoxemia
- Increase gas exchange, improve lung perfusion, reduce the risk for further clot formation, and prevent complications.
  Nonsurgical Management
- Oxygen therapy
  1. Apply oxygen by nasal cannula or by mask.
  2. For the severely hypoxemic patient intubation with mechanical ventilation may be required.
  3. *Monitor* the patient continually for any changes in status.
     - Oxygen saturation continually
     - Vital signs, lung sounds, and cardiac status
  4. Assess for and document increasing or decreasing:
     - Dyspnea
     - Dysrhythmias
     - Distended neck veins
     - Abnormal lung sounds
     - Peripheral perfusion
- Drug therapy
  1. Anticoagulants keep the embolus from enlarging and prevent the formation of new clots.
  2. Fibrinolytic drugs, such as alteplase, are used for the treatment of PE when specific criteria are met, such as shock, hemodynamic collapse, or instability.

National Patient Safety Goals
Heparin Therapy

Heparin comes in a variety of concentrations in vials that have differing amounts, which contributes to possible drug errors. In accordance with The Joint Commission's National Patient Safety Goals (NPSGs), check the prescribed dose carefully and ensure that the correct concentration is being used to prevent overdosing or underdosing.

Surgical Management
- *Embolectomy* is the surgical or percutaneous removal of the embolus.
- *Inferior vena cava filtration* with placement of a retrievable vena cava device prevents further emboli from reaching the lungs in some patients with ongoing risk for PE.

Managing Hypotension
- Hypotension is related to inadequate circulation to the left ventricle and/or reduced circulation from bleeding due to anticoagulant or antifibrinolytic therapy.
- IV fluid therapy involves giving crystalloid solutions to restore plasma volume and prevent shock.
- Drug therapy with vasopressors is used when hypotension persists despite fluid resuscitation. Common IV agents are norepinephrine, epinephrine, or dopamine.

Minimizing Bleeding
- Monitor the patient's response to anticoagulant and antifibrinolytic therapy to reduce the risk for unintended hemorrhage from excess anticoagulation or recurrent clot formation from inadequate anticoagulation therapy.
  1. Inspect skin and mucous membranes for bleeding and petechiae.
  2. Assess hemoglobin, hematocrit, platelets, and coagulation test results; maintain values in safe range.
  3. Examine stools, urine, drainage, and vomit for gross blood, and test for occult blood in hemoglobin drops.

Care Coordination and Transition Management
- The patient with PE is discharged after hypoxemia and hemodynamic instability have been resolved and adequate anticoagulation has been achieved.
- Anticoagulation therapy usually continues after discharge.
- Patients with extensive lung damage may have reduced activity tolerance.
- Teach the patient and family about:
  1. Bleeding precautions
  2. Activities to reduce the risk for VTE
  3. Need for follow-up care

Evaluate Outcomes: Evaluation
- Evaluate the care of the patient with PE on the basis of the identified priority patient problems. The expected outcomes are that the patient:
  1. Attains and maintains adequate *gas exchange* and oxygenation
  2. Does not experience hypovolemia and shock
  3. Remains free from bleeding episodes

See Chapter 26 in the main text for more information on pulmonary embolus.

PYELONEPHRITIS: ELIMINATION CONCEPT EXEMPLAR

Overview

- Pyelonephritis is a bacterial *infection* of the kidney and renal pelvis and interferes with urinary *elimination.*
- Pyelonephritis can be acute or chronic.
  1. Acute pyelonephritis is an active bacterial infection.
  2. Chronic pyelonephritis results from repeated or continued upper UTIs, usually in patients with anatomic abnormalities of the urinary tract, urinary stasis, or obstruction with reflux.

P

Interprofessional Collaborative Care

Recognize Cues: Assessment

- Obtain patient information about:
  1. History of urinary tract and kidney infections
  2. History of diabetes mellitus or other conditions associated with immunocompromise
  3. History of stone disease or other structural or functional abnormalities of the genitourinary tract

 KEY FEATURES

Acute Pyelonephritis

- Fever
- Chills
- Tachycardia and tachypnea
- Flank, back, or loin pain
- Tenderness at the costovertebral angle (CVA)
- Abdominal, often colicky, discomfort
- Nausea and vomiting
- General malaise or fatigue
- Burning, urgency, or frequency of urination
- Nocturia
- Recent cystitis or treatment for urinary tract infection (UTI)

KEY FEATURES

Chronic Pyelonephritis

- Hypertension
- Inability to conserve sodium
- Decreased urine-concentrating ability, resulting in nocturia
- Tendency to develop hyperkalemia and acidosis

- Diagnostic testing may include:
  1. Urinalysis and urine for culture and sensitivity
  2. WBC count with differential; basic metabolic panel for kidney function
  3. X-ray, CT, or cystourethrogram to diagnose stones or obstruction

Analysis: Analyze Cues and Prioritize Hypotheses
- The priority collaborative problems for the patient with pyelonephritis are:
  1. *Pain* (flank and abdominal) due to *inflammation* and *infection*
  2. Potential for chronic kidney disease (CKD) due to kidney tissue destruction

Generate Solutions and Take Actions: Planning and Implementation
Managing Pain
- Acetaminophen is preferred over NSAIDs because it does not interfere with kidney autoregulation of blood flow.
- Drug therapy with antibiotics is ordered to treat the infection.
- Surgical interventions can correct structural problems causing urine reflux or obstruction of urine outflow or can remove the source of infection.

Preventing Chronic Kidney Disease
- Specific antibiotics are ordered to treat the infection. Stress the importance of completing the drug therapy as directed.
- Maintain sufficient perfusion to the kidneys to prevent hypotensive or hypertensive kidney injury.
- For the patient with a chronic need for indwelling urinary catheter, replace the catheter and closed drainage system to reduce bioburden.

Care Coordination and Transition Management
- Health teaching includes:
  1. Information about pyelonephritis, its causes, and therapy
  2. Antibiotic self-administration, including effects, side effects, and the importance of following the prescribed duration of therapy
  3. Planning and implementing healthy choices for fluid intake
  4. Describing the plan for posttreatment follow-up, including knowledge of recurrent symptoms
  5. Management of an indwelling urinary catheter if needed for a chronic condition or following a surgical intervention

Evaluate Outcomes: Evaluation

- Evaluate the care of the patient with pyelonephritis based on the identified priority patient problems. Expected outcomes may include that the patient will:
  1. Report that *pain* is controlled
  2. Be knowledgeable about the disease, its treatment, and interventions to prevent or reduce CKD progression

See Chapter 59 in the main text for more information on pyelonephritis.

P

RAYNAUD PHENOMENON/DISEASE

- *Raynaud phenomenon* is caused by vasospasm of the arterioles and arteries of the upper and lower extremities, usually unilaterally.
  1. Causes painful vasospasms of arteries and arterioles in extremities, especially digits
  2. Occurs more often in women

Interprofessional Collaborative Care

- Health teaching emphasizes methods to minimize vasoconstriction.
  1. Smoking cessation and caffeine reduction
  2. Minimizing exposure to cold by wearing warm clothes, socks, and gloves and maintaining a warm indoor ambient temperature
  3. Stress management

  See Chapter 30 in the main text for more information on Raynaud phenomenon/disease.

RESPIRATORY FAILURE, ACUTE

- A near match in the lungs between air movement or ventilation (V) and blood flow or **perfusion** (Q) is needed for adequate pulmonary **gas exchange**. When either ventilation or perfusion is mismatched with the other in a lung or lung area, gas exchange is reduced, and respiratory failure can result (Rogers, 2023).
- Acute respiratory failure can be defined in three ways, based on the underlying problem.
  1. *Ventilatory failure* occurs when air movement into/out of the lungs is inadequate. As a result, too little oxygen reaches the alveoli and carbon dioxide is retained.
  2. *Oxygenation failure* is a problem in which air moves in and out of lungs without difficulty but does not oxygenate the pulmonary blood sufficiently. Generally, lung blood flow (**perfusion**) is decreased.
  3. *Combined ventilatory and oxygenation failure* involves hypoventilation and impairment of oxygenation at the alveolar-capillary membrane. This type of respiratory failure leads to a more profound hypoxemia than either ventilatory failure or oxygenation failure alone.
- Regardless of the underlying cause, the patient in acute respiratory failure is always hypoxemic.

Interprofessional Collaborative Care
Recognize Cues: Assessment

- Assess for and document:
  1. Dyspnea (the hallmark of respiratory failure)
  2. Changes in the respiratory rate or pattern
  3. Abnormal lung sounds
  4. Pulse oximetry (Spo_2) may show decreased oxygen saturation, but end-tidal CO_2 ($ETco_2$ or $PETco_2$) monitoring may be more valuable for monitoring the patient with acute respiratory failure (ARF).
  5. Review arterial blood gas (ABG) values to accurately identify the degree of hypoxia and hypercarbia.

Take Actions: Interventions

- Management of acute respiratory failure of any origin includes:
  1. Applying oxygen therapy to keep the Pao_2 greater than 60 mm Hg
  2. Implementing invasive or noninvasive mechanical ventilation if other measures do not increase oxygenation
  3. Administering drugs as prescribed to dilate the bronchioles and decrease inflammation to promote *gas exchange*
  4. Assisting the patient to find a position of comfort that allows easier breathing, usually a more upright position
  5. Assisting the patient to use relaxation, diversion, and guided imagery to reduce anxiety
  6. Instituting energy-conserving measures of minimal self-care and no unnecessary procedures
  7. Encouraging deep-breathing techniques or the use of an incentive spirometer to increase oxygen intake or reduce carbon dioxide retention

See Chapter 26 in the main text for more information on respiratory failure (acute).

REHABILITATION NURSING CARE

- The practice of rehabilitation nursing is recognized as the specialty of managing care of people with disabilities and chronic health conditions across the life span.
- Patients with chronic and disabling health conditions need the integration of rehabilitation nursing concepts into their care, regardless of setting, to prevent further disability, maintain function, and restore individuals to optimal functioning in their community. This desired outcome requires care coordination and collaboration with the interprofessional health care team.

- Rehabilitation care occurs on a continuum.
- Services decrease across the continuum from the inpatient rehabilitation facility (IRF) or skilled nursing facility (SNF) to home health to outpatient ambulatory programs.

Rehabilitation Post–COVID-19

The evidence regarding COVID-19 is continually evolving, and the long-term effects are still developing. Some patients experience a variety of persistent symptoms after the acute COVID-19 infection. Symptoms include (but are not limited to) fatigue, chest discomfort, dyspnea, cough, decreased concentration, and memory problems, as well as psychological symptoms such as anxiety and depression (Mikkelsen & Abramoff, 2023).

Many patients who have either recovered from severe COVID-19 or are now experiencing post-COVID persistent symptoms require rehabilitation care. As the demand for acute care for COVID-19 begins to decrease, the resources to provide longer support are developing. Post-COVID rehabilitative care should be started within 30 days of the initial infection and requires significant screening prior to initiating rehabilitation (Mikkelsen & Abramoff, 2023). Currently, more than 60 hospitals and health systems have launched post-COVID care units (Carbajal & Gleeson, 2022).

PATIENT-CENTERED CARE: VETERAN HEALTH
Combat Disability

Combat in war is another source of major disability. Many military men and women who served in recent wars, such as those in Iraq and Afghanistan, have one or more physical or mental health disabilities, most commonly traumatic brain injury (TBI), single or multiple limb amputations, and post-traumatic stress disorder (PTSD). In addition, a large population of veterans is living with disabilities from wars of the past. These disabilities require months to years of follow-up rehabilitation after returning to the community.

- *Rehabilitation nurses* in the inpatient setting coordinate the collaborative plan of care and function as the patient's case manager. Nurses also create a rehabilitation milieu, which includes:
  1. Allowing time for patients to practice self-management skills
  2. Encouraging patients and providing emotional support
  3. Promoting self-esteem (e.g., bowel training)
  4. Making the inpatient unit a more homelike environment

Nurse's Role in the Rehabilitation Team

- Advocates for the patient and family
- Creates a therapeutic rehabilitation milieu
- Provides and coordinates whole-person patient care in a variety of health care settings, including the home
- Collaborates with the rehabilitation team to establish expected patient outcomes to develop a plan of care
- Coordinates rehabilitation team activities to ensure implementation of the plan of care
- Acts as a resource to the rehabilitation team who has specialized knowledge and the clinical skills needed to care for patients with chronic and disabling health problems
- Communicates effectively with all members of the rehabilitation team, including the patient and family
- Plans continuity of care when the patient is discharged from the health care facility
- Evaluates the effectiveness of the interprofessional plan of care for the patient and family

Adapted from Association of Rehabilitation Nurses. (2014). *Standards and scope of rehabilitation nursing practice* (6th ed.). Glenview, IL: Author.

Assessment of Patients in Rehabilitation Settings

Body System	Relevant Data
Cardiovascular system	Chest pain Fatigue Fear of heart failure
Respiratory system	Shortness of breath or dyspnea Activity tolerance Fear of inability to breathe
Gastrointestinal system and nutrition	Oral intake, eating pattern Anorexia, nausea, and vomiting Dysphagia Laboratory data (e.g., serum prealbumin level) Weight loss or gain Bowel elimination pattern or habits Change in stool (constipation or diarrhea) Ability to get to toilet

Continued

Assessment of Patients in Rehabilitation Settings—cont'd

Body System	Relevant Data
Renal-urinary system	Urinary pattern Fluid intake Urinary incontinence or retention Urine culture and urinalysis
Neurologic system	Motor function Sensation Perceptual ability Cognitive abilities
Musculoskeletal system	Functional ability Range of motion Endurance Muscle strength
Integumentary system	Risk for skin breakdown Presence of skin lesions

Interprofessional Collaborative Care

Recognize Cues: Assessment

- An essential component of rehabilitation assessment and evaluation is the assessment of functional ability.
    1. *Functional ability* refers to the ability to perform **activities of daily living (ADLs),** such as bathing, dressing, eating, using the toilet, and ambulating.
    2. **Instrumental activities of daily living (IADLs)** refer to activities necessary for living in the community, such as using the telephone, shopping, preparing food, and housekeeping. Functional assessment tools are used to assess a patient's abilities.

Analyze Cues and Prioritize Hypotheses: Analysis

- Regardless of age or specific disability, these priority patient problems are common. Additional problems depend on the patient's specific chronic condition or disability. The priority collaborative problems for patients with chronic and disabling health conditions typically include:
    1. Decreased mobility due to neuromuscular impairment, sensory-perceptual impairment, and/or persistent (chronic) pain
    2. Decreased functional ability due to neuromuscular impairment and/or impairment in perception or cognition

3. Risk for pressure injury due to altered sensation and/or altered nutritional state

4. Urinary incontinence or urinary retention due to neurologic dysfunction and/or trauma or disease affecting spinal cord nerves

5. Changes in bowel function due to neurologic impairment, inadequate nutrition, or decreased mobility

Generate Solutions and Take Actions: Planning and Implementation
Increasing Mobility

- Most problems requiring rehabilitation relate to decreased or impaired mobility.
- Before assisting patients with mobility, nurses must understand the importance of safe patient-handling and mobility practices (SPHM).

    1. Maintain a wide, stable base with your feet.
    2. Place the bed at the correct height—waist level while providing direct care and hip level when moving patients.
    3. Keep the patient or work directly in front of you to prevent your spine from rotating.
    4. Keep the patient as close to your body as possible to prevent reaching.
    5. Utilize the appropriate safe patient-handling equipment.

R

! NURSING SAFETY PRIORITY

Action Alert

Assess the patient and the situation before any transfer. Orthostatic, or postural, hypotension is a common problem and may contribute to falls. If the patient moves from a lying to a sitting or standing position too quickly, the patient's blood pressure may drop; as a result, the patient can become dizzy or faint. This problem is worsened by antihypertensive drugs, especially in older adults. To prevent this situation, help the patient change positions slowly, with frequent pauses to allow the blood pressure to stabilize. If needed, measure blood pressure with the patient in the lying, sitting, and standing positions to examine the differences. *Orthostatic hypotension* is indicated by a drop of more than 20 mm Hg in systolic pressure or 10 mm Hg in diastolic pressure between positions. Notify the health care provider and the therapists about this change.

If the patient has problems maintaining blood pressure while out of bed, the physical therapist may start the patient on a tilt table to gradually increase tolerance. A low blood pressure is a particularly common problem for patients with quadriplegia because they have a delayed blood flow to the brain and upper part of the body.

- The person with a mobility limitation must be assessed for the level of assistance needed for the specific mobility activity (e.g., bed to chair).
- The necessary safe patient-handling equipment (e.g., stand-assist device, total lift assistance, friction-reducing surface) must be used to prevent **work-related musculoskeletal disorders (MSDs),** most often back and shoulder injuries, which can often be prevented.

Increasing Functional Ability

- ADLs, or self-care activities, include eating, bathing, dressing, grooming, and toileting.
  1. Encourage the patient to perform as much self-care as possible.
  2. Collaborate with the occupational therapist (OT) to identify ways in which self-care activities can be modified so that the patient can perform them as independently as possible and with minimal frustration.
  3. Most facilities have developed restorative nursing programs and have coordinated these programs with rehabilitation therapy and activities therapy.
  4. A variety of devices are available for patients with chronic conditions and disabilities for assisting with self-care.

Examples and Uses of Common Assistive/Adaptive Devices

Device	Use
Buttonhook	Threaded through the buttonhole to enable patients with weak finger mobility to button shirts Alternative uses include serving as pencil holder or cigarette holder
Extended shoehorn	Assists in the application of shoes for patients with decreased mobility Alternative uses include turning light switches off or on while patient is in a wheelchair
Plate guard and spork (spoon and fork in one utensil)	Applied to a plate to assist patients with weak hand and arm mobility to feed themselves; spork allows one utensil to serve two purposes

Examples and Uses of Common Assistive/ Adaptive Devices—cont'd	
Device	**Use**
Gel pad	Placed under a plate or a glass to prevent dishes from slipping and moving Alternative uses include placement under bathing and grooming items to prevent them from moving
Foam buildups	Applied to eating utensils to assist patients with weak hand grasps to feed themselves Alternative uses include application to pens and pencils to assist with writing or over a buttonhook to assist with grasping the device
Hook-and-loop fastener (Velcro) straps	Applied to utensils, a buttonhook, or a pencil to slip over the hand and provide a method of stabilizing the device when the patient's hand grasp is weak
Long-handled reacher	Assists in obtaining items located on high shelves or at ground level for patients who are unable to change positions easily
Elastic shoelaces or Velcro shoe closure	Eliminates the need for tying shoes

R

Preventing Pressure Injury
- The best intervention to prevent pressure injury and maintain tissue integrity is frequent position changes in combination with adequate skin care and sufficient nutritional intake.
  1. Teach staff to assist with turning and repositioning at least every 2 hours if the patient is unable to reposition independently.
  2. Patients who sit for prolonged periods in a wheelchair need to be repositioned at least every 1 to 2 hours.
  3. Adequate skin care is an essential component of prevention.
     - If a patient is incontinent, use topical barrier creams or ointments to help protect the skin from moisture.
  4. Use pressure-relieving devices and adequate nutrition to prevent new skin breakdown.

Establishing Urinary Continence
- Neurologic disabilities often interfere with successful bladder control. These disabilities result in two basic functional types of neurogenic bladder: overactive (e.g., reflex or spastic bladder) and underactive (e.g., hypotonic or flaccid bladder).
  1. *Overactive (spastic) bladder* causes incontinence with sudden voiding.

2. *Underactive (flaccid) bladder* causes urinary retention and overflow (dribbling).
- Teach bladder management techniques, including triggering techniques, intermittent catheterization, and consistent toileting (timed voiding).
- Mild overactive bladder may be treated with antispasmodics such as oxybutynin, solifenacin, or tolterodine.

PATIENT-CENTERED CARE: OLDER ADULT HEALTH
Urinary Antispasmodic Drugs

> When urinary antispasmodic drugs are used in older adults, observe for, document, and report hallucinations, delirium, or other acute cognitive changes caused by the anticholinergic effects of the drugs.

Establishing Bowel Continence
- Neurologic problems often affect the patient's bowel pattern by causing a reflex (spastic) bowel, a flaccid bowel, or an uninhibited bowel.
  1. Establish a bowel retraining program with adequate fluid intake, a consistent toileting schedule, dietary modification, time for bowel evacuation, and, if needed, drug therapy such as a laxative (bisacodyl) or stool softener.
  2. Collaborate with patients with a chronic condition to schedule bowel elimination as close as possible to their previous routine.

PATIENT CENTERED CARE: OLDER ADULT HEALTH
Preventing Constipation

> Many rehabilitation patients, especially older adults, are at high risk for constipation. Encourage fluids (at least 8 glasses a day) and 20 to 35 g of fiber in the diet. Teach patients to eat two to three daily servings of whole grains, legumes, and bran cereals, and five daily servings of fruits and vegetables. Do not offer a bedpan when toileting. Instead, be sure that the patient sits upright on a bedside commode or bathroom toilet to facilitate defecation.

Care Coordination and Transition Management
- Care coordination and transition management begin at the time of the patient's admission. If the patient is transferred from a hospital to an IRF or SNF, orient the patient to the change in

routine and emphasize the importance of self-care. When the patient is admitted, a case manager and/or OT/PT should assess the patient's current living situation at home.

1. Before discharge, the home must be assessed to ensure accessibility for the patient, given a new mobility impairment. If a patient will use a wheelchair after discharge, the patient may need home modifications.
2. The OT and PT should teach the patient to perform ADLs independently.
3. After discharge to the home, various health care resources (e.g., physical therapy, home care nursing, vocational counseling) are available to the patient with chronic conditions and disabilities.
4. Assess the need for additional care and support throughout the hospitalization, and coordinate with the case manager and health care provider in arranging for home services.

Evaluate Outcomes: Evaluation

- The patient and rehabilitation team evaluate the effectiveness of interdisciplinary interventions based on common patient problems. Expected outcomes may include that the patient will:
  1. Prevent complications of decreased *mobility*
  2. Perform self-care and other self-management skills independently or with minimal assistance, possibly using assistive/adaptive devices
  3. Have intact skin and underlying tissues
  4. Establish urinary *elimination* without infection, incontinence, or retention
  5. Have regular evacuation of stool without constipation or incontinence

See Chapter 7 in the main text for more information on rehabilitation nursing care.

RETINAL HOLES, TEARS, AND DETACHMENTS

- A *retinal hole* is a break in the retina, usually caused by trauma or aging.
- A *retinal tear* is a jagged and irregularly shaped break, often caused by traction on the retina.
- A *retinal detachment* is the separation of the retina from the epithelium. Detachments are classified by the nature of their development.

Interprofessional Collaborative Care
Recognize Cues: Assessment
- Subjective signs are sudden:
  1. Bright flashes of light (*photopsia*) or floating dark spots in the affected eye
  2. The sensation of a curtain being pulled over part of the visual field
  3. No pain
- Ophthalmoscopic signs
  1. Gray bulges or folds in the retina
  2. Possibly a hole or tear at the edge of the detachment

Take Actions: Interventions
- For detachment, surgical repair is needed to place the retina in contact with the underlying structures. A common repair procedure is scleral buckling.
  1. Preoperative care includes applying prescribed topical drugs to inhibit pupil constriction and accommodation, and allaying fears about visual loss.
  2. Standard postoperative care includes the following:
     - Monitor the patient's vital signs and check the eye patch and shield for any drainage.
     - If gas or oil has been placed in the eye, teach the patient to keep their head in the position prescribed by the surgeon to promote reattachment.
     - Remind the patient to avoid activities that increase intraocular pressure (IOP).
     - Teach the patient to avoid reading, writing, and close work such as sewing during the first week after surgery because these activities cause rapid eye movements and promote detachment.
     - Teach the patient the signs and symptoms of infection and detachment (sudden reduced visual acuity, eye pain, pupil that does not respond to light by constricting) and the need to notify the surgeon immediately if symptoms occur.

See Chapter 39 in the main text for more information on retinal holes, tears, and detachments.

ROTATOR CUFF INJURIES

- The function of the rotator cuff is to stabilize the head of the humerus during shoulder abduction.
- It may be injured by substantial trauma or the accumulation of many small tears related to aging, repetitive motions, or falls.

Interprofessional Collaborative Care

- Symptoms include shoulder pain and the inability to achieve or maintain abduction of the arm at the shoulder.
- Conservative management for patients with a partial-thickness tear involves the use of nonsteroidal antiinflammatory drugs (NSAIDs), intermittent steroid injections, physical therapy, sling or immobilizer support, and ice or heat applications while the injury heals.
- Surgical cuff repair may be needed for patients who do not respond to conservative treatment over a 3- to 6-month period and for those who have a complete tear.

R

See Chapter 44 in the main text for more information on rotator cuff injuries.

SEIZURE DISORDERS

- A seizure is an abnormal, sudden, excessive, uncontrolled electrical discharge of neurons within the brain that may result in alterations in consciousness, motor or sensory ability, or behavior.
- Epilepsy is defined as a chronic disorder in which repeated unprovoked seizure activity occurs.
- There are three major categories and associated subclasses of seizures.
  1. *Generalized seizures* involve both cerebral hemispheres.
     - *Tonic-clonic seizure* is characterized by stiffening or rigidity of the muscles (tonic phase), followed by rhythmic jerking of the extremities (clonic phase). Immediate unconsciousness occurs, and the patient may be incontinent of urine or feces and may bite his or her tongue.
     - *Clonic* seizures last several minutes and cause muscle contraction and relaxation.
     - *Tonic* seizures are characterized by stiffening of the muscles, loss of consciousness, and autonomic changes lasting 30 seconds to several minutes.
     - The *myoclonic seizure* causes a brief jerking or stiffening of the extremities that may occur singly or in groups. Lasting for just a few seconds, the contractions may be symmetric (both sides) or asymmetric (one side).
     - In an *atonic (akinetic) seizure,* the patient has a sudden loss of muscle tone, lasting for seconds, followed by **postictal** (after the seizure) confusion. In most cases, these seizures cause the patient to fall, which may result in injury. This type of seizure tends to be most resistant to drug therapy.
  2. Partial (also called *focal* or *local*) seizures begin in one cerebral hemisphere.
     - The patient with a *simple partial seizure* remains conscious throughout the episode.
       - Before the seizure takes place, an **aura** (unusual sensation) may occur, such as a "déjà vu" (already seen) phenomenon, perception of an offensive smell, or sudden onset of pain.
       - During the seizure, the patient may have one-sided movement of an extremity, experience unusual sensations, or have autonomic symptoms. Autonomic changes include a change in heart rate, skin flushing, and epigastric discomfort.

- *Complex partial seizures* may cause loss of consciousness (**syncope**), or a blackout, for 1 to 3 minutes.
  - Characteristic automatisms (e.g., lip smacking, patting) may occur, as in absence seizures. The patient is unaware of the environment and may wander at the start of the seizure. In the period after the seizure, the patient may have **amnesia** (loss of memory).
  3. **Unclassified,** or **idiopathic, seizures** account for about half of all seizure activity. They occur for no known reason and do not fit into the generalized or partial classifications.
- *Status epilepticus* is one seizure that lasts longer than 5 minutes or repeated seizures over the course of 30 minutes. It is a neurologic emergency and must be treated promptly, or brain damage and possibly death from anoxia, cardiac dysrhythmias, or lactic acidosis may occur. Seizures lasting longer than 10 minutes can cause death!
- Seizures caused by head injury, substance abuse, high fever, metabolic disorders, or electrolyte disturbances are not considered epilepsy.
- Genetic, structural, and metabolic abnormalities contribute to the occurrence of seizures.

S

PATIENT-CENTERED CARE: OLDER ADULT HEALTH

Seizures

Complex partial seizures are most common among older adults. These seizures are difficult to diagnose because symptoms appear similar to dementia, psychosis, or other neurobehavioral disorders, especially in the postictal stage (after the seizure). New-onset seizures in older adults are typically associated with conditions such as hypertension, cardiac disease, diabetes mellitus, stroke, dementia, and recent brain injury.

Interprofessional Collaborative Care
Recognize Cues: Assessment
- Obtain patient information about:
  1. Frequency, duration, and pattern of occurrence for seizure activity
  2. Description of preictal symptoms and postictal activity (aura, motor activity, sequence of progression, eye signs, consciousness, respiratory patterns) and events surrounding the seizure
  3. Current drugs, including dosage, frequency of administration, and the time at which the drug was last taken
  4. Adherence with the antiepileptic drug schedule and reasons for noncompliance if a diagnosis of epilepsy has been made

Take Actions: Interventions
Nonsurgical Management

- Administer antiepileptic drugs, and monitor the patient's response with serum levels for effectiveness. Anticipate multiple drug-drug interactions with antiepileptic drugs and other medications.
- When providing care for the patient during a seizure:
  1. Protect the patient from injury by removing environmental hazards.
  2. Do not force anything into the patient's mouth.
  3. Turn the patient to the side to prevent aspiration and keep the airway clear.
  4. Loosen any restrictive clothing.
  5. Maintain the airway, and suction as needed.
  6. Do not restrain the patient; rather, guide the patient's movements.
  7. Document onset and cessation of seizure activity: date, time, and duration.
  8. Report sequence and type of movement and whether more than one activity occurs to the neurologist.
  9. At the completion of the seizure:
     - Take vital signs.
     - Perform a neurologic assessment.
     - Allow the patient to rest.

! NURSING SAFETY PRIORITY
Action Alert

Seizure precautions include ensuring that oxygen and suctioning equipment with an airway are readily available. If the patient does not have an IV access, insert a saline lock, especially if the patient is at significant risk for generalized tonic-clonic seizures. The saline lock provides ready access if IV drug therapy must be given to stop the seizure activity.

- Follow agency policy for the implementation of seizure precautions.
  1. Keep oxygen, suctioning equipment, and an airway available at the bedside.
  2. Maintain IV access (a saline lock) for patients at risk for tonic-clonic seizures.
  3. Keep the bed in the low position. The use of padded side rails is controversial; side rails are rarely the source of significant injury and the use of padded side rails may embarrass the patient and family.

- Status epilepticus is a medical emergency.
  1. The drugs of choice for treating status epilepticus are IV lorazepam or diazepam. Diazepam rectal gel can be used instead.

✚ NURSING SAFETY PRIORITY
Critical Rescue

Convulsive status epilepticus must be treated promptly and aggressively! Establish an airway, and notify the primary health care provider or Rapid Response Team immediately if this problem occurs! *Establishing an airway is the priority for this patient's care.* Intubation by an anesthesia provider or respiratory therapist may be necessary. Administer oxygen as indicated by the patient's condition. If not already in place, establish IV access with a large-bore catheter and start 0.9% sodium chloride. The patient is usually placed in the intensive care unit for continuous monitoring and management.

Surgical Management
- Several procedures may be performed when traditional methods fail to maintain seizure control.
  1. Vagal nerve stimulation involves surgically implanting a vagal nerve-stimulating device below the left clavicle to control partial seizures.
- Routine perioperative care is involved, with the addition of assessing neurologic status with vital signs postoperatively.

Care Coordination and Transition Management
- Promote self-management with education for the patient and family.
  1. Emphasize the importance of taking all drugs consistently as prescribed (even if seizures have stopped) and monitoring for effects and side effects; dosage or effectiveness may change over time or with the occurrence of comorbid conditions.
  2. Review the components of a balanced diet; remind the patient that alcohol should be avoided.
  3. Discuss the role of rest, time management, and stress management in health promotion.
  4. Explore the utility of keeping a seizure diary to determine whether there are factors that tend to be associated with seizure activity.
  5. Review restrictions (if any), such as driving or operating dangerous equipment and participating in certain physical activities or sports.

6. Teach the value of follow-up visits with the health care provider.
7. Offer information about a medical alert bracelet or necklace.
- Inform the patient that state laws prohibit discrimination against people who have epilepsy.

See Chapter 36 in the main text for more information on seizure disorders.

✳ SHOCK, HYPOVOLEMIC: PERFUSION CONCEPT EXEMPLAR

Overview
- The basic problem of hypovolemic shock is a loss of vascular volume, resulting in a decreased mean arterial pressure (MAP) and, in some cases, a loss of circulating red blood cells (RBCs).
- The main trigger leading to hypovolemic shock is a sustained decrease in MAP from decreased circulating blood volume.
- Decreased tissue perfusion and oxygenation lead to anaerobic cellular metabolism, with subsequent increases in serum lactate.
- Uncorrected hypovolemic shock progresses in four stages as poor cellular oxygenation continues.
  1. The initial stage is when decreased tissue *perfusion* occurs. The cause of the decrease in perfusion is relative to the type of shock. With hypovolemic shock perfusion decreases because of decreased intravascular volume. There are no obvious clinical signs of shock in this stage.

❗ NURSING SAFETY PRIORITY
Action Alert

Be aware that increased heart and respiratory rates or a slight *increase* in diastolic blood pressure are often the first signs of shock.

2. The compensatory stage of shock occurs when decreased tissue *perfusion* continues and triggers neural, endocrine, and chemical compensatory mechanisms to maintain MAP and supply oxygen to vital organs. Signs and symptoms of this stage include changes resulting from decreased tissue *perfusion*. Subjective changes include thirst and anxiety. Objective changes include restlessness, tachycardia, increased respiratory rate, decreased urine output, falling systolic blood pressure, rising diastolic blood pressure, narrowing pulse pressure, cool

extremities, and a decrease in oxygen saturation. ***Comparing these changes with the values and observations obtained earlier is critical to identifying this stage of shock.***

3. The progressive stage of shock occurs when compensatory mechanisms are functioning but can no longer deliver sufficient oxygen, even to vital organs.

❗ NURSING SAFETY PRIORITY

Action Alert

> The progressive stage of shock is a life-threatening emergency. Vital organs tolerate this situation for only a short time before developing multiple organ dysfunction syndrome (MODS) with permanent damage. Immediate interventions are needed to reverse the effects of this stage of shock. The patient's life usually can be saved if the conditions causing shock are corrected within 1 hour or less of the onset of the progressive stage. Continuously monitor vital signs, physical signs, urine output, and laboratory results and compare with earlier findings to assess therapy effectiveness and determine when therapy changes are needed.

---

4. The *refractory stage of shock* occurs when too much cell death and tissue damage result from too little oxygen reaching the tissues; in addition, the body experiences a buildup of toxic metabolites and destructive enzymes that are not removed due to poor perfusion. The body can no longer respond effectively to interventions, and shock continues. Despite aggressive interventions, multiple organ dysfunction syndrome (MODS) occurs, and death is an expected outcome.

Interprofessional Collaborative Care

• Recognizing hypovolemic shock is a major nursing responsibility. Identify patients at risk for dehydration, and assess for early signs and symptoms. This is especially important for those who have reduced cognition or mobility or who are on NPO status.

Recognize Cues: Assessment

• Assess patient history for risk factors associated with hypovolemic shock (fluid intake, urine output, recent illness or trauma).
• Assess for:
  1. Cardiovascular changes
     • Decreased MAP
     • Increased heart rate
     • Narrowed pulse pressure
     • Slow capillary refill in nail beds/reduced peripheral pulses

> **! NURSING SAFETY PRIORITY**
>
> *Action Alert*
>
> Because changes in systolic blood pressure are not always present in the initial stage of shock, use changes in pulse rate and quality as the main indicators of shock presence or progression.

2. Respiratory changes
   - Increased respiratory rate
   - Shallow depth of respirations
   - Decreased Pao_2 or peripheral oxygenation (Spo_2)

Laboratory Profile

Hypovolemic Shock

Test	Normal Range for Adults	Significance of Abnormal Findings
pH (arterial)	7.35–7.45	Decreased: insufficient tissue oxygenation causing anaerobic metabolism and acidosis
Pao_2	80–100 mm Hg	Decreased: anaerobic metabolism
$Paco_2$	35–45 mm Hg	Increased: anaerobic metabolism
Lactic acid (lactate) (arterial)	3–7 mg/dL (0.3–0.8 mmol/L)	Increased: anaerobic metabolism with buildup of metabolites
Hematocrit	*Females:* 37%–47% (0.37–0.47 volume fraction) *Males:* 42%–52% (0.42–0.52 volume fraction)	Increased: fluid shift, dehydration Decreased: hemorrhage
Hemoglobin	*Females:* 12–16 g/dL (7.4–9.9 mmol/L) *Males:* 14–18 g/dL (8.7–11.2 mmol/L)	Increased: fluid shift, dehydration Decreased: hemorrhage
Potassium	3.5–5.0 mEq/L or mmol/L	Increased: dehydration, acidosis
Serum creatinine	*Females:* 0.5–1.2 mg/dL *Males:* 0.6–1.3 mg/dL	Increased: dehydration, urinary tract obstruction, abnormal muscle breakdown, kidney disease
Serum BUN	10–20 mg/dL (3.6–7.1 mmol/L)	Increased: dehydration, urinary tract obstruction, abnormal muscle breakdown, kidney disease, GI bleeding

BUN, Blood urea nitrogen; *Paco_2,* partial pressure of arterial carbon dioxide; *Pao_2,* partial pressure of arterial oxygen.

Data from Pagana, K., Pagana, T. J., & Pagana, T. (2022). *Mosby's manual of diagnostic and laboratory tests* (7th ed.). St. Louis: Elsevier.

3. Central nervous system changes
   - Early
     - Anxiety and restlessness
     - Increased thirst
   - Late
     - Lethargy to coma
     - Generalized muscle weakness
     - Sluggish pupillary response to light
4. Kidney changes
   - Decreased urine output (less than 30 mL/hr or 0.5 mL/kg/hr) is a sensitive indicator of early shock.
5. Skin and mucous membrane changes
   - Cool, pale/ash gray, mottled, or cyanotic changes

Analyze Cues and Prioritize Hypotheses: Analysis

- The priority collaborative problem for patients with hypovolemic shock is:
  1. Inadequate **perfusion** due to active fluid volume loss and hypotension

Generate Solutions and Take Actions: Planning and Implementation

- Interventions for patients in hypovolemic shock focus on reversing the shock, restoring fluid volume to the normal range, and preventing complications.
- Monitoring is critical to determine whether the patient is responding to therapy or whether shock is progressing and a change in intervention is needed. Surgery may be needed to correct some causes of shock.

Nonsurgical Management

- Oxygen therapy is useful whenever shock is present. It can be delivered by mask, hood, nasal cannula, nasopharyngeal tube, endotracheal tube, or tracheostomy tube. Maintain O_2 saturations at 90% to 96% (Schmidt & Mandel, 2023). Supplemental oxygen with normal oxygen saturations is no longer recommended because it may be associated with increased mortality risk (Chu et al., 2018).
- IV fluid resuscitation is initiated as prescribed.
  1. Crystalloids and colloids are often used for volume replacement.
  2. If the patient is bleeding, anticipate infusing packed RBCs, plasma, plasma fractions, and clotting factors.
  3. Drug therapy is used when the patient does not respond to the replacement of fluid volume and blood products and can include intravenous vasoconstricting agents such as norepinephrine.

S

BEST PRACTICE FOR PATIENT SAFETY AND QUALITY CARE

The Patient in Hypovolemic Shock

- Ensure a patent airway.
- Insert an IV catheter or maintain an established catheter. A large-bore catheter is suggested.
- Correct hypoxemia by administering oxygen to maintain O_2 saturation at 90% to 96%; supplemental oxygen is no longer recommended if saturation is normal (Schmidt & Mandel, 2023).
- Elevate the patient's feet, keeping the head flat or elevated to no more than a 30-degree angle.
- Examine the patient for overt bleeding.
- If overt bleeding is present, apply direct pressure to the site.
- Administer drugs as prescribed.
- Do not leave the patient.

! NURSING SAFETY PRIORITY

Action Alert

Use only normal saline for infusion with blood or blood products because the calcium in Ringer's lactate induces ***clotting*** of the infusing blood.

- Additional nursing interventions include assessing the patient's response to therapy.
  1. Until shock is controlled, monitor the following every 15 minutes:
     - Blood pressure, pulse pressure, and MAP
     - Heart rate and pulse quality
     - Skin and mucosal color
     - Urine output
     - LOC
     - Respiratory rate and Spo_2

Surgical Management

- Surgical intervention in addition to nonsurgical management may be needed to correct the cause of shock.
  1. Such procedures include vascular repair, surgical hemostasis of major wounds, closure of bleeding ulcers, and electrocoagulation topical application of procoagulation agents such as thrombin and fibrin glue, and injection therapy such as epinephrine.

Care Coordination and Transition Management

- Hypovolemic shock is a complication of another condition and is resolved before patients are discharged from the acute care setting.
- Because surgery and many other invasive procedures now occur on an ambulatory care basis, more patients at home are at increased risk for hypovolemic shock.
- Teach patients and family members the early indicators of shock (increased thirst, decreased urine output, light-headedness, sense of apprehension) and to seek immediate medical attention if they appear.

Evaluate Outcomes: Evaluation

- Evaluate the care of the patient with hypovolemic shock. The expected outcome is that the patient's vascular volume will be restored with normal tissue perfusion.

See Chapter 31 in the main text for more information on shock, hypovolemic.

✸ SHOCK, SEPTIC: INFECTION CONCEPT EXEMPLAR

Overview

- Sepsis is an extreme response to *infection* that can cause tissue damage, organ failure, and death if not treated promptly and appropriately. Septic shock is a subset of sepsis that is associated with a much higher risk of death than in sepsis alone (Singer et al., 2016). Septic shock is associated with both systemic inflammatory response syndrome (SIRS) and sepsis with multiorgan dysfunction syndrome (MODS) (Urden et al., 2022).
- Sepsis is defined as a life-threatening organ dysfunction brought on by a dysregulated response to infection.
- *Septic shock* is a term used to describe a subset of sepsis in which circulatory, cellular, and metabolic abnormalities substantially increase the risk of death over that associated with sepsis alone (Singer et al., 2016).
- If infection escapes local control, then sepsis develops. As the bacteria increase, widespread inflammation known as systemic inflammatory response syndrome (SIRS) is triggered.
  1. Failure to recognize and intervene in early sepsis is a major factor for progression to septic shock and death.

2. Nurses and all other health care professionals have a responsibility to identify cues that indicate sepsis before it progresses to organ failure.
3. The Surviving Sepsis Campaign (2021) recommends using SIRS, NEWS, or MEWS over qSOFA as a single sepsis screening tool. The use of qSOFA can assist with identifying patients at high risk for sepsis and with predicting risk of death from sepsis (Dugar et al., 2020; Ward et al., 2021).

Sequential Organ Failure Assessment (SOFA)[a] and Quick Sequential Organ Failure Assessment (qSOFA)

To calculate the SOFA score the following laboratory values are needed: bilirubin, creatinine, coagulation studies, and arterial blood gases. These laboratory values combined with clinical assessment data are then scored from 0 (normal function) to 4 (organ failure). The higher the cumulative score, the greater the patient's risk. A score of 2 or higher in any system indicates an increased risk for organ failure, poor outcome, or death (Makic & Bridges, 2018). The following parameters are considered abnormal, and each would receive a score of 2 or higher:

- Respiratory: Pao_2/Fio_2 <300 mm Hg
- Coagulation: Platelets <100 × $10^3/mm^3$
- Liver: Bilirubin ≥2 mg/dL
- Cardiovascular: Hypotension requiring vasopressor support
- Central nervous system: Glasgow Coma Scale score ≤12
- Renal: Creatinine ≥2 mg/dL, or urine output <500 mL/day

Quick Sequential Organ Failure Assessment (qSOFA)

The Quick Sequential Organ Failure Assessment (qSOFA) can alert clinicians to the need for further assessment for organ dysfunction (Makic & Bridges, 2018). There are three parameters, and patients are assigned one point for each abnormal parameter. Abnormal parameters include:

- Systolic blood pressure ≤100 mm Hg
- Respiratory rate ≥22 breaths/min
- Any change in mental status

Non-ICU patients with a score of 2 or 3 require additional assessment using the SOFA and are at risk for an extended ICU stay or death.

The qSOFA has poor sensitivity and should be used to assist with identifying high-risk patients for sepsis and predicting risk of death from sepsis (Dugar et al., 2020; Ward et al., 2021).

---

[a]Adapted from Makic, M., & Bridges, E. (2018). Managing sepsis and septic shock: Current guidelines and definitions. *The American Journal of Nursing, 118*(2), 34–39; and Singer, M., Deutschman, C. S., Seymour, C. W., Shankar-Hari, M., Annane, D., Bauer, M., et al. (2016). The Third International Consensus Definitions for Sepsis and Septic Shock (Sepsis-3). *JAMA: The Journal of the American Medical Association, 315*(8), 801–810.
Fio_2, Fraction of inspired oxygen; Pao_2, partial pressure of oxygen.

Interprofessional Collaborative Care
Recognize Cues: Assessment

- Early detection of sepsis is a key component of saving lives. Nursing assessment plays a critical role in the detection of subtle changes that can occur, indicating sepsis or a progression to septic shock. When sepsis is recognized and treated quickly, chances of recovery are good. Once a patient progresses to septic shock, in which circulatory, cellular, and metabolic abnormalities are occurring, the risk of death substantially increases (Lester et al., 2018).
- Obtain patient information about recent illness, trauma, procedures, allergies, infections, or chronic health problems that may contribute to decreased perfusion
- Document:
  1. Swelling, skin discoloration, or severe localized pain that may indicate an internal hemorrhage or infection
  2. Appearance of any wounds, particularly wounds with surrounding inflammation, pus, or odor
- Communicate trend information regularly to the health care provider about cardiovascular changes, particularly blood pressure (SBP, MAP, and pulse pressure), heart rate, peripheral pulse quality, and presence of coolness in extremities
- Record respiratory changes.
  1. Increased rate
  2. Decreased depth
  3. Spo_2
  4. Acute respiratory distress syndrome (ARDS) can occur in septic shock.
- Record and communicate urine changes.
  1. Decreased urine output
  2. Increased urine concentration
- Document skin perfusion changes.
  1. Cool or clammy sensation
  2. Pallor/ash gray skin or cyanosis, especially oral mucous membranes
  3. Slow or sluggish capillary refill
  4. Blood may ooze from the gums or other mucous membranes.
- Recognize and communicate central nervous system (CNS) changes.
  1. Decreasing alertness, orientation, or cognition and increasing confusion (level of consciousness [LOC])
  2. Restlessness or apprehension
- Identify and communicate significant laboratory changes.
  1. Hallmarks of sepsis are a rising serum procalcitonin level, an increasing serum lactate level, a normal or low total white blood cell (WBC) count, and a decreasing segmented neutrophil level with a rising band neutrophil level.

Analyze Cues and Prioritize Hypotheses: Analysis

- The priority collaborative problems for patients with sepsis and septic shock are:
  1. Widespread **infection** due to altered immunity
  2. Potential for organ dysfunction due to inappropriate **clotting**, poor **perfusion**, and poor **gas exchange** from widespread **infection**

Generate Solutions and Take Actions: Planning and Implementation

- Interventions for sepsis and septic shock focus on identifying the problem as early as possible, correcting the conditions causing it, and preventing complications.

Drug Therapy

- The use of a sepsis resuscitation bundle for treatment of sepsis within 1 hour is the standard of practice.

Hour-1 Bundle for Management of Sepsis

Within 1 hour:
1. Measure lactate level.[a]
2. Obtain blood cultures before administering antibiotics.
3. Administer broad-spectrum antibiotics.
4. Begin rapid administration of 30 mL/kg crystalloid for hypotension or lactate ≥4 mmol/L.
5. Apply vasopressors if hypotensive during or after fluid resuscitation to maintain a mean arterial pressure ≥65 mm Hg.

[a] Remeasure lactate if the initial lactate is elevated (>2 mmol/L).
Data from Surviving Sepsis Campaign. (2021). https://sccm.org/SurvivingSepsisCampaign/Guidelines/Adult-Patients.

- *Oxygen therapy* is useful whenever poor tissue perfusion and poor gas exchange are present.
  1. The patient with septic shock is more likely to be mechanically ventilated.
- Antibiotic therapy is initiated within 1 hour of suspected septic shock; broad-spectrum antibiotics are administered intravenously.
- The stress of severe sepsis can cause adrenal insufficiency. Adrenal support may involve providing the patient with low-dose corticosteroids during the treatment period.
- *Blood replacement therapy* is used when poor clotting with hemorrhage occurs and may include clotting factors, platelets, fresh frozen plasma (FFP), or packed red blood cells.
- During severe sepsis, patients have microvascular abnormalities and form many small clots. Heparin therapy with fractionated heparin is used to limit inappropriate clotting and prevent the excessive consumption of clotting factors.

Care Coordination and Transition Management

- Identified sepsis should be resolved before patients are discharged from the acute care setting.
- Because more patients are receiving treatment on an ambulatory care basis and are being discharged earlier from acute care settings, more patients at home are at increased risk for sepsis.
- Protecting frail patients from infection and sepsis at home is an important nursing function.
- Teach about the importance of self-care strategies, such as good hygiene, handwashing, balanced diet, rest and exercise, skin care, and mouth care.

Evaluate Outcomes: Evaluation

- Evaluate the care of the patient with sepsis or septic shock. The expected outcome is that the patient will maintain normal aerobic cellular metabolism.

 See Chapter 31 in the main text for more information on shock, septic.

S

✳ SICKLE CELL DISEASE: PERFUSION CONCEPT EXEMPLAR

Overview

- *Sickle cell disease* (SCD) is a genetic disorder in which a mutation in the gene for the beta chains of hemoglobin causes chronic anemia, pain, disability, organ damage, increased risk for *infection*, and early death as a result of poor blood perfusion.
- The SCD genetic mutation results in the formation of abnormal hemoglobin chains that distort the cell into an abnormal (sickle-shape) form during low oxygen states. RBCs affected by abnormal hemoglobin chains are also fragile and sticky, leading to a reduced circulating time and clumping in small vessels.
  1. SCD is an autosomal recessive genetic disorder. Inheritance of two sickle-type alleles results in more than 80% to 100% of hemoglobin chain formed abnormally.
  2. *Sickle cell trait* (AS) is the inheritance of one normal and one abnormal gene for hemoglobin formation. The symptoms of AS are milder when precipitating conditions (hypoxemia-causing situations) are present because less hemoglobin is abnormal.
- Episodes of vascular occlusion from sickled, clumped RBCs cause poor perfusion, leading to potential organ damage from ischemia and infarction.
- Conditions that cause sickling include hypoxia, dehydration, infections, venous stasis, pregnancy, alcohol consumption, high altitudes, low environmental or body temperatures, acidosis, strenuous exercise, and anesthesia.

Interprofessional Collaborative Care

- SCD is a chronic disease that reduces **perfusion**, and complications can worsen over time. Patients must self-manage continually at home or in other residential settings. When crises or other acute complications occur, patients are cared for in an acute care environment, usually on a medical-surgical unit.

Recognize Cues: Assessment

- Obtain patient information about:
  1. Family history
  2. Previous sickling occurrences and crises, with precipitating events and treatments
  3. Onset of pain and events leading to current symptoms
- Signs and symptoms from RBC destruction or anemia
  1. Skin changes (pallor/ash gray skin, jaundice, or cyanosis)
  2. Priapism, a prolonged penile erection, can occur in men with SCD.
  3. Organ damage or systemic dysfunction from poor perfusion, such as acute or chronic kidney disease, heart failure, lung damage, cirrhosis/liver damage, jaundice from RBC destruction (elevated serum bilirubin), joint swelling, bone necrosis, muscle damage, disability (dependent activities of daily living [ADLs]), open wounds, stroke, or seizure
- Symptoms related to acute chest syndrome, a life-threatening condition associated with respiratory infection, fat embolism, and pulmonary debris from sickled cells. Symptoms are cough, dyspnea, abnormal lung sounds, and CXR infiltrate similar to pneumonia.
- The diagnosis of SCD is based on the percentage of hemoglobin S (HbS) on electrophoresis.

Analyze Cues and Prioritize Hypotheses: Analysis

- The priority collaborative problems for the patient with sickle cell disease include:
  1. **Pain** due to poor tissue **perfusion** and joint destruction with low oxygen levels
  2. Potential for **infection**, sepsis, multiple organ dysfunction (MODS), and death

Generate Solutions and Take Actions: Planning and Implementation
Managing Pain

- Severe pain can cause/prolong crisis.
  1. Morphine and hydromorphone are common agents used to manage pain with sickle cell crisis for the first 48 hours.

2. Moderate pain may be managed with oral doses of opioids or NSAIDs.
3. Administer hydroxyurea to reduce sickling episodes and pain.
4. L-glutamine oral powder, known as Endari, is composed of the amino acid glutamine. Higher levels of glutamine in RBCs appear to lower oxidative stress in these cells. This cellular response to glutamine both decreases sickling rates and increases RBC life spans.
5. Crizanlizumab is a monoclonal antibody that prevents adhesion and reduces the frequency of vaso-occlusive crisis.
6. Provide hydration by the oral or IV route to reduce the duration of pain episodes.

> ### ! NURSING SAFETY PRIORITY
> **Action Alert**
>
> Hydroxyurea is a teratogen (agent that can cause birth defects). Teach sexually active women of childbearing age that a pregnancy test will be done before this drug is started. Also, they must adhere to strict contraceptive measures while taking it and for at least 1 month after it is discontinued.

S

Preventing Sepsis, Multiple Organ Dysfunction, and Death
* Monitor vital signs, temperature, and other indicators of perfusion impairment regularly to detect early signs of organ damage.
    1. Monitor temperature and complete blood count (CBC) with differential, along with lung sounds and urine output characteristics, for early indicators of infection.
    2. Anoxic damage to the spleen can contribute to immunosuppression and risk for infections.
    3. Use oxygen therapy and optimize perfusion to prevent or minimize multiorgan dysfunction because of occlusion and ischemia during sickling episodes.
    4. Administer therapeutic or prophylactic antibiotics, and evaluate patient response to drugs.

Care Coordination and Transition Management
* Provide and reinforce self-management education, including:
    1. Avoiding activities that lead to hypoxia and hypoxemia
    2. Recognition of early symptoms of crisis and steps to seek help or intervene
    3. Implications of an inheritable condition
    4. Opportunities for social support and other forms of support and community resources

👥 PATIENT AND FAMILY EDUCATION

Prevention of Sickle Cell Crisis

- Drink at least 3 to 4 L of liquids every day.
- Avoid consuming alcoholic beverages and illicit substances.
- Avoid smoking cigarettes or using tobacco or nicotine in any form.
- Practice deep breathing to facilitate **gas exchange**.
- Avoid strenuous physical exercise.
- Avoid exposure to hot and cold temperature extremes.
- Avoid getting overheated or overexposure to the sun.
- Wear socks, hats, gloves, and a coat when going outside on cold days to avoid getting too cold.
- Avoid airplanes with unpressurized passenger cabins.
- Avoid traveling to areas of high altitudes.
- When you are not in crisis, engage in mild, low-impact exercise three times a week.
- See your primary health care provider for regular checkups.
- Be sure to get an influenza immunization and COVID-19 immunization every year.
- Ask your primary health care provider about receiving the pneumonia vaccine.
- Contact your primary health provider at the first sign of illness or infection.
- Be sure all your health care providers know that you have sickle cell disease, especially the anesthesia provider and radiologist.
- Consider genetic counseling before becoming sexually active.
- For additional support, contact your local chapter of the Sickle Cell Foundation.

🪶 *See Chapter 34 in the main text for more information on sickle cell disease and trait.*

SKIN INFECTIONS

- Skin infections can be bacterial, viral, or fungal.
- *Folliculitis* is an inflammation of the hair follicles. Lesions appear as pustules and papules with surrounding erythema/hyperpigmentation.
- *Furuncles* (boils) are deeper follicle infections that appear red and are firm and painful.
- *Cellulitis* is a generalized infection and involves the deeper connective tissue.

- Viral skin infections are commonly caused by the herpes simplex virus (HSV) and include type I infections (common cold sore) and type II infections (genital herpes). A second viral infection manifested in skin but that is actually an infection of the nerve is herpes zoster (shingles). Viral infections differ from bacterial infections in two ways.
  1. After the first infection, the virus remains in the body in a dormant state in the nerve ganglia and the patient has no symptoms.
  2. Reactivation stimulates the virus to travel the pathways of sensory nerves to the skin, where lesions reappear.
- Many fungal infections also affect the skin.
  1. Superficial dermatophyte infections can occur anywhere on the body but are usually seen on the foot.
     - Tinea pedis ("athlete's foot")
  2. *Candidiasis,* also known as *yeast infection,* is another common superficial fungal infection of skin and mucous membranes.
     - Risk factors include immunosuppression, long-term antibiotic therapy, diabetes mellitus, and obesity.
     - The incidence is higher in hot, humid climates.
     - Infected skin (most often in skinfolds, such as under the breasts) has a moist, red, irritated appearance, usually with itching and burning.
- Parasitic skin infections include lice, scabies, and bedbugs.
  1. Lice infestation or pediculosis can occur in the scalp or pubic area, or be generalized on the body. Both the parasite and eggs must be destroyed.
     - The most common manifestation is itching.
     - Treatment is chemical killing of lice with topical sprays, creams, and shampoos, with an active ingredient of permethrin or malathion.
     - Oral agents such as ivermectin can be used.
     - Clothing and bed linens that have touched the infected body part should be washed in hot water and detergent.
     - Social contacts may also need treatment.
  2. Scabies is a mite infestation passed on by close personal contact or contact with infested bedding. Intense itching and curved or linear ridges on the skin are the common manifestations. Egg and mites can be seen under a microscope from skin scrapings.
     - Treatment involves the use of a topical scabicide with permethrin or oral or topical ivermectin.
     - Laundry of clothes, personal items, and linen with hot water and detergent is also necessary to eliminate mites.

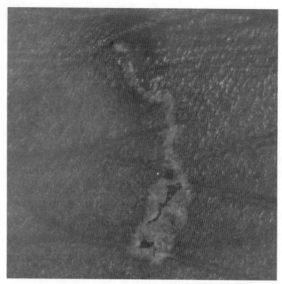

Scabies. Note the lines, indicating burrowing of the organism under the skin.

3. Bedbugs are parasites that live on human blood, but they do not cause infection. The bite can itch, but it is NOT an infection. Humans do not harbor or carry the mite.
   - Management can include a topical antihistamine for itch relief. Topical insecticides are not used.
   - The environment in which the bites occurred (e.g., home, hotel, or transport) will need extensive pest control by experts to eradicate the bedbugs.
- Prevention of skin infections, especially bacterial and fungal infections, involves avoiding the offending organism and good personal hygiene to remove the organism before infection can occur.

Interprofessional Collaborative Care
- Depending on the type of infection and existence of associated health issues, patients with minor skin infections are generally treated on an outpatient basis. For more severe infections, hospitalization for IV antibiotics may be recommended.

Recognize Cues: Assessment
- Obtain patient information about:
  1. Recent history of skin trauma
  2. Living conditions, home sanitation, personal hygiene habits, and leisure or sport activities

3. Whether fever and malaise are also present
4. Lesion locations, especially skinfolds, lips, mouth, or genital region
5. Whether the patient has ever had chicken pox or shingles
6. Whether the patient has received the shingles prevention vaccine
- Assess for and document the condition of the skin, including local or general:
  1. Redness/hyperpigmentation
  2. Warmth
  3. Itching
  4. Location of areas of inflammation, rash, or infection
  5. Presence of:
     - Blisters or vesicles
     - Pustules
     - Papules
     - Single or multiple lesions

Take Actions: Interventions

- Priority nursing interventions focus on patient and family education to prevent infection spread to other body areas or to other people.
- Nursing interventions include:
  1. Skin care instructions
     - Showering daily with soap to keep the skin clean
     - Keeping the skin dry between treatments
     - Positioning for optimal air circulation to the area
  2. Prevention of transmission
     - Using handwashing and antimicrobial hand solutions to prevent cross-contamination
     - Isolating the patient if infections are colonized with bacteria resistant to antibiotic therapy (e.g., methicillin-resistant *Staphylococcus aureas*)
     - Teaching patients to avoid sharing personal items such as hairbrushes, articles of clothing, or footwear
     - Teaching patients to avoid skin-to-skin and sexual contact when infectious skin lesions are present
- Drug therapy is specific to the type and cause of skin infection and can include:
  1. Topical agents for superficial infections and mild bacterial infections
  2. Systemic antibiotic therapy for extensive infections, especially if fever or lymphadenopathy is present
  3. Antiviral agents such as acyclovir, valacyclovir, or famciclovir
  4. Antifungal agents

See Chapter 21 in the main text for more information on skin infections.

✳ SPINAL CORD INJURY: MOBILITY CONCEPT EXEMPLAR

Overview
- Spinal cord injuries (SCIs) are classified as complete or incomplete.
    1. *Complete* if the spinal cord is damaged in a way that eliminates all innervation below the level of injury, and total motor and sensory loss occurs
    2. *Incomplete* (more common), allowing some function or movement below the level of injury
- Trauma is the leading cause of SCI.
- The causes of SCI can be divided into primary and secondary mechanisms of injury. Five primary mechanisms may result in an SCI:
    1. **Hyperflexion:** a sudden and forceful acceleration (movement) of the head forward, causing extreme flexion of the neck (e.g., motor vehicle accidents or diving accidents)

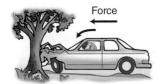

Hyperflexion injury of the cervical spine

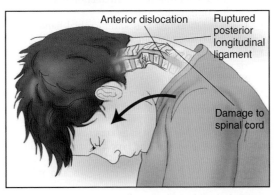

Hyperflexion injury of the cervical vertebrae. (From Leonard, P. C. [2022]. *Building a medical vocabulary: With Spanish translations* [11th ed.]. St. Louis: Elsevier.)

2. **Hyperextension:** the head is suddenly accelerated and then decelerated (e.g., motor vehicle collisions in which the vehicle is struck from behind or falls when the patient's chin is struck)

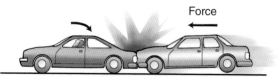

Hyperextension injury of the cervical spine

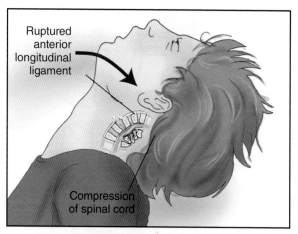

Hyperextension injury of the cervical vertebrae. (From Leonard, P. C. [2022]. *Building a medical vocabulary: With Spanish translations* [11th ed.]. St. Louis: Elsevier.)

3. **Axial loading or vertical compression:** injuries resulting from diving accidents, falls onto the buttocks, or a jump in which a person lands on the feet

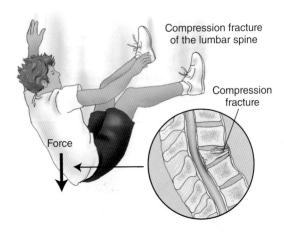

Compression fracture of the lumbar spine

Compression fracture

Force

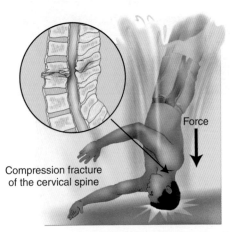

Force

Compression fracture of the cervical spine

Vertical compression of the cervical spine and the lumbar spine. (From Leonard, P. C. [2022]. *Building a medical vocabulary: With Spanish translations* [11th ed.]. St. Louis: Elsevier.)

4. Excessive rotation: results from injuries that are caused by turning the head beyond the normal range.
5. Penetrating trauma: classified by the speed of the penetrating object. Low-speed injuries cause damage directly at the site or local damage to the spinal cord. In contrast, high-speed injuries, such as a gunshot wound, cause both direct and indirect damage.
- Secondary injury worsens the primary injury. Secondary injuries include:
  1. Hemorrhage
  2. Ischemia
  3. Hypovolemia
  4. Local edema
  5. Impaired tissue perfusion from neurogenic shock (a medical emergency)

Interprofessional Collaborative Care
- The initial and priority assessment focuses on the patient's ABCs (**a**irway, **b**reathing, and **c**irculation). After an airway is established, assess the patient's breathing pattern.

Recognize Cues: Assessment
- Obtain information about:
  1. How the injury occurred and the probable mechanism of injury
  2. The patient's position and location immediately after the injury
  3. Symptoms that occurred after the injury and what changes have occurred since
  4. Type of immobilization devices used
  5. Medical treatment given at the scene of the injury or in the emergency department
  6. Medical history, with particular attention to a history of arthritis of the spine, congenital deformities, cancer, previous injury to the back or spinal cord, and respiratory problems
- Assess for and document:
  1. Adequacy of airway, breathing, and circulation
     - The patient with a cervical SCI is at high risk for respiratory compromise because the cervical spinal nerves (C3 to C5) innervate the phrenic nerve controlling the diaphragm.
  2. Vital signs and indication of hemorrhage or other non-CNS injury
  3. Indications of a head injury, such as a change in LOC, abnormal pupil size and reaction to light, and change in behavior or ability to respond to directions

S

4. Evidence of spinal shock, characterized by complete but temporary loss of motor, sensory, reflex, and autonomic function that often lasts less than 48 hours but may continue for several weeks

5. Sensory perception and mobility, to determine the level of injury and establish baseline data for future assessment
   - The level of injury is the lowest neurologic segment with intact or normal motor and sensory function. **Tetraplegia** (also called *quadriplegia*) (paralysis) and **quadriparesis** (weakness) involve all four extremities, as seen with cervical cord and upper thoracic injury. **Paraplegia** (paralysis) and **paraparesis** (weakness) involve only the lower extremities, as seen in lower thoracic and lumbosacral injuries or lesions.

✚ NURSING SAFETY PRIORITY

Critical Rescue

In *acute* SCI, monitor for a decrease in **sensory perception** from baseline, especially in a proximal (upward) dermatome and/or new loss of motor function and **mobility**. The presence of these changes is considered an emergency and requires immediate communication with the Rapid Response Team or primary health care provider, using SBAR or other agency-approved protocol for notification. Document these assessment findings in the electronic health record.

6. Change in thermoregulatory capacity, with the patient's body tending to assume the temperature of the environment (hypothermia)

7. Breathing problems resulting from an interruption of spinal innervation to the respiratory muscles, assessing for atelectasis and/or pneumonia symptoms

8. Evaluation of the patient's abdomen for manifestations of internal bleeding, distention, or paralytic ileus; paralytic ileus is manifested by decreased or absent bowel sounds and distended abdomen, usually 72 hours or longer after injury

9. Bladder fullness and/or urinary tract infection. Autonomic dysfunction initially causes an areflexic (neurogenic) bladder (no reflex ability for bladder contraction), which later leads to urinary retention. The patient is at risk for urinary tract infection (UTI) from an indwelling urinary catheter, intermittent catheterizations, or bladder distention, stasis, and/or overflow.
   - **Autonomic dysreflexia (AD)**, sometimes referred to as *autonomic hyperreflexia*, is a potentially life-threatening condition in which noxious visceral or cutaneous stimuli (such as from a full bladder or bowel) cause a sudden, massive, uninhibited reflex sympathetic discharge in people with high-level SCI.

10. Coping strategies used to deal with illness, difficult situations, or disappointments; initial hospitalization after SCI lasts for 3 or more months to include rehabilitation

Analyze Cues and Prioritize Hypotheses: Analysis

- The priority collaborative problems for patients with an *acute* spinal cord injury (SCI) include:
    1. Potential for respiratory distress/failure due to aspiration, decreased diaphragmatic innervation, and/or decreased *mobility*
    2. Potential for cardiovascular instability (e.g., shock and autonomic dysreflexia) due to loss or interruption of sympathetic innervation or hemorrhage
    3. Potential for secondary spinal cord injury due to hypoperfusion, edema, or delayed spinal column stabilization
    4. Decreased *mobility* and *sensory perception* due to spinal cord damage and edema

Generate Solutions and Take Actions: Planning and Implementation
Managing the Airway and Improving Breathing

- Manage the airway and improve breathing related to risk for aspiration or lack of diaphragmatic innervation.
    1. Manage respiratory secretions with assisted coughing, positioning, and suctioning.
    2. Implement strategies to prevent ventilator-associated pneumonia (VAP).
    3. Coordinate the cough effort of the tetraplegic patient with an assistant who uses an upward thrust to the diameter during forceful exhalation ("quad cough" or "assist cough").

> ### ! NURSING SAFETY PRIORITY
> **Action Alert**
>
> Assess breath sounds every 2 to 4 hours during the first few days after SCI, and document and report any adventitious or diminished sounds. Monitor vital signs with pulse oximetry. Watch for changes in respiratory pattern or airway obstruction. Intervene per agency or primary health care provider (PHCP) protocol when there is a decrease in oxygen saturation (Spo_2) to below 95%.

Monitoring for Cardiovascular Instability

- Monitor for cardiovascular instability (e.g., shock, autonomic dysreflexia) related to loss or interruption of sympathetic innervation or hemorrhage.
    1. Maintain adequate hydration through IV therapy and oral fluids as appropriate, depending on the patient's overall condition.

2. Dextran, a plasma expander, may be used to increase capillary blood flow within the spinal cord and prevent or treat hypotension.
3. Atropine sulfate is used to treat bradycardia if the pulse rate falls below 50 to 60 beats/min.

➕ NURSING SAFETY PRIORITY

Critical Rescue

Monitor the patient with acute spinal cord injury at least hourly for indications of **neurogenic shock**:
- Temperature dysregulation, including warm, flushed skin
- Symptomatic bradycardia, including reduced level of consciousness and deceased urine output
- Hypotension with systolic blood pressure (SBP) <90 or mean arterial pressure (MAP) <65 mm Hg

Notify the Rapid Response Team or primary health care provider immediately if these symptoms occur because this is an emergency! Similar to interventions for any type of shock, neurogenic shock is treated symptomatically by providing fluids to the circulating blood volume, adding vasopressor IV therapy, and providing supportive care to stabilize the patient.

➕ NURSING SAFETY PRIORITY

Critical Rescue

If the patient experiences AD, raise the head of the bed *immediately* to help reduce the blood pressure as the first action. Notify the Rapid Response Team or primary health care provider immediately for drug therapy to quickly reduce blood pressure as indicated. Determine the cause of AD, and manage it promptly.

Preventing Secondary Spinal Cord Injury
- During the immediate care of the patient with a suspected or confirmed cervical spine injury, a hard cervical collar, such as the Miami J or Philadelphia collar, is placed immediately and maintained until a specific order indicates that it can be removed.

BEST PRACTICE FOR PATIENT SAFETY AND QUALITY CARE

Emergency Care of the Patient Experiencing Autonomic Dysreflexia: Immediate Interventions

- Place patient in a sitting position (first priority!), or return to a previous safe position.
- Assess for and remove/manage the cause:
  - Check for urinary retention or catheter blockage:
  - Check the urinary catheter tubing (if present) for kinks or obstruction.
  - If a urinary catheter is not present, check for bladder distention and catheterize immediately if indicated. Consider using anesthetic ointment on tip of catheter before catheter insertion to reduce urethral irritation.
- Determine whether a urinary tract infection or bladder calculi (stones) are contributing to genitourinary irritation.
- Check the patient for fecal impaction or other colorectal irritation, using anesthetic ointment at rectum; disimpact if needed.
- Examine skin for new or worsening pressure injury symptoms.
- Monitor blood pressures every 10 to 15 minutes.
- Give nifedipine or nitrate as prescribed to lower blood pressure as needed. (Patients with recurrent autonomic dysreflexia may receive clonidine or other centrally acting alpha-agonist agent prophylactically [Burchum & Rosenthal, 2022].)

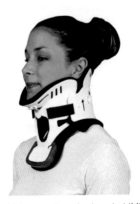

Patient with a spinal cord injury wearing a hard cervical (Miami J) collar. (Found in Ostendorf, W. R., et al. [2020]. *Nursing interventions and clinical skills* [7th ed.]. St. Louis: Elsevier. From Össur Americas.)

- The patient may be placed in fixed skeletal traction to realign the vertebrae, facilitate bone healing, and prevent further injury, often after surgical stabilization. The most commonly used device for immobilization of the *cervical spine* is the **halo fixator** device, also called a halo crown, which is worn for 6 to 12 weeks.
- Until the spinal column is stabilized, a jaw-thrust maneuver is preferable to a head-tilt maneuver to open the airway should the patient need an airway intervention.

Drug Therapy for SCI
- Centrally acting skeletal muscular relaxants may help control severe muscle spasticity.
- Intrathecal baclofen therapy may be used and is administered via an implanted infusion pump directly into the cerebrospinal fluid.

Managing Decreased Mobility
- Patients with SCI are especially at risk for pressure ulcers, thromboembolism, contractures, orthostatic hypotension, and fractures related to osteoporosis. The following interventions may be used to decrease risks:
  1. Frequent and therapeutic positioning not only helps prevent complications but also provides alignment to prevent further SCI or irritability.
  2. Assess the condition of the patient's skin, especially over pressure points, with each turn or repositioning.
  3. Turning may be performed manually, or the patient may be placed on an automatic rotating bed.
  4. Reposition patients frequently (every 1 or 2 hours). When sitting in a chair, the patient is repositioned or taught how to reposition more often than every hour.
  5. Prevent VTE, including using interventions of intermittent pneumatic compression stockings and low-molecular-weight heparin (LMWH).
  6. Collaborate with the rehabilitation team to teach or reinforce mobility skills.

Care Coordination and Transition Management
- Most patients are discharged to a rehabilitation setting, where they learn processes to enable self-care, mobility, and bladder and bowel management.
  1. Psychosocial adaptation is a crucial factor in determining the success of rehabilitation.
     - Assist the patient to verbalize feelings and fears about body image, self-concept, role performance, and self-esteem.

- Talk to the patient about the expected reactions of those outside the hospital environment.
- Help to set and reinforce realistic goals for managing self-care while promoting independence and decision making daily.
- Provide opportunities for emotional and spiritual support.
- Sexuality can be a major concern; work closely with the rehabilitation interprofessional team to address concerns about intercourse and reproduction.

2. Collaborate with the patient, family, case manager, and rehabilitation professionals to assess the home environment to ensure accessibility access and plan for vocational adaptation or education.
3. Ensure that the patient can correctly use all adaptive devices ordered for home use.
4. Teach the patient and family, in collaboration with health care team members:
   - Mobility skills
   - Pressure ulcer prevention
   - ADL skills
   - Bowel and bladder program
   - Education about sexuality and referral for counseling to promote sexual health
   - Prevention of AD with appropriate bladder, bowel, and skin care practices and recognition of early signs or symptoms of autonomic dysreflexia

Evaluate Outcomes: Evaluation

- Evaluate the care of the patient with an SCI based on the identified priority patient problems. The expected outcomes are that the patient:
  1. Exhibits no deterioration in neurologic status
  2. Maintains a patent airway, a physiologic breathing pattern, and adequate ventilation
  3. Does not experience a cardiovascular event (e.g., shock, hemorrhage, autonomic dysreflexia) or receives prompt treatment if an event occurs
  4. Does not experience secondary spinal cord injury, including VTE and heterotopic ossification
  5. Is free from complications of decreased *mobility*

See Chapter 37 in the main text for more information on spinal cord injury.

✳ STOMATITIS: TISSUE INTEGRITY CONCEPT EXEMPLAR

Overview

- **Stomatitis** is a broad term that refers to inflammation within the oral cavity. It may present in many different ways. Painful, inflamed ulcerations (called *aphthous ulcers* or *canker sores*) that erode **tissue integrity** of the mouth are one of the most common forms of stomatitis.

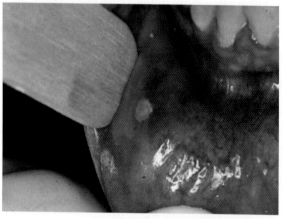

Aphthous ulcer. (From Auerbach, P. S., et al. [2017]. *Auerbach's Wilderness medicine* [7th ed.]. Philadelphia: Elsevier.)

- Primary stomatitis, the most common type, includes **aphthous** (noninfectious) **stomatitis,** herpes simplex stomatitis, and traumatic ulcers.
- Secondary stomatitis results from infection by opportunistic viruses, fungi, or bacteria in patients who are immunocompromised.
  1. A common type of secondary stomatitis is caused by *Candida albicans.*
  2. Long-term antibiotic therapy destroys other normal flora and allows the *Candida* to overgrow. The result can be **candidiasis,** also called *moniliasis,* a fungal infection that is very painful. Candidiasis is also common in those undergoing immunosuppressive therapy, such as chemotherapy, radiation, and corticosteroids.
  3. Oral hygiene can discourage the frequency and severity of stomatitis, although it may not completely prevent all occurrences.

Interprofessional Collaborative Care

Recognize Cues: Assessment

- Assess for:
  1. History of recent infection
  2. Nutritional changes
  3. Oral trauma
  4. Hygiene habits
  5. Stress

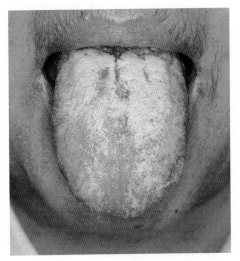

Oral candidiasis. (From Millsop, J. W., & Fazel, N. [2016]. Oral candidiasis. *Clinics in Dermatology, 34*[4], 487–494. doi:10.1016/j.clindermatol.2016.02.022.)

- Document the course of the current symptoms, and determine whether stomatitis has occurred in the past.
- While examining the mouth, wear gloves, use a penlight to ensure adequate lighting, and use a tongue blade to aid the examination of the oral cavity.
- In cases of oral candidiasis, white plaquelike lesions appear on the tongue, palate, pharynx (throat), and buccal mucosa (inside the cheeks). When these patches are wiped away, the underlying surface is red, sore, and painful, and *tissue integrity* is compromised.
- Assess the mouth for lesions, coating, and cracking.
  1. Document characteristics of the lesions, including their location, size, shape, odor, color, and drainage.
- For definitive diagnosis, the primary health care provider may prescribe swallowing studies.

! NURSING SAFETY PRIORITY
Action Alert

Airway obstruction, aspiration pneumonia, and malnutrition can result from dysphagia. Assess for signs and symptoms, such as coughing or choking when swallowing, a sensation of food "sticking" in the pharynx, or difficulty swallowing. If dysphagia is suspected, use the PASS acronym for quick assessment: Is it **P**robable that the patient will have swallowing difficulty? **A**ccount for previous swallowing problems. **S**creen for signs and symptoms. Obtain a **S**peech-language pathologist referral (Azer & Kshirsager, 2022). Report signs and symptoms to the primary health care provider, and institute aspiration prevention interventions.

Analyze Cues and Prioritize Hypotheses: Analysis

* The priority collaborative problems for the patient with stomatitis include:
    1. Impaired *tissue integrity* due to oral and/or esophageal lesions
    2. *Pain* due to oral and/or esophageal lesions

Generate Solutions and Take Actions: Planning and Implementation
Preserving Tissue Integrity

* Instruct the patient to:
    1. Use a soft-bristled brush to gently clean teeth, gums, and the oral cavity.
    2. Rinse the mouth often with sodium bicarbonate solution, warm saline, or hydrogen peroxide solution. Avoid alcohol-based commercial mouthwashes.
    3. Take drug therapy as prescribed, which may include clotrimazole troches, nystatin suspension, and chlorhexidine.

Minimizing Pain

* Manage oral pain by teaching the patient to:
    1. Use topical agents (2% viscous lidocaine).
    2. Modify diet to avoid salty, spicy, acidic, and other irritating foods.

◆ NURSING SAFETY PRIORITY
Drug Alert

Teach patients to use viscous lidocaine with extreme caution. Lidocaine causes a topical anesthetic effect so that patients may not easily feel burns from hot liquids. As sensation in the mouth and throat decreases, the risk for aspiration rises.

Care Coordination and Transition Management
- Teach appropriate administration of home medications, such as swish and swallow versus swish and spit (rinse only).
- Teach the patient about dietary choices that will not irritate the oral cavity.

Evaluate Outcomes: Evaluation
- Evaluate the care of the patient with stomatitis based on the identified priority patient problems. The expected outcomes include that the patient will:
    1. Have healthy oral mucosa without inflammation or infection
    2. Experience minimized or absence of *pain*.

 See Chapter 46 in the main text for more information on stomatitis.

✳ STROKE: PERFUSION CONCEPT EXEMPLAR

Overview
- Stroke is caused by an interruption of *perfusion* to any part of the brain. The National Stroke Association uses the term *brain attack* to describe a stroke to convey the urgency for activation of the emergency medical system for care.
- Strokes may be classified as:
    1. *Acute ischemic stroke,* which is caused by the occlusion of a cerebral or carotid artery; types of ischemic strokes include the following:
        - A *thrombotic stroke,* which is commonly associated with the development of atherosclerosis of the blood vessel wall. Signs and symptoms occur over minutes to hours.
        - An *embolic stroke,* which is caused by a thrombus or group of thrombi that travel to the cerebral arteries through the carotid artery and block the artery, resulting in ischemia. Sudden, rapid development of focal neurologic deficits occurs. Embolic strokes are associated with atrial fibrillation, coronary disease, and heart valve disease or repair.
    2. *Hemorrhagic stroke,* in which the integrity of the vessel wall is interrupted and bleeding occurs into the brain tissue (intracerebral) or spaces surrounding the brain (ventricular, subdural, subarachnoid); causes include hypertension, ruptured aneurysm, and arteriovenous malformation (AVM).
        - An *aneurysm* is the abnormal ballooning of an artery, which may become stretched or thinned and rupture.
        - *AVM* is a thin-walled, dilated vessel that results in an abnormal communication between the arterial and venous vessels without a capillary network.

S

- *Vasospasm,* a sudden and periodic constriction of a cerebral artery, often follows a cerebral hemorrhage caused by aneurysm or AVM rupture.

Healthy People 2030: Improving Stroke Outcomes

A major goal of the *Healthy People 2030* initiative is to improve cardiovascular health and reduce deaths from heart disease and stroke. Specific objectives to help meet these goals include the following:
- Increase the proportion of adult stroke survivors who participate in rehabilitation services
- Reduce stroke death

Another objective addresses the need to increase blood pressure and cholesterol control to help reduce the incidence of stroke and, therefore, reduce stroke death. Nurses have a vital role in helping to meet these objectives through patient and family education and coordinating transitions in care.

Interprofessional Collaborative Care
Recognize Cues: Assessment
- Although an accurate history is important in the diagnosis of a stroke, the first priority is to ensure that the patient is transported to a stroke center.
  1. A stroke center is designated by The Joint Commission (TJC) for its ability to rapidly recognize and effectively treat strokes.
- Obtain patient information about:
  1. Time of symptom onset
  2. Progression and severity of symptoms, including the presence of TIA previously
  3. LOC, orientation, and other measures of cognitive function
  4. Motor status: gait, balance, reading and writing abilities
  5. Sensory status: speech, hearing, vision
  6. Medical history with attention to identifying risk factors, such as hypertension, hyperlipidemia, cardiovascular disease, diabetes, smoking, sedentary lifestyle, alcohol use, obesity, high fat diet, conditions that alter coagulation, and the presence of atrial fibrillation (dysrhythmia)
  7. Social history, with attention to identifying sources of support
  8. Current drugs and nonprescribed drugs, especially anticoagulants, aspirin, vasodilators, and illegal drugs

✚ NURSING SAFETY PRIORITY

Critical Rescue

In the ED, assess the stroke patient within 10 minutes of arrival. This same standard applies to patients already hospitalized for other medical conditions who have a stroke. The priority is assessment of the ABCs—**a**irway, **b**reathing, and **c**irculation. Many hospitals have designated stroke teams and centers that are expert in acute stroke assessment and management.

- Assess for and document:
  1. Neurologic function using a standard stroke screening tool such as the National Institutes of Health Stroke Scale (NIHSS), including:
     - LOC
     - Orientation
     - Motor ability
     - Pupil size and reaction to light, extraocular movement, visual field deficits, ptosis (drooping eyelid)
     - Speech and language
  2. Vital signs
  3. Blood glucose
  4. Additional assessment for ongoing care, including:
     - Cognition, memory, judgment, and problem-solving and decision-making abilities
     - Ability to concentrate and attend to tasks
     - Range of motion (ROM), proprioception, head and trunk control, balance, gait, coordination, bowel and bladder control
     - Sensory status (response to touch and painful stimuli; ability to distinguish between two tactile stimuli presented simultaneously; ability to read, write, and follow verbal directions; and ability to name objects and use them correctly)
     - Speech pattern (rhythm, clarity, aphasia)
     - Visual system (homonymous hemianopsia, bitemporal hemianopsia, amaurosis fugax)
     - Cranial nerve function
     - Cardiac system (dysrhythmias and murmurs)
     - Coping mechanisms or personality changes
  5. Emotional lability and screen for depression
  6. Nutritional status
  7. Social support, financial status, and occupation

- Diagnostic tests
  1. For definitive evaluation of a suspected stroke, a *computerized tomography perfusion (CTP) scan* and/or *computerized tomography angiography (CTA)* is used to assess the extent of ischemia of brain tissue. Cerebral aneurysms or AVM may also be identified.
  2. Magnetic resonance imaging (MRI) and related multimodal imaging demonstrate ischemia earlier than CT scan and are used to identify the presence of hemorrhage or a cerebral aneurysm. Results also help differentiate stroke from other pathologic changes that mimic a stroke.
  3. CBC, serum electrolytes, and coagulation factors
  4. Carotid ultrasound
  5. ECG and echocardiography to determine whether cardiac disease or dysrhythmia is a contributing factor to stroke

Analyze Cues and Prioritize Hypotheses: Analysis

- Depending on stroke severity and/or response to immediate management, the priority collaborative problems for patients with stroke may include:
  1. Inadequate **perfusion** to the brain due to interruption of arterial blood flow and a possible increase in intracranial pressure (ICP)
  2. Decreased **mobility** and possible need for assistance to perform ADLs due to neuromuscular or cognitive impairment
  3. Aphasia and/or dysarthria due to decreased circulation in the brain or facial muscle weakness
  4. **Sensory perception** deficits due to altered neurologic reception and transmission

Generate Solutions and Take Actions: Planning and Implementation
Improving Cerebral Perfusion
Nonsurgical Management

- The two major treatment modalities for patients with acute ischemic stroke are IV fibrinolytic therapy and endovascular interventions.

⬥ NURSING SAFETY PRIORITY
Drug Alert

In addition to frequent monitoring of vital signs, carefully observe for signs of intracerebral hemorrhage and other signs of bleeding during administration of fibrinolytic drug therapy.

- Monitor for neurologic changes or complications before, during, and after medical interventions.
    1. Perform a neurologic assessment at least every 2 to 4 hours, checking:
        - Verbal ability, orientation
        - Eye opening, pupil size, and reaction to light
        - Motor response
    2. Monitor vital signs with neurologic checks. Assess for signs of increased intracranial pressure (ICP).

✚ NURSING SAFETY PRIORITY

Critical Rescue

Be alert for symptoms of increased ICP, and report any deterioration in the patient's neurologic status to the health care provider immediately. The first sign of increased ICP is a declining LOC.

    3. Perform a cardiac assessment.
        - Monitor the patient for dysrhythmias; auscultate the heart and palpate peripheral pulses to identify new irregular heart rhythms in the absence of a cardiac monitor.
    4. Position the backrest to promote cerebral perfusion. In the presence of ischemic stroke, a flat backrest may be preferred initially.
- Drug therapy
    1. Fibrinolytic therapy may be used for an acute ischemic stroke.
        - Currently, the U.S. Food and Drug Administration (FDA) approves administration of alteplase within 3 hours of stroke onset. The American Stroke Association endorses extension of that time frame to 4.5 hours to administer this fibrinolytic for patients *unless* they fall into one or more of these categories (Powers et al., 2019):
            - Age older than 80 years
            - Anticoagulation regardless of international normalized ratio (INR)
            - Imaging evidence of ischemic injury involving more than one-third of the brain tissue supplied by the middle cerebral artery
            - Baseline National Institutes of Health Stroke Scale score greater than 25
            - History of both stroke and diabetes
            - Evidence of active bleeding
        - Endovascular procedures to improve *perfusion* include intra-arterial thrombolysis using drug therapy, mechanical

embolectomy (surgical blood clot [thrombosis] removal), and carotid stent placement. *Intra-arterial thrombolysis* has the advantage of delivering the fibrinolytic agent directly into the thrombus within 6 hours of the stroke onset.

2. Anticoagulant therapy and antiplatelet therapy may be prescribed, depending on the health care provider's preference, following ischemic stroke or TIA.
   - Antiplatelet drugs include the use of aspirin and/or clopidogrel and are the standard of care for treatment following acute ischemic strokes and for preventing future strokes (Powers et al., 2019).

3. Other drugs used to treat symptoms associated with stroke include:
   - Calcium channel blockers (nimodipine), which may be administered to treat vasospasm or chronic spasm of the vessel that inhibits blood flow to the area
   - Stool softeners, analgesics for pain, and antianxiety drugs

---

 KEY FEATURES

Increased Intracranial Pressure (ICP)

- Decreased level of consciousness (LOC) (earliest sign)
- Behavioral changes: restlessness, irritability, and confusion
- Headache
- Nausea and vomiting (may be projectile)
- Aphasia
- Change in speech pattern/**dysarthria**
- Change in sensorimotor status:
  - Pupillary changes: dilated and nonreactive pupils ("blown pupils") or constricted and nonreactive pupils (very late sign)
  - Cranial nerve dysfunction
  - **Ataxia**
- Seizures (usually within first 24 hours after stroke)
- **Cushing's triad**: (very late sign)
  - Severe hypertension
  - Widened pulse pressure
  - Bradycardia
- Abnormal posturing (very late sign):
  - Decerebrate
  - Decorticate

Promoting Mobility and ADL Ability

- In collaboration with the rehabilitation therapists, assess the patient's functional ability for bed ***mobility*** skills and ADL ability, and implement early progressive rehabilitation.
- Follow agency guidelines for screening for swallowing difficulties; this may be a component of the stroke care protocol.
  1. The best practice for all suspected and diagnosed stroke patients is to maintain NPO status until their swallowing ability is assessed!
- Implement venous thromboembolism (VTE) prophylaxis.
- Collaborate with the physical therapist (PT) and occupational therapist (OT) to manage flaccid or spastic limbs.

Promoting Effective Communication

- Language or speech problems are usually the result of a stroke involving the dominant hemisphere. The left cerebral hemisphere is the speech center in most patients.
  1. Present one idea or thought in a sentence (e.g., "I am going to help you get into the chair").
  2. Use simple one-step commands rather than asking patients to do multiple tasks.
  3. Speak slowly but not loudly; use cues or gestures as needed.
  4. Avoid "yes" and "no" questions for patients with expressive aphasia.
  5. Use alternative forms of communication if needed, such as a computer, handheld mobile device, communication board, or flash cards (often with pictures).

Managing Changes in Sensory Perception

- Unilateral neglect, or neglect syndrome, occurs most commonly in patients who have had a right cerebral stroke.
  1. Help the patient adapt to these disabilities by using frequent verbal and tactile cues and by breaking down tasks into discrete steps.
  2. Always approach the patient from the unaffected side, which should face the door of the room!
- Hemianopsia, in which the vision of one or both eyes is affected, places the patient at additional risk for injury, especially falls.
  1. Teach the patient to turn their head from side to side to expand the visual field.
  2. The scanning technique is also useful when the patient is eating or ambulating.

S

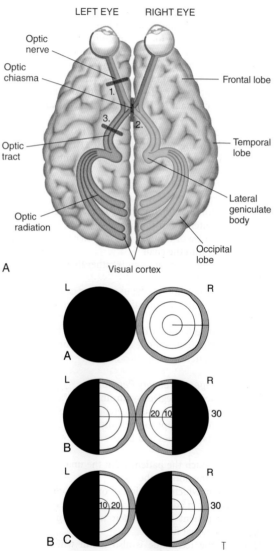

(A) Site of lesions causing visual loss. 1, Total blindness left eye. 2, Bitemporal hemianopsia. 3, Left homonymous hemianopsia. (B) Visual fields corresponding to lesions shown in (A): 1, Total blindness left eye. 2, Bitemporal hemianopsia. 3, Left homonymous hemianopsia. (From Ball, J. W., et al. [2023]. *Seidel*'s Guide to physical examination [10th ed.]. St. Louis: Elsevier.)

- With a right-sided stroke, patients may have an inability to recognize their physical impairment or a lack of proprioception (position sense).
  1. Teach the patient to touch and use both sides of the body.
  2. When dressing, remind the patient to dress the affected side first.
- The patient with a left hemisphere lesion generally has memory deficits and may show significant changes in the ability to carry out simple tasks.
  1. Assist with memory problems, reorient the patient to the month, year, day of the week, and circumstances surrounding hospital admission.
  2. Establish a routine or schedule that is as structured, repetitious, and consistent as possible.
  3. Provide information in a simple, concise manner.

Care Coordination and Transition Management

- Provide a detailed plan of care at the time of discharge for patients to be transferred to a rehabilitation center or long-term care facility.
- If possible, a case manager should be assigned to help coordinate plans for the patient discharged to the home setting. The case manager should collaborate with the home health agency and with physical and occupational therapists to:
  1. Identify and suggest corrections of hazards in the home before discharge.
  2. Ensure that the patient and family can correctly use all adaptive devices ordered for home use.
  3. Arrange follow-up appointments as needed.
- Teaching for self-management includes:
  1. Providing drug information as needed
     - Discharge with antithrombotic therapy is one of The Joint Commission's core measures for patients with ischemic stroke.
     - Provide both written and verbal instruction at discharge.
  2. Reinforcing mobility skills (in collaboration with other therapists) such as:
     - How to safely climb stairs, transfer from bed to chair, and get into and out of a car
     - How to use adaptive equipment
  3. Teaching the family that depression and emotional or mood changes may occur
     - Depression is usually self-limited, but counseling or antidepressants may be needed.
     - Advise the family to avoid being overprotective.
     - Assist the family and patient to develop realistic and achievable goals.

Evaluate Outcomes: Evaluation.

- Evaluate the care of the patient with stroke based on the identified priority patient problems. The expected outcomes are that the patient:
  1. Has adequate cerebral *perfusion* to avoid long-term disability
  2. Maintains blood pressure and blood glucose within a safe, prescribed range
  3. Performs self-care and *mobility* activities independently, with or without assistive devices
  4. Learns to adapt to *sensory perception* changes, if present
  5. Communicates effectively or develops strategies for effective communication as needed
  6. Has adequate nutrition and avoids aspiration

⮞ *See Chapter 38 in the main text for more information on stroke (brain attack).*

SYNDROME OF INAPPROPRIATE ANTIDIURETIC HORMONE

- Syndrome of inappropriate antidiuretic hormone (SIADH) occurs when ADH (also known as vasopressin) is secreted even when plasma osmolality is low or normal, resulting in water retention and fluid overload.
- Water is retained, which results in dilutional hyponatremia (a decreased serum sodium level) and expansion of the extracellular fluid volume.

Interprofessional Collaborative Care
Recognize Cues: Assessment

- Obtain patient information about:
  1. Medical history. Assess for conditions that are associated with SIADH.
- Assess for fluid overload, electrolyte derangements, pulmonary edema, and heart failure.
  1. Increased pulse quality (bounding central and peripheral pulses)
  2. Increased neck vein distention
  3. Presence of crackles in lungs
  4. Increasing peripheral edema
  5. Altered serum sodium, potassium, calcium, phosphate, and magnesium levels
  6. Reduced and concentrated urine output
  7. Lethargy or decreased mental status
  8. Neuromuscular changes related to electrolyte imbalance, especially hyponatremia

Conditions Causing the Syndrome of Inappropriate Antidiuretic Hormone

Malignancies
- Small cell lung cancer
- Pancreatic, duodenal, and GU carcinomas
- Thymoma
- Hodgkin lymphoma
- Non-Hodgkin lymphoma

Pulmonary Disorders
- Viral and bacterial pneumonia
- Lung abscesses
- Active tuberculosis
- Pneumothorax
- Chronic lung diseases
- Mycoses
- Positive-pressure ventilation

CNS Disorders
- Trauma
- Infection
- Tumors (primary or metastatic)
- Strokes
- Porphyria
- Systemic lupus erythematosus

Drugs
- Exogenous ADH
- Chlorpropamide
- Vincristine
- Cyclophosphamide
- Carbamazepine
- Opioids
- Tricyclic antidepressants
- General anesthetics
- Fluoroquinolone antibiotics

ADH, Antidiuretic hormone; *CNS,* central nervous system; *GU,* genitourinary.

Take Actions: Interventions
- Fluid restriction; intake may be restricted to 500 to 1000 mL/24 hr.
- Assess therapy for fluid excretion and sodium replacement.
    1. Measure intake and output; anticipate a goal that output is greater than intake.
    2. Weigh the patient daily.
    3. Monitor serum electrolytes and osmolality.
- Drug therapy may include:
    1. Administering ADH antagonists to promote water loss without urinary sodium excretion: tolvaptan (oral) or conivaptan (IV)

⬥ NURSING SAFETY PRIORITY
Drug Alert

Administer tolvaptan or conivaptan only in the hospital setting, so serum sodium levels can be monitored closely for the development of hypernatremia and other complications.

2. Using loop diuretics if heart failure results from fluid overload
3. Hypertonic saline (i.e., 3% sodium chloride [3% NaCl]) infusions

- Provide a safe environment when serum sodium is below 120 mEq/L.
  1. Initiate seizure precautions.
  2. Increase patient surveillance to prevent falls or harm during a period of disorientation.

See Chapter 54 in the main text for more information on syndrome of inappropriate diuretic hormone (SIADH).

SYPHILIS

- Syphilis is a complex sexually transmitted infection (STI) that can become systemic and can cause serious complications, including death.
- The causative organism is a spirochete called *Treponema pallidum.*
- The infection is usually transmitted by sexual contact and blood exposure, but transmission can occur through close bodily contact such as touching or kissing where there are open lesions (e.g., on the breast, genitals, or lips, or in the oral cavity (Hicks & Clement, 2022a).
- Untreated syphilis is divided into two categories—early and late— and progresses through four stages: primary (localized chancre), secondary (systemic illness), early latent (seropositive yet without symptoms), and tertiary (symptomatic infection).
  1. Neurosyphilis can occur at any time in any stage; patients with this form of the disease may experience meningitis, vision or hearing loss, and brain and spinal cord dysfunction.
- The appearance of an ulcer called a **chancre** is the first sign of *primary* syphilis.
  1. It develops at the site of entry (inoculation) of the organism from 12 days to 12 weeks days after exposure (3 weeks is average) (Rogers, 2023).
  2. During this highly infectious stage, the chancre begins as a small papule, approximately 1 to 2 centimeters in diameter with a raised margin (Hicks & Clement, 2022a).
  3. Within 3 to 7 days, it breaks down into its typical appearance: a painless, indurated, smooth, weeping lesion. Regional lymph nodes enlarge, feel firm, and are not painful.
  4. Without treatment, the chancre usually disappears within 3 to 6 weeks (Hicks & Clement, 2022a). However, the organism spreads throughout the body, and the patient is still infectious.

- *Secondary* syphilis develops in approximately 25% of untreated infected individuals within a few months (Hicks & Clement, 2022a). During this stage, syphilis is a systemic disease because the spirochetes circulate throughout the bloodstream, and it is commonly mistaken for influenza. Signs and symptoms include malaise, low-grade fever, headache, muscular aches, sore throat, hoarseness, generalized adenopathy, joint pain, and a generalized rash (Rogers, 2023).
- *Tertiary, or late,* syphilis is uncommon because of the widespread availability of antibiotics (Rogers, 2023).

PATIENT-CENTERED CARE: GENDER HEALTH

Risk for Syphilis

Men who have sex with men (MSM) are at high risk for contracting primary and secondary syphilis (Centers for Disease Control and Prevention, 2023). Do not assume that people have only had sexual experiences congruent with their noted sexual orientation, as this limits the accuracy of the nurse's risk assessment. Collect an appropriate sexual history for all patients, and design a plan of care based on that specific information.

Interprofessional Collaborative Care
Recognize Cues: Assessment
- Assess the following:
  1. Patient history specific to ulcers and rash
  2. Sexual history with risk assessment
- Conduct a physical examination, including inspection and palpation.
  1. Wear gloves while palpating any lesions because of the highly contagious treponemes that are present.
  2. Observe for and document rashes of any type because of the variable presentation of secondary syphilis.
- Diagnosis of primary or secondary syphilis is confirmed by a finding of *T. pallidum* on microscopic examination, by a positive Venereal Disease Research Laboratory (VDRL) serum test, or by a positive rapid plasma reagin (RPR) test result.
- Latent and tertiary syphilis may be confirmed by the fluorescent treponemal antibody absorption (FTA-ABS) test or the micro-hemagglutination assay for *T. pallidum* (MHA-TP) (Hicks & Clement, 2022b).

Take Actions: Interventions
- Antibiotic therapy with benzathine penicillin given intramuscularly (IM) is the treatment for all stages of syphilis. A prolonged

course of intravenous antibiotics for the late latent stage may be required.

- Provide education about safe sex practices.
- It is essential to teach patients to follow up at 6, 12, and 24 months after their initial treatment.
- Inform patients that the disease will be reported to the local health authority and that all information will be held in strict confidence.
- Encourage the patient to provide accurate information for this follow-up to ensure that all at-risk partners are treated appropriately.
- Provide a setting that offers privacy and encourages open discussion.

 See Chapter 65 in the main text for more information on syphilis.

SYSTEMIC LUPUS ERYTHEMATOSUS: IMMUNITY ✳ CONCEPT EXEMPLAR

Overview

- **Systemic lupus erythematosus (SLE)** is a chronic and progressive autoimmune disorder in which inflammatory and immune attacks occur against multiple self tissues and organs.
- Although chronic and progressive in nature, symptoms associated with SLE may be present constantly, at a reduced level *(remission)*, or as an acute episode of increased symptoms known as a "flare," or exacerbation.

Interprofessional Collaborative Care

- The onset of SLE is usually slow, and the symptoms may be so mild, general, and vague that diagnosis often is difficult and delayed. The average time from initial mild symptoms to actual diagnosis is 54 months (Kapsala et al., 2022). Progression of the disorder can be delayed when it is diagnosed and managed earlier in its course. Exacerbations (flares) accelerate organ damage.

Recognize Cues: Assessment

- Assess for and document:
  1. Past medical history
  2. Key features of SLE

KEY FEATURES

Systemic Lupus Erythematosus (SLE)

Musculoskeletal
- Arthralgias and arthritis
- Osteoporosis

Integumentary
- Alopecia
- Coin-shaped lesions (discoid rash) on the face, scalp, and sun-exposed areas, which leave scarring
- Mucocutaneous lesions
- Photosensitivity and rash development after sun exposure

Immune
- Chronic fatigue
- Generalized inflammation
- Increased number of infections
- Intermittent unexplained low-grade fever

Cardiovascular
- Pericarditis
- Raynaud phenomenon (hands that appear intermittently cyanotic, then reddened/hyperpigmented when exposed to cold)
- Vasculitis

Renal
- Glomerulonephritis

Gastrointestinal
- Esophagitis

Sensory
- Peripheral neuropathies
- Retinal vasculopathy

Hematologic
- Anemia
- Leukopenia

Data from Rogers, J. L. (2023). *McCance and Huether's Pathophysiology: The biologic basis for disease in adults and children* (9th ed.). St. Louis: Elsevier; Wallace, D., & Gladman, D. (2023). Clinical manifestations and diagnosis of systemic lupus erythematosus in adults. *UpToDate*. Retrieved May 3, 2023, from https://www.uptodate.com/contents/clinical-manifestations-and-diagnosis-of-systemic-lupus-erythematosus-in-adults.

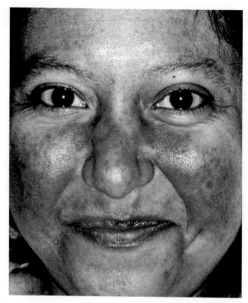

The characteristic "butterfly" rash of systemic lupus erythematosus.

- Diagnostic tests include the following:
  1. Classic laboratory assessment for diagnosis of SLE is based on the presence of circulating autoantibodies to components of cellular nuclei, as well as general indicators of *inflammation*, such as the erythrocyte sedimentation rate and serum complement levels for C3 and C4.
  2. No single laboratory test is used to definitively diagnose the disorder.

Analyze Cues and Prioritize Hypotheses: Analysis

- The priority collaborative problems for patients with systemic lupus erythematosus (SLE) are:
  1. Persistent *pain* due to chronic *inflammation*
  2. Fatigue due to chronic *inflammation*
  3. Potential for organ failure due to chronic inflammation and/or vasculitis

Generate Solutions and Take Actions: Planning and Implementation
Managing Persistent Pain

- Drug therapy may include:
  1. Corticosteroids such as prednisone

2. Acetaminophen and NSAIDs to help moderate daily joint and muscle pain
3. Some states recognize SLE as a qualifying (eligible) condition for their state's medical cannabis program.

Managing Fatigue

- Fatigue associated with SLE is chronic and often occurs at the point in life when adults are expected to be most active and productive in their career and family roles.
  1. Recommend ways of conserving energy.
  2. Plan rest times intermittently throughout the day.
  3. Prepare meals ahead of time that can easily be reheated.
  4. Give yourself permission to say "no" to activities that consume energy that you don't want to engage in.
  5. Avoid nicotine in any form.

Preventing Organ Failure

- Drug therapy for SLE often involves a combination of general and selective immunosuppressive agents.
  1. Corticosteroids such as prednisone remain a cornerstone of treatment for SLE.

NURSING SAFETY PRIORITY

Drug Alert

Teach patients taking long-term corticosteroids to never stop taking this type of drug abruptly because a life-threatening adrenal crisis can result. If the patient becomes ill and cannot tolerate the oral corticosteroid, teach the patient to immediately contact the rheumatology health care provider to discuss other treatment options.

2. *Antimalarial drugs,* such as hydroxychloroquine and chloroquine, are frequently used for the treatment of SLE. Many patients experience remission while taking this type of drug.
   - Teach patients who are given hydroxychloroquine or chloroquine to have frequent eye examinations with visual field testing (before starting the drug and every 6 months thereafter).
3. *Immunosuppressives* such as cyclophosphamide, azathioprine, mycophenolate mofetil, voclosporin, and methotrexate are sometimes used to keep the body from attacking itself.
4. *Nonsteroidal antiinflammatory drugs(NSAIDs),* such as ibuprofen, naproxen, indomethacin, nabumetone, and celecoxib, are used to treat pain and inflammation.

5. *Monoclonal antibodies* have been used successfully to help control many other autoimmune disorders. These drugs, usually given intravenously or subcutaneously, block specific proinflammatory cytokines that stimulate immune attacks on self tissues.

🔖 NURSING SAFETY PRIORITY

Drug Alert

All immunosuppressant drugs reduce protective *immunity* to some degree. Patients who are prescribed long-term therapy with glucocorticoids should be taught about the potential for new infections and how to avoid these.

- Teach the patient lifestyle changes, which include:
  1. Minimizing exposure to sunlight and other forms of ultraviolet light by:
     - Wearing long sleeves and wide-brimmed hats
     - Using sun-blocking agents with a sun protective factor of at least 30
  2. Cleaning the skin with a mild soap and avoiding harsh, perfumed products
  3. Using moisturizers and sun protectants

Care Coordination and Transition Management
- Teach the patient about:
  1. Informing the provider at the onset of symptoms that signal exacerbation
  2. Monitoring for infection, particularly the onset of fever
  3. Protecting joints and conserving energy
  4. Risks related to pregnancy and contraception options for those with lupus
  5. Resources such as the Lupus Foundation
  6. Drug therapy information for scheduling, side effects, and any precautions

Evaluate Outcomes: Evaluation
- Evaluate the care of the patient with SLE based on the identified priority patient problems. The expected outcomes of care are that the patient will:
  1. Adhere to the prescribed long-term SLE management plan to reduce incidence of complications associated with SLE
  2. Have pain managed at a level they deem acceptable
  3. Maintain energy to participate in activities important to them
  4. Experience longer periods of remission with low SLE activity

🔖 *See Chapter 17 in the main text for more information on systemic lupus erythematosus.*

THROMBOCYTOPENIA

- Thrombocytopenia is a reduction in platelets; platelets are essential in clotting.
- Some conditions associated with low platelets include hematopoietic disease (anemia, leukemia, and myelodysplastic syndromes), thrombotic thrombocytopenic purpura (an abnormality of platelet clumping associated with inadequate clumping during trauma or surgery), heparin-induced thrombocytopenia (an immune-mediated response that targets platelets after heparin exposure), and autoimmune thrombocytopenia purpura.
- Treatment is generally focused on the prevention of bleeding and on close monitoring and replacement of platelets or blood products during bleeding.

THROMBOCYTOPENIA PURPURA

- **Thrombocytopenic purpura** is the destructive reduction of circulating platelets after normal platelet production.
- Common types are:
  1. *Immune thrombocytopenia purpura (ITP),* formerly called idiopathic thrombocytopenic purpura
  2. Thrombotic thrombocytopenia purpura (TTP)
  3. Heparin-induced thrombocytopenia (HIT)
- Although symptoms are similar, the causes and management vary.

Interprofessional Collaborative Care
Recognize Cues: Assessment
- Assess for and document:
  1. Large bruises or petechial rash on the arms, legs, upper chest, and neck
  2. Mucosal bleeding
  3. Anemia
  4. Neurologic impairment as a result of an intracranial bleeding-induced stroke
  5. Laboratory findings: decreased platelet count, large numbers of megakaryocytes in the bone marrow, presence of antiplatelet antibodies in the blood, low hematocrit and low hemoglobin levels, and abnormalities in the structure of the spleen

Take Actions: Interventions

- The decreased platelet count increases the patient's risk for poor *clotting* and excessive bleeding. Interventions include protection from bleeding episodes and therapy for the different underlying conditions.

 See Chapter 34 in the main text for more information on thrombocytopenia purpura.

TOXIC SHOCK SYNDROME

- Toxic shock syndrome (TSS) can result from leaving a tampon, contraceptive sponge, or diaphragm in the vagina.
- Other conditions associated with TSS include surgical wound infection, minor trauma, and viral infection.
- Toxic shock syndrome can be fatal.
- In menstrual-related infection, menstrual blood provides a growth medium for the bacteria, which produces endotoxins that cross the vaginal mucosa to the bloodstream.

Interprofessional Collaborative Care
Recognize Cues: Assessment

- Assess for:
  1. Abrupt onset of a high fever
  2. Headache, myalgia, and flulike symptoms
  3. Hypotension
  4. Diffuse macular rash, which often looks like a sunburn

Take Actions: Interventions

- Management includes:
  1. Removal of the infection source
  2. Management of fluids and electrolyte imbalances, avoiding hypotension
  3. Intravenous (IV) antibiotics and other measures included in the management of sepsis and septic shock
- Patient education focuses on prevention by teaching all women about the proper use of tampons, internal contraceptive devices such as vaginal sponges and diaphragms, and prompt treatment of gynecologic infections.

PATIENT AND FAMILY EDUCATION

Prevention of Toxic Shock Syndrome

- Wash your hands before inserting a tampon.
- Do not use a tampon if it is dirty.
- Insert the tampon carefully to avoid injuring the delicate tissue in your vagina.
- Change your tampon every 3 to 6 hours.
- Use perineal pads ("sanitary napkins") (instead of tampons) at night.
- Avoid the use of insertable contraceptive devices.
- Call your primary health care provider if you experience a sudden onset of high temperature, vomiting, or diarrhea.
- Do not use tampons at all if you have had toxic shock syndrome.

 See Chapter 63 in the main text for more information on toxic shock syndrome.

TRACHEOSTOMY

- Tracheotomy is a surgical incision into the trachea to create an airway to help maintain *gas exchange*. Tracheostomy is the tracheal *stoma* (opening) in the neck that results from the tracheotomy. A tracheotomy can be an emergency procedure or a scheduled surgery.
- Indications for tracheostomy include:
  1. Acute airway obstruction
  2. Airway protection
  3. Laryngeal or facial trauma or burns
  4. Airway involvement during head or neck surgery
  5. Inability to wean from mechanical ventilation

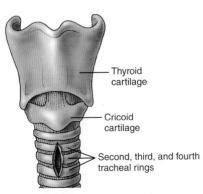

Thyroid cartilage

Cricoid cartilage

Second, third, and fourth tracheal rings

A vertical tracheal incision for a tracheostomy.

- Many types of tracheostomy tubes are available. Selection is based on patient needs.
  1. A tracheostomy tube may have a cuff and may have an inner cannula. A cuffed tube is used for patients receiving mechanical ventilation. The cuff is a small balloon surrounding the outside of the tracheostomy tube. When inflated to the proper size and pressure, the cuff comes into contact with the trachea and seals it off so that all air movement occurs within the tracheostomy tube, not around it.

Interprofessional Collaborative Care
Recognize Cues: Assessment

- The initial tracheotomy to form a tracheostomy is usually performed in an acute care setting. When the tracheostomy is permanent, care of the patient often occurs in the home or in long-term care and community settings.

Assessment of the Patient with a Tracheostomy

- Note the quality, pattern, and rate of breathing and compare with the patient's baseline. Tachypnea can indicate hypoxia, and dyspnea can indicate secretions in the airway.
- Assess for cyanosis, especially around the lips, which could indicate hypoxia.
- Check the patient's oxygen saturation with pulse oximetry.
- If oxygen is prescribed, ensure that the patient is receiving the correct amount, with the correct equipment and humidification.
- Assess the tracheostomy site for color, consistency, and amount of secretions in the tube or externally.
- If the tracheostomy is sutured in place, assess for redness/hyperpigmentation, swelling, or drainage from suture sites.
- If the tracheostomy is secured with ties, assess the condition and security of the ties. Change if they are moist or dirty.
- Assess the skin around the tracheostomy and neck for impaired *tissue integrity*, including behind the neck, from the ties, or from excess secretions.
- Assess behind the faceplate for the size of the space between the outer cannula and the patient's tissue and whether any secretions have collected in this area.
- If the tube is cuffed, check cuff pressure or collaborate with the respiratory therapist to confirm cuff pressure.
- Auscultate the lungs.
- Ensure that a second (emergency) tracheostomy tube and obturator are available.

Take Actions: Interventions
Providing Tracheostomy Care
- Tracheostomy care keeps the tube free of secretions, maintains a patent airway, and provides wound care. It is performed whether or not the patient can clear secretions.

❗ NURSING SAFETY PRIORITY
Action Alert

Prevent decannulation during tracheostomy care by keeping the old ties or holder on the tube while applying new ties or holder, or by keeping a hand on the tube until it is securely stable. (This is best performed with the assistance of a coworker. Some hospitals require a second licensed person during tracheostomy care for the first 72 hours posttracheostomy.)

⟫ BEST PRACTICE FOR PATIENT SAFETY AND QUALITY CARE
Tracheostomy Care

- Assemble the necessary equipment and maintain Standard Precautions.
- Suction the tracheostomy tube if necessary.
- Remove old dressings and excess secretions.
- Set up a sterile field.
- Remove and clean the inner cannula. Use half-strength hydrogen peroxide (if prescribed) to clean the cannula and sterile saline to rinse it. If the inner cannula is disposable, remove the cannula and replace it with a new one.
- Clean the stoma site and then the tracheostomy plate with half-strength hydrogen peroxide followed by sterile saline. Ensure that none of the solutions enters the tracheostomy.
- Change tracheostomy ties if they are soiled. Secure new ties in place before removing soiled ones to prevent accidental decannulation. If a knot is needed, tie a square knot that is visible on the side of the neck. Only one finger should be able to be placed between the tie tape and the neck.
- Document the type and amount of secretions and the general condition of the stoma and surrounding skin tissue integrity. Document the patient's response to the procedure.

- Mucosal ischemia occurs when the pressure exerted by the cuff on the mucosa exceeds the capillary perfusion pressure. To reduce tracheal damage, keep the cuff pressure less than 30 cm H_2O (22 mm Hg).
- The tracheostomy tube bypasses the nose and mouth, which normally humidify and warm the inspired air. If humidification and warming are inadequate, tracheal damage can occur.
  1. Humidify the air as ordered.
  2. Continually assess for a fine mist emerging from the tracheostomy collar or T-piece during ventilation.

! NURSING SAFETY PRIORITY

Action Alert

Keep the temperature of the air entering a tracheostomy between 98.6°F and 100.4°F (37°C and 38°C), and never exceed 104°F (40°C).

Maintaining Communication
- The patient can speak when there is a cuffless tube, when a fenestrated tracheostomy tube is in place, and when the fenestrated tube is capped or covered.
- Until natural speech is feasible, teach about other communication means, such as:
  1. A writing tablet
  2. A board with pictures and letters
  3. Communication "flash cards"
  4. Hand signals
  5. Smartphones
  6. Use of *yes* or *no* questions

Ensuring Nutrition
- Swallowing can be a major problem for the patient with a tracheostomy tube in place.
- In a normal swallow, the larynx lifts and moves forward to prevent food and saliva from entering. The tracheostomy tube sometimes tethers the larynx in place, making it unable to move effectively. The result is difficulty in swallowing.

Suctioning
- Suctioning maintains a patent airway and promotes *gas exchange* by removing secretions when the patient cannot cough adequately.

Provide Bronchial and Oral Hygiene
- Good oral hygiene keeps the airway patent, prevents *infection* from bacterial overgrowth, and promotes comfort.
- Avoid using glycerin swabs or mouthwash that contains alcohol for oral care because these products dry the mouth.
- Apply lip balm or water-soluble jelly to prevent cracked lips and promote comfort.

Care Coordination and Transition Management
- By the time of discharge, the patient should be able to provide self-care, including tracheostomy care, nutrition care, suctioning, and communication.

- Instruct the patient to use a shower shield over the tracheostomy tube when bathing to prevent water from entering the airway.
- Teach the patient to cover the opening loosely during the day with a small cotton cloth to protect the opening and filter the air entering the stoma.

⟩ BEST PRACTICE FOR PATIENT SAFETY AND QUALITY CARE

Preventing Aspiration While Swallowing

- Avoid serving meals when the patient is fatigued.
- Provide smaller and more frequent meals.
- Provide adequate time; do not "hurry" the patient.
- Closely supervise the self-feeding patient.
- Keep suctioning equipment close at hand and turned on.
- Avoid water and other "thin" liquids, as well as the use of straws.
- Thicken all liquids, including water.
- Thin liquids may be permitted after a swallowing evaluation by a speech/language pathologist.
- Avoid foods that generate thin liquids during the chewing process, such as fruit.
- Position the patient in the most upright position possible.
- When possible, completely (or at least partially) deflate the tube cuff during meals.
- Suction after cuff deflation to clear the airway and allow comfort during the meal.
- Feed each bite or encourage the patient to take each bite slowly.
- Encourage the patient to "dry swallow" after each bite ("double swallowing") to clear residue from the throat.
- Avoid consecutive swallows of liquids.
- Provide controlled small volumes of liquids, using a spoon.
- Tell the patient to "tuck" the chin down and move the forehead forward while swallowing.
- Allow patients to indicate when they are ready for the next bite.
- If coughing occurs, stop the feeding until the patient indicates that the airway is clear.
- Assess respiratory rate, ease of swallowing, pulse oximetry, and heart rate during feeding.

BEST PRACTICE FOR PATIENT SAFETY AND QUALITY CARE

Suctioning the Artificial Airway

- Assess the need for suctioning.
- Wash hands. Don protective eyewear. Maintain Standard Precautions.
- Explain to the patient that sensations such as shortness of breath and coughing are to be expected but that any discomfort will be very brief.
- Check the suction source. Occlude the suction source, and adjust the pressure dial to between 80 and 120 mm Hg to prevent hypoxemia and trauma to the mucosa.
- Set up a sterile field.
- Preoxygenate the patient with 100% oxygen for 30 seconds to 3 minutes (at least three hyperinflations) to prevent hypoxemia. Synchronize hyperinflations with inhalation.
- Quickly insert the suction catheter until resistance is met. *Do not apply suction during.*
- Routine instillation of normal saline is **not** supported. **Gas exchange** is impaired due to hypoxia, and there is an increased risk for **infection**.
- Withdraw the catheter 0.4 to 0.8 inch (1 to 2 cm), and begin to apply suction. Apply continuous suction and use a twirling motion of the catheter during withdrawal to avoid impairing tissue integrity. *Never suction longer than 10 to 15 seconds.*
- Hyperoxygenate for 1 to 5 minutes or until the patient's baseline heart rate and oxygen saturation are within normal limits.
- Repeat as needed for up to three total suction passes.
- Document secretion characteristics and patient responses.

PATIENT-CENTERED CARE: OLDER ADULT HEALTH

Self-Management of Tracheostomy and Oxygen Therapy

Older patients who have vision problems or difficulty with upper arm movement may have difficulty self-managing tracheostomy care and oxygen therapy. Teach them to use magnifying lenses or glasses to ensure the proper setting on the oxygen gauge. Assess their ability to reach and manipulate the tracheostomy. If possible, work with a family member who can provide assistance during tracheostomy care.

See Chapter 26 in the main text for more information on tracheostomy.

TRAUMATIC BRAIN INJURY: COGNITION CONCEPT ✳ EXEMPLAR

Overview

- A traumatic brain injury (TBI) is damage to the brain from an external mechanical force that leads to impaired *cognition, mobility, sensory perception,* or psychosocial function.
- Impairment can be temporary or permanent.
- The type of force and the mechanism of injury contribute to TBI.
  1. An *acceleration* injury is caused by an external force contacting the head, suddenly placing the head in motion.
  2. A *deceleration* injury occurs when the moving head is suddenly stopped or hits a stationary object.

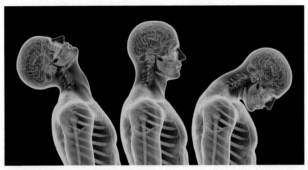

Acceleration-deceleration injury. (Used with permission from istockphoto, 2016, angelhell.)

- Primary brain damage occurs at the time of injury and results from the physical stress (force) within the tissue caused by blunt or penetrating force. A primary brain injury may be categorized as focal or diffuse.
- Secondary injury to the brain includes any processes that occur *after* the initial injury and worsen or negatively influence patient outcomes. Secondary injuries result from physiologic, vascular, and biochemical events that are an extension of the primary injury.
- Damage to brain tissue depends on the location, degree, and mechanism of injury.
  1. TBI can be classified as mild, moderate, or severe, depending on the initial Glasgow Coma Scale (GCS) score, which has implications for both treatment and prognosis.

2. It may be also described by the degree of apparent damage to the brain.
   - A *concussion* is a mild type of traumatic brain injury that temporarily changes how the brain functions as a result of mechanical force or trauma. It may or may not be associated with a brief loss of consciousness.
   - The most common secondary injury from mild TBI, such as a concussion, is **postconcussion syndrome**. In this syndrome, the patient reports that headaches, impaired *cognition*, and dizziness continue to occur for weeks to months after the initial brain injury.
- Increased intracranial pressure
   1. The cranial contents include brain tissue, blood, and cerebrospinal fluid (CSF). These components are encased in the relatively rigid skull. Within this space, there is little room for any of the components to expand or increase in volume. *A normal level of intracranial pressure (ICP) is 10 to 15 mm Hg.*
   2. A sustained ICP of greater than 20 mm Hg is considered detrimental to the brain because neurons begin to die.
   3. *Increased ICP is the leading cause of death from head trauma in patients who reach the hospital alive.* It occurs when compliance no longer takes place and the brain cannot accommodate further volume changes.
- The types of hemorrhage that occur after a TBI are epidural, subdural, and intracerebral.

✚ NURSING SAFETY PRIORITY

Critical Rescue

After the initial injury, symptoms of neurologic impairment from hemorrhage can progress very quickly, with potentially life-threatening ICP elevation and irreversible structural damage to brain tissue. Monitor the patient suspected of epidural bleeding frequently (every 5 to 10 minutes) for changes in neurologic status. The patient can become quickly and increasingly symptomatic. *A loss of consciousness from an epidural hematoma is a neurosurgical emergency!* Notify the primary health care provider or Rapid Response Team immediately if these changes occur. Carefully document your assessments, and identify any trends.

- In the presence of increased intracranial pressure (ICP), the brain tissue may shift (herniate), creating additional neuron damage.
   1. All herniation syndromes are potentially life-threatening, and the Rapid Response Team or primary health care provider must be notified immediately when they are suspected!

Interprofessional Collaborative Care
Recognize Cues: Assessment
- Obtain patient information about:
  1. When, where, and how the injury occurred
  2. The patient's level of consciousness (LOC) immediately after the injury and on admission to the hospital or unit and whether there have been any changes or fluctuations
  3. Presence of seizure activity at the scene of injury
  4. Medical and social history, especially presence of alcohol or drug use
  5. Hand dominance

✚ NURSING SAFETY PRIORITY
Critical Rescue

The upper cervical spinal nerves innervate the diaphragm to control breathing. Monitor all TBI patients for respiratory problems and diaphragmatic breathing, as well as for diminished or absent reflexes in the airway (cough and gag). Hypoxia and hypercapnia are best detected through arterial oxygen levels (partial pressure of arterial oxygen [Pao_2]), oxygen saturation (Spo_2), and end-tidal volume carbon dioxide measurement ($ETco_2$). Observe chest wall movement and listen to breath sounds. Provide respiratory support, including oxygen therapy and bed positioning. Report any sign of respiratory problems immediately to the Rapid Response Team or primary health care provider!

- Assess for:
  1. Airway patency and breathing pattern: RR, depth, and quality with Spo_2
  2. Signs and symptoms of hypovolemic shock or hemorrhage, which may indicate additional traumatic injuries such as abdominal bleeding or bleeding into soft tissue around major fractures
  3. HR and rhythm, BP, peripheral pulses, and core temperature
  4. Baseline and ongoing neurologic status with a standard assessment tool such as the GCS
     - *The most important variable to assess with any brain injury is LOC!* A decrease or change in LOC is typically the *first* sign of deterioration in neurologic status.
     - Decreased or garbled verbal response to auditory or tactile stimulus; new aphasia
     - Inability to follow commands; confusion
     - Pupils that are large, pinpoint, or ovoid, and nonreactive to light (indicates cranial nerve dysfunction, especially III, IV, and VII; may indicate brain stem dysfunction)

- Decreased or absent motor strength in the extremities; hemiparesis or hemiplegia
- Reports of severe headache, nausea, or vomiting
- Seizure activity
- Drainage of CSF from the ear or nose ("halo sign")

✚ **NURSING SAFETY PRIORITY**

Critical Rescue

Check pupils of TBI patients for size and reaction to light, particularly if the patient is unable to follow directions, to assess changes in level of consciousness. *Document any changes in pupil size, shape, and reactivity, and notify the Rapid Response Team or primary health care provider immediately because these changes could indicate an increase in ICP!*

---

5. Indications of posttraumatic sequelae in the patient who experienced a traumatic brain injury (symptoms may persist for weeks or months)
   - Persistent headache
   - Weakness
   - Dizziness
   - Loss of memory
   - Personality and behavioral changes
   - Problems with perception, reasoning abilities, and concept formation
6. Changes in personality, behavior, and abilities, such as:
   - Increased incidence of temper outbursts, risk-taking behavior, depression, and denial of disability
   - Becoming more talkative and developing a very outgoing personality
   - Decreased ability to learn new information, to concentrate, and to plan
   - Impaired memory, especially recent or short-term memory; this should not be confused with problems of aphasia
- Diagnostic studies may include:
  1. The primary health care provider immediately requests a CT of the brain to identify the extent and scope of injury. This diagnostic test can identify the presence of an injury that requires surgical intervention, such as an epidural or subdural hematoma.
  2. An *MRI* may be done to detect subtle changes in brain tissue and show more specific detail of the brain injury.

Analyze Cues and Prioritize Hypotheses: Analysis

- The priority collaborative problems for patients with TBI vary greatly, depending on the severity of the event. The most common problems include:
  1. Potential for decreased cerebral tissue *perfusion* due to primary event and/or secondary brain injury
  2. Potential for decreased *cognition, sensory perception*, and/or *mobility* due to primary or secondary brain injury
  3. Traumatic stress due to primary event and/or secondary injury

Generate Solutions and Take Actions: Planning and Implementation

Maintaining Cerebral Tissue Perfusion

- Assess vital signs with a standard neurologic assessment every 1 to 2 hours to detect early signs of decreased levels of consciousness, poor perfusion, hypovolemia, and dangerous elevations of BP that may cause further brain damage. Cardiac monitoring to detect cardiac dysrhythmias may be implemented. Report derangements immediately.
- Position the patient to avoid extreme flexion or extension of the neck, which interferes with CSF outflow. Maintain the head in a midline, central position; logroll the patient and elevate the back rest 30 degrees unless contraindicated; use reverse Trendelenburg's position if spinal cord injury is still being evaluated.
- Maintain the Pao$_2$ at 80 to 100 mm Hg to prevent secondary brain injury.
- Administer drug therapy.
  1. Administer hypertonic saline or osmotic diuretics (mannitol) to reduce cerebral edema.
     - Use a filter to eliminate microscopic crystals when removing mannitol from its vial.
  2. Opioids such as fentanyl may be used if the patient is mechanically ventilated to decrease *pain* and control restlessness and agitation that causes increased ICP.
  3. Propofol and midazolam (GABA-receptor agonists) provide sedation to decrease ICP, but are not as effective for pain control.

Maintaining or Managing Cognition, Sensory Perception, and Mobility

- *Cognitive rehabilitation* is a way of helping brain-injured patients regain function in areas that are essential for a return to independence and a reasonable quality of life, but these services are not widely available.
- Always introduce yourself before any interaction.
- Keep explanations of procedures and activities short and simple, and give them immediately before and throughout patient care.

- To the extent possible, maintain a sleep-wake cycle with scheduled rest periods.
- Orient the patient to time (day, month, and year) and place, and explain the reason for the hospitalization.
- Sensory stimulation is done to facilitate a meaningful response to the environment. Present visual, auditory, or tactile stimuli one at a time, and explain the purpose and the type of stimulus presented.

PATIENT AND FAMILY EDUCATION
Mild Traumatic Brain Injury

- For a headache, give acetaminophen every 4 hours as needed.
- Avoid giving the patient sedatives, sleeping pills, or alcoholic beverages for at least 24 hours after TBI unless the primary health care provider instructs otherwise.
- Do not allow the patient to engage in strenuous activity for at least 48 hours.
- Teach caregivers to be aware that balance disturbances in the patient cause safety concerns and that they should provide for monitored or assisted movement.
- If any of these symptoms occur, take the patient back to the emergency department or call 911 *immediately*:
  - Seizure
  - Severe or worsening headache
  - Persistent or severe nausea or vomiting
  - Blurred vision
  - Clear drainage from the ear or nose
  - Increasing weakness
  - Slurred speech
  - Progressive sleepiness
  - Unequal pupil size
- Keep follow-up appointments with the primary health care provider.

Managing Traumatic Stress
- Trauma-informed care is an approach to health care involving understanding, acceptance, and support for victims of trauma through positive adaptation and healing.
- Effective nursing care requires an understanding of the patient's lived trauma experience.

Care Coordination and Transition Management
- The patient with a *mild* brain injury recovers at home after discharge from the emergency department (ED) or hospital.

- Most patients with *moderate to severe TBI* are discharged with varied long-term physical and cognitive disabilities. Changes in personality and behavior are very common. The family must learn to cope with the patient's increased fatigue, irritability, temper outbursts, depression, loneliness, and memory problems. Patients often require constant supervision at home, and families may feel socially isolated.
  1. Respite care may be needed to help family members cope with feelings of isolation, increased responsibility, financial or emotional stress, or role reversal; refer them to support groups.
  2. The patient may experience a sense of isolation and loneliness because personality and behavioral changes make it difficult to resume or maintain preinjury social contacts; provide referrals to counseling and community resources, such as the local chapter of the Brain Injury Association of America or the Brain Injury Association of Canada.
- The patient with a *severe* brain injury requires long-term case management and ongoing rehabilitation after hospitalization. Behavioral interventions are used by cognitive and brain injury rehabilitation specialists to help both the patient and family members develop adaptive strategies.

Evaluation Outcomes: Evaluation
- Evaluate the care of the patient with TBI based on the identified priority problems. Expected outcomes are that the patient:
  1. Maintains cerebral tissue *perfusion*
  2. Learns to adapt to altered *mobility* and *sensory perception* changes, if any
  3. Has minimal alterations in *cognition* or understands how to compensate for *cognition* changes when necessary

See Chapter 38 in the main text for more information on traumatic brain injury.

TRAUMA, ESOPHAGEAL

- Trauma to the esophagus can result from blunt injuries, chemical burns, surgery or endoscopy (rare), or the stress of continuous severe vomiting.
- Trauma may affect the esophagus directly, impairing swallowing and nutrition, or create problems and complications in the lungs or mediastinum.

Common Causes of Esophageal Perforation

- Straining
- Seizures
- Trauma
- Foreign objects
- Instruments or tubes
- Chemical injury
- Complications of esophageal surgery
- Ulcers

Interprofessional Collaborative Care

Recognize Cues: Assessment

- Assess for and document:
  1. Airway patency, breathing
  2. Chest pain
  3. Dysphagia
  4. Vomiting, hematemesis
  5. Results of x-ray examination, CT, and endoscopy

Take Actions: Interventions

- Treatment includes:
  1. Maintaining NPO status to prevent further leakage of esophageal secretions
  2. Maintaining NG or gastrostomy tube drainage to heal ("rest") the esophagus
  3. Administering total parenteral nutrition (TPN) during esophageal rest
  4. Administering broad-spectrum antibiotics, corticosteroids, and analgesics
- Surgery may be needed to remove the damaged tissue. A resection or replacement of the damaged esophageal segment with small bowel tissue may be required.

See Chapter 46 in the main text for more information on trauma, esophageal.

TRAUMA, FACIAL

- Facial trauma is described by the specific bones (e.g., mandibular, maxillary, orbital, or nasal fractures) and the side of the face involved.
  1. Mandibular (lower jaw) fractures can occur at any point on the mandible and are the most common facial fractures.
  2. The rich blood supply of the face leads to extensive bleeding and bruising with facial trauma.

Interprofessional Collaborative Care
Recognize Cues: Assessment
- The priority action when caring for a patient with facial trauma is airway assessment for *gas exchange*.
- Assess for:
    1. Signs and symptoms of airway obstruction, including:
        - Stridor
        - Shortness of breath
        - Anxiety and restlessness or decreased consciousness
        - Hypoxia and decreased oxygen saturation
        - Hypercarbia
    2. Soft tissue edema
    3. Facial asymmetry
    4. Pain
    5. Leakage of spinal fluid through the ears or nose
    6. Vision and eye movement
    7. Bruising behind the ears in the mastoid area ("battle sign")

Take Actions: Interventions
- The priority action is to establish and maintain a patent airway.
    1. Provide suction at the bedside.
    2. Anticipate the need for emergency intubation, tracheotomy, or cricothyroidotomy.
- Other interventions include:
    1. Controlling hemorrhage
    2. Assessing for the extent of injury
    3. Establishing IV access and initiating fluid resuscitation
    4. Assisting in the stabilization of fractures
    5. Administering prescribed antibiotics
    6. For mandibular fixation with plates, teaching the patient about:
        - Oral care with an irrigating device
        - Soft diet or dental liquid diet restrictions
        - How to cut the wires if emesis occurs

T

✚ NURSING SAFETY PRIORITY
Critical Rescue

Instruct patients with mandibular fixation to keep wire cutters with them at all times to prevent aspiration if vomiting occurs.

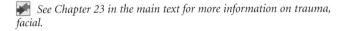 *See Chapter 23 in the main text for more information on trauma, facial.*

TRAUMA, KIDNEY

- Trauma to one or both kidneys may occur with penetrating wounds or blunt injuries to the back, flank, or abdomen or with urologic procedures.
- Traumatic kidney injury is classified into five grades, based on the severity of the injury. Grade 1 consists of low-grade injury in the form of kidney bruising, and grade 5 represents the most severe variety, associated with shattering of the kidney and tearing of its blood supply.

Interprofessional Collaborative Care
Recognize Cues: Assessment

- Obtain patient information about:
  1. The mechanism of injury, including the events surrounding the trauma
  2. History of kidney or urologic disease, including previous surgical intervention
  3. History of diabetes or hypertension
- Assess for and document the following:
  1. Take the patient's blood pressure, apical and peripheral pulses, respiratory rate, and temperature.
  2. Inspect both flanks for bruising, asymmetry, or penetrating injuries. Also inspect the abdomen, chest, and lower back for bruising or wounds.
  3. Percuss the abdomen for distention.
  4. Inspect the urethra for blood.
  5. Urine output hourly and abnormal urine, especially blood in the urine
  6. Decreased serum hemoglobin and hematocrit values

Take Actions: Interventions

- Treatment may include fluids and drugs to support perfusion:
  1. Fluid therapy is used to restore circulating blood volume and ensure adequate kidney blood flow. During fluid restoration, give fluids at the prescribed rate, and monitor the patient for signs of shock.
  2. Drug therapy is used for bleeding prevention or control.
- Interventional radiology techniques may be used to drain fluid around the urinary tract or to stent or embolize a renal artery.
- Surgical interventions such as nephrectomy or vascular repair may be required.

See Chapter 59 in the main text for more information on trauma, kidney.

TRAUMA, LARYNGEAL

- Laryngeal trauma occurs with a crushing or direct blow, fracture, or by prolonged endotracheal intubation.
- Symptoms include dyspnea, aphonia, hoarseness, subcutaneous emphysema, and hemoptysis.
- Management consists of assessing the effectiveness of gas exchange.
  1. The primary health care provider performs a direct visual examination of the larynx by laryngoscopy or fiberoptic laryngoscopy to determine the extent of the injury.
  2. Maintaining a patent airway is a priority.

✚ NURSING SAFETY PRIORITY
Critical Rescue

Assess the patient for signs of respiratory difficulty (tachypnea, nasal flaring, anxiety, sternal retraction, shortness of breath, restlessness, decreased oxygen saturation, decreased level of consciousness, stridor). If any signs are present, respond by staying with the patient and instructing other trauma team members or the Rapid Response Team to prepare for an emergency intubation or tracheotomy.

- Surgical intervention is necessary for lacerations of the mucous membranes, cartilage exposure, or paralysis of the cords.
- An artificial airway may be needed.

See Chapter 23 in the main text for more information on trauma, laryngeal.

TUBERCULOSIS, PULMONARY

- **Tuberculosis (TB)** is a highly communicable disease caused by *infection* with *Mycobacterium tuberculosis.*
- The organism is transmitted by aerosolization (airborne route) from an infected person during coughing, laughing, sneezing, whistling, or singing.
- When the bacillus is inhaled into a susceptible site in the bronchi or alveoli, it multiplies freely, causing an exudative pneumonitis.
- Cell-mediated immunity develops 2 to 10 weeks after infection and is manifested by a positive reaction to a tuberculin skin test.

- Secondary TB is a reactivation of the disease in a previously infected person; this can happen when *immunity* is reduced.

Interprofessional Collaborative Care
Recognize Cues: Assessment
- Obtain patient information about:
  1. Persistent cough
  2. Unintended weight loss
  3. Anorexia
  4. Night sweats
  5. Fever or chills
  6. Dyspnea or hemoptysis
  7. Past exposure to TB
  8. Country of origin and travel to foreign countries
  9. History of bacillus Calmette-Guérin (BCG) vaccination
- Assess for and document:
  1. Lung sounds: dullness with percussion over involved lung fields, bronchial breath sounds, crackles, wheezes
  2. Fatigue, lethargy, anorexia, weight loss
  3. Fever, night sweats
  4. Cough, with or without purulent sputum that may be streaked with blood
- There are two types of tests available for infection with tuberculosis—skin testing and blood testing.
- Blood analysis with the QuantiFERON-TB Gold (QFT-G) or T-SPOT TB test show how the patient's immune system responds to the TB bacterium.
- A purified protein derivative (PPD; Mantoux) two-step test is a common, reliable screening test.

Take Actions: Interventions
Decreasing Drug Resistance and Infection Spread
- Administer combination antimicrobial therapy that occurs in an initial phase (8 weeks) and in a continuation phase (18 weeks); drug therapy can last as long as 2 years when a multidrug-resistant infecting TB organism is present.
- Teach that strict adherence to the prescribed antimicrobial regimen is crucial for suppressing TB, and develop adherence strategies with the patient.
- Patients with multidrug-resistant TB infection or those who are unable to adhere to the therapy independently can be prescribed directly observed therapy.

⬭ NURSING SAFETY PRIORITY

Drug Alert

> The first-line drugs used as therapy for tuberculosis all can damage the liver. Warn the patient not to drink any alcoholic beverages for the entire duration of TB therapy.

- Place the hospitalized patient with active TB in airborne (infection control) precautions. The room should be well ventilated with at least six exchanges of fresh air per minute. All health care workers must use a personal respirator when caring for the patient.
- The community-dwelling person will need to stay home, avoid crowds, and ensure that others are not exposed to droplets of sputum (e.g., cover mouth, dispose of tissues in dedicated container).
- Encourage household members or other close contacts to undergo TB testing.
- When three consecutive sputum cultures are negative for TB, the individual is no longer considered infectious and can return to former activities.

 See Chapter 25 in the main text for more information on tuberculosis.

TUMORS, BRAIN

- Brain tumors can arise anywhere within the brain structures and are named according to the cell or tissue where they are located.
- *Primary tumors* originate within the CNS.
- *Secondary tumors (metastatic tumors)* spread to the brain from cancers in other body areas, such as the lungs, breast, kidney, and GI tract.
- Regardless of location, tumors can expand and invade, infiltrate, compress, and displace normal brain tissue. Similar to the pathophysiologic changes that occur in patients with TBI, these changes can lead to cerebral edema or brain tissue inflammation, increased intracranial pressure (ICP), and neurologic deficits (focal or diffuse). In some cases, pituitary dysfunction can result.
- *Supratentorial tumors* are located within the cerebral hemispheres, and *infratentorial tumors* are located in the brain stem structures and cerebellum.

Interprofessional Collaborative Care

Recognize Cues: Assessment

- Obtain patient information about general symptoms of a brain tumor, including:
  1. Headaches that are usually more severe on awakening in the morning
  2. Nausea and vomiting
  3. Vision changes (blurred or double vision)
  4. Seizures
  5. Changes in mentation or personality
  6. Specific neurologic deficits
- Supratentorial (cerebral) tumors usually result in paralysis, seizures, memory loss, cognitive impairment, language impairment, or vision problems.
- Infratentorial tumors produce ataxia, autonomic nervous system dysfunction, vomiting, drooling, hearing loss, and vision impairment.
- Diagnosis is based on the patient's history, neurologic assessment, clinical examination, and results of neurodiagnostic testing.

Take Actions: Interventions

- Management depends on tumor size and location, patient symptoms and general condition, and whether the tumor is primary or has recurred.

Nonsurgical Management

- Drug therapy to treat the malignant or metastatic tumor may include the following:
  1. Chemotherapy may be given alone, in combination with radiation therapy and surgery, and with tumor progression. More than one agent may be given orally, IV, intra-arterially, or intrathecally through an Ommaya reservoir placed in a cranial ventricle.
  2. Direct drug delivery to the tumor using a disk-shaped drug wafer (carmustine) can be placed directly into the cavity created during surgical tumor removal (interstitial chemotherapy).
  3. Analgesics, such as codeine and acetaminophen, are given for headaches.
  4. Dexamethasone may be prescribed for the control of cerebral edema.
  5. Levetiracetam or other antiepileptic drugs (AEDs) may be prescribed to prevent seizure activity.
- General management issues for the care of patients undergoing chemotherapy are presented under *Cancer.*
- Stereotactic radiosurgery (SRS) is an alternative to traditional surgery. Techniques used may include:
  1. Modified linear accelerator using accelerated x-rays (LINAC)
  2. Particle accelerator using beams of protons (cyclotron)

3. Isotope seeds implanted in the tumor (brachytherapy)
4. Gamma knife, using a single high dose of ionized radiation to focus multiple beams of gamma radiation produced by the radioisotope cobalt 60
5. CyberKnife
6. Treating Fields (TTFields) is a new technological modality that delivers regional low-intensity, intermediate frequency–specific, alternating electrical fields to a solid tumor.

Surgical Management

- A **craniotomy** (surgical incision into the cranium to access the brain) may be performed to remove the tumor, improve symptoms related to the lesion, or decrease the tumor size (debulk).
- Small tumors that are easily located may be removed by *minimally invasive surgery (MIS)*.
- Stereotactic surgery using a rigid head frame can be done for tumors that are easily reached. This procedure requires only burr holes and local anesthesia because the brain has no sensory neurons for pain.
- In traditional open craniotomy, the patient's head is placed in a skull fixation device, and a piece of bone (bone flap) is removed to expose the tumor area. The tumor is removed, the bone flap is replaced, and a drain or monitoring device may be inserted.
- Provide preoperative care, including:
  1. Allowing the patient to express anxiety and concerns about:
     - Surgery into the brain
     - Possibility of neurologic deficits
     - Changes in appearance and self-image
  2. Teaching the patient and family about what to expect immediately after surgery and throughout the recovery period
- Provide postoperative care. The focus of postoperative care is to monitor the patient to detect changes in status and prevent or minimize complications, especially increased intracranial pressure (ICP).
  1. Assess neurologic (LOC) and vital signs every 15 to 30 minutes for the first 4 to 6 hours after surgery and then every hour.
  2. Ensure appropriate positioning.
     - After supratentorial surgery:
       - Elevate the head of the bed 30 degrees.
       - Avoid extreme hip or neck flexion.
       - Maintain the head in a midline, neutral position.
       - Place the patient on the nonoperative side.
     - After infratentorial (brain stem) craniotomy:
       - Keep the patient flat or at 10 degrees (according to primary health care provider prescription).
       - Position the patient on either side for 24 to 48 hours.
  3. Maintain NPO status until the patient is awake and alert.

T

4. Monitor the head dressing every 1 to 2 hours for:
   - Amount, type, and color of drainage
   - Suction of drains maintained as prescribed

! NURSING SAFETY PRIORITY

Action Alert

Assess neurologic and vital signs every 15 to 30 minutes for the first 4 to 6 hours after a craniotomy and then every hour. If the patient is stable for 24 hours, the frequency of these checks may be decreased to every 2 to 4 hours, depending on agency policy and the patient's condition. *Report immediately and document new neurologic deficits, particularly a decreased level of consciousness (LOC), motor weakness or paralysis, aphasia, decreased sensory perception, and sluggish pupil reaction to light!* Personality changes such as agitation, aggression, or passivity can also indicate worsening neurologic status.

+ NURSING SAFETY PRIORITY

Critical Rescue

After craniotomy, monitor the patient's dressing for excessive amounts of drainage. Report a saturated head dressing or drainage greater than 50 mL/8 hr immediately to the surgeon! *Monitor frequently for signs of increasing ICP!*

Postoperative Complications of Craniotomy

Early Postoperative Complications	Late Postoperative Complications
• Increased intracranial pressure (ICP)	• Wound infection
• Hematomas	• Meningitis
• Subdural hematoma	• Fluid and electrolyte
• Epidural hematoma	imbalances
• Subarachnoid hemorrhage	• Dehydration
• Hypovolemic shock	• Hyponatremia
• Hydrocephalus	• Hypernatremia
• Respiratory complications	• Seizures
• Atelectasis	• Cerebrospinal fluid
• Hypoxia	(CSF) leak
• Pneumonia	• Cerebral edema
• Neurogenic pulmonary edema	

5. Monitor for postoperative complications.
6. Monitor for signs of increased ICP, including:
   - Severe headache
   - Deteriorating LOC
   - Restlessness and irritability
   - Dilated or pinpoint pupils that are slow to react or nonreactive to light

Care Coordination and Transition Management

- Assist the family to make the environment safe for the prevention of falls (e.g., remove scatter rugs, install grab bars in the bathroom).
- When needed, work with the case manager or discharge planner to help the family select a facility with experience in providing care for neurologically impaired patients.
- Teach patients and families about:
  1. Seizure precautions and what to do if a seizure occurs
  2. Drug therapy and where to call if adverse drug events occur
  3. The importance of recommended follow-up health care appointments
- Refer the patient and family to support groups and community resources, such as the American Brain Tumor Association, the National Brain Tumor Society, the American Cancer Society, home care agencies, and hospice services or palliative care services (for those who are terminally ill).

See Chapter 38 in the main text for more information on tumor, brain.

✳ ULCERS, PEPTIC: INFECTION CONCEPT EXEMPLAR

Overview
- Peptic ulcer disease (PUD) results when GI mucosal defenses become impaired and no longer protect the epithelium from the effects of acid and pepsin.
- Types of peptic ulcers include:
  1. *Gastric ulcer,* which occurs when there is a break in the mucosal barrier and hydrochloric acid injures the stomach, usually near the antrum; gastric emptying is often delayed with gastric ulceration, worsening the injury
  2. *Duodenal ulcer,* a chronic break in the duodenal mucosa that extends through the muscularis mucosa and most commonly occurs in the upper portion of the duodenum; it is characterized by high gastric acid secretion and is the most common type of peptic ulcer
  3. *Stress ulcer,* which occurs with acute and chronic diseases or major trauma; bleeding resulting from gastric erosion is the principal manifestation, and multiple lesions occur in the proximal portion of the stomach, beginning with the area of ischemia and evolving into erosions
- Many ulcers are caused by *Helicobacter pylori* **infection**. The most common route of *H. pylori* infection transmission is either oral-to-oral (stomach contents are transmitted from mouth to mouth) or fecal-to-oral (from stool to mouth) contact.
- Complications of PUD include:
  1. Gastrointestinal (GI) bleeding
  2. Perforation
  3. Pyloric obstruction
  4. Intractable disease

Interprofessional Collaborative Care
Recognize Cues: Assessment
- Obtain patient information about:
  1. Symptoms, including epigastric **pain**, abdominal tenderness, cramps, indigestion, nausea, or vomiting and their onset, duration, location, and frequency, as well as aggravating and alleviating factors, including meal and sleep patterns
  2. Tobacco, alcohol, caffeine, and intake of foods known to cause gastric irritation

3. Medical history focusing on GI problems, particularly *H. pylori* infection
4. Prescribed and over-the-counter (OTC) drugs, such as corticosteroids and NSAIDs
5. Recent severe, serious, complex, or traumatic illness
6. Presence of chronic disease and recent changes in flares or medications

- Assess for and document:
  1. Epigastric *pain* and tenderness; rigid, boardlike abdomen accompanied by rebound tenderness (if perforation occurred)
  2. Secretions (emesis, sputum, stool, urine, and nasogastric drainage) for frank or occult blood
  3. Color, amount, and character of stools; note the presence of melena or occult blood
  4. Vital signs, including orthostatic blood pressure indicating hypovolemia or bleeding

KEY FEATURES

Upper GI Bleeding

- Bright red or coffee-ground vomitus (**hematemesis**)
- **Melena** (tarry or dark sticky) stools
- Decreased hemoglobin and hematocrit
- Decreased blood pressure
- Increased heart rate
- Weak peripheral pulses
- Acute confusion (in older adults)
- Vertigo
- Dizziness or light-headedness
- Syncope (loss of consciousness)

U

- Diagnostic studies may include:
  1. Hemoglobin and hematocrit levels to determine occult or severity of GI bleeding
  2. Testing for *H. pylori*
  3. Esophagogastroduodenoscopy (EGD), which is the major diagnostic test for PUD; direct visualization of the ulcer crater by EGD allows the health care provider to take specimens for *H. pylori* testing and for biopsy and cytologic studies for ruling out gastric cancer

Analyze Cues and Prioritize Hypotheses: Analysis

- The priority collaborative problems for the patient with peptic ulcer disease include:
  1. Acute or persistent **pain** due to gastric and/or duodenal ulceration
  2. Potential for upper GI bleeding due to gastric and/or duodenal ulceration or perforation

Generate Solutions and Take Actions: Planning and Implementation

Managing Acute Pain or Persistent Pain

- PUD causes significant discomfort that impacts many aspects of daily living. Interventions to manage pain focus on drug therapy and dietary changes.
- Administer drugs to eliminate *H. pylori* infection; a common approach is triple therapy for 10 to 14 days:
  1. Proton pump inhibitor (PPI) such as lansoprazole
  2. Two antibiotics, such as metronidazole and tetracycline or clarithromycin and amoxicillin
- Other drugs to promote healing are:
  1. Bismuth subsalicylate, which inhibits *H. pylori* from binding to the mucosal lining and stimulates mucosal protection and prostaglandin production
  2. Histamine-2 (H_2) blockers, which stop histamine-stimulated gastric acid secretion
  3. Sucralfate, which binds to and protects the mucosa, preventing further digestive damage from acid and pepsin
  4. Antacids, which buffer gastric acid and slow the formation of pepsin
- Prevent recurrence with complementary and integrative health therapies that reduce stress, including hypnosis and imagery.
- The role of diet in the management of ulcer disease is controversial.
  1. There is no evidence that dietary restriction reduces gastric acid secretion or promotes tissue healing, although a bland diet may assist in relieving pain symptoms.
  2. Food itself acts as an antacid by neutralizing gastric acid for 30 to 60 minutes. An increased rate of gastric acid secretion, called *rebound,* may follow.

Managing Upper GI Bleeding

- For patients with persistent upper GI bleeding, embolization during endoscopy is done. An interventional radiologist may complete a catheter-directed embolization for small or persistent bleeding. For patients with a perforation, a surgical intervention may be needed to remove the ulcer site.

✚ NURSING SAFETY PRIORITY

Critical Rescue

Recognize that your priority for care of the patient with upper GI bleeding is to maintain **a**irway, **b**reathing, and **c**irculation (ABCs). Respond to these needs by providing oxygen and other ventilatory support as needed, starting two large-bore IV lines for replacing fluids and blood, and monitoring vital signs, hematocrit, and oxygen saturation (Pezzotti, 2020).

- The patient is at risk for fluid volume deficit (hypovolemia), anemia, and hemorrhagic shock.
  1. Management of hypovolemia and hemorrhage includes:
     - Monitoring vital signs with urine output to detect hypovolemia. Fluid replacement in older adults should be closely monitored to prevent fluid overload.
     - Recording intake and output, including output from bleeding or vomiting
     - Monitoring serum electrolytes, coagulation factors, hematocrit, and hemoglobin and reporting abnormal values to the provider in a timely manner
     - Replacing fluids with intravenous (IV) fluids such as normal saline or lactated Ringer's solution
     - Transfusing blood products safely in the presence of symptomatic anemia or hypoxemia from low hemoglobin
     - Inserting an NG tube to ascertain the presence of blood in the stomach, assess the rate of bleeding, prevent gastric dilation, and provide lavage or removal of blood in the stomach
     - Keeping the patient NPO during periods of active bleeding

! NURSING SAFETY PRIORITY

Action Alert

After esophagogastroduodenoscopy (EGD), monitor vital signs, heart rhythm, and oxygen saturation per agency protocol until they return to baseline. In addition, frequently assess the patient's ability to swallow saliva. The patient's gag reflex may initially be absent after an EGD because of anesthetizing (numbing) of the throat with a spray before the procedure. *After the procedure, do not allow the patient to have food or liquids until the gag reflex has returned!*

Care Coordination and Transition Management

- Instruct the patient about symptoms that should be brought to the attention of the health care provider, such as persistent abdominal **pain**, bloody stools, and signs of hypovolemia.
- Instruct the patient to avoid NSAIDs unless under the care of a health care provider, who may prescribe concurrent acid-reducing medication.
- Help the patient plan ways to make needed lifestyle changes.

! NURSING SAFETY PRIORITY

Action Alert

Teach the patient who has peptic ulcer disease to seek immediate medical attention if experiencing any of these symptoms:
1. Sharp, sudden, persistent, and severe epigastric or abdominal pain
2. Bloody or black stools
3. Bloody vomit or vomit that looks like coffee grounds

Evaluate Outcomes: Evaluation

- Evaluate the care of the patient with peptic ulcer disease (PUD) based on the identified priority patient problems. The expected outcomes are that the patient:
  1. Does not have active PUD or *H. pylori* **infection**
  2. Verbalizes relief or control of **pain**
  3. Adheres to the drug regimen and lifestyle changes to prevent recurrence and heal the ulcer
  4. Does not experience an upper GI bleed; if bleeding occurs, it will be promptly and effectively managed

See Chapter 47 in the main text for more information on ulcers, peptic.

❋ UNDERNUTRITION: NUTRITION CONCEPT EXEMPLAR

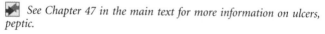

Overview

- Undernutrition is a multinutrient problem.
- **Protein-energy undernutrition (PEU),** formerly known as protein-calorie malnutrition (PCM), has two common forms:
  1. **Marasmus:** a malnutrition of calories, in which body fat and protein are wasted. Serum proteins are often preserved.
  2. **Kwashiorkor:** a lack of protein quantity and quality in the presence of adequate calories. Body weight is more normal, and serum proteins are low.
- Starvation, a complete lack of nutrients, is an acute and severe form of PEU, which usually occurs when food is unavailable.

Interprofessional Collaborative Care
Recognize Cues: Assessment
- Obtain information about the patient's:
  1. Usual daily food intake, and timing of eating
  2. Food preferences (including cultural considerations)
  3. Eating behaviors/patterns
  4. Change in appetite
  5. Recent weight changes
  6. Economic status that may influence access to, or purchase of, food
- Collaborate with the registered dietitian nutritionist to assess:
  1. Usual daily food intake
  2. Eating behaviors
  3. Change in appetite
  4. Recent weight changes

! NURSING SAFETY PRIORITY
Action Alert

Assess for difficulty or pain in chewing or swallowing. Unrecognized dysphagia is a common problem among older adults, and can cause undernutrition, dehydration, and aspiration pneumonia.

- Interpret laboratory data carefully with regard to the total patient. Laboratory data can supply objective data that can support subjective data and identify deficiencies.

Analyze Cues and Prioritize Hypotheses: Analysis
- The priority collaborative problem for the patient with undernutrition is:
  1. Weight loss due to inability to access, ingest or digest food, or absorb nutrients

Generate Solutions and Take Actions: Planning and Implementation
Improving Nutrition
- Collaborate with the registered dietitian nutritionist to set caloric and protein intake goals.
- Adapt meal choices and times to reflect the patient's preferences.
- Provide nutritional supplements.
- Administer vitamins and minerals as prescribed to avoid nutrient deficits.
- Maintain a daily calorie count, and weigh the patient daily. Evaluate whether nutrients consumed are sufficient to meet basal and stress-related energy needs.

- Evaluate nutritional indices at least weekly: skin intactness, weight, serum albumin, electrolytes, renal function, hemoglobin and hematocrit, and white blood cell (WBC) count.

Promoting Nutritional Intake

Environment
- Remove bedpans, urinals, and emesis basins from the environment.
- Eliminate or decrease offensive odors as much as possible.
- Decrease environmental distractions as much as possible.
- Administer pain medication and/or antiemetics for nausea at least 1 hour before mealtime.

Comfort
- Allow the patient to toilet before mealtime.
- Provide mouth care before mealtime.
- Ensure that eyeglasses and hearing aids are in place, if appropriate, during meals.
- Remind assistive personnel (AP) to have the patient sit in a chair, if possible, at mealtime.

Function
- Ensure that meals are visually appealing, appetizing, and at appropriate temperatures.
- If needed, open cartons and packages and cut up food.
- Observe during meals for food intake, and document the percentage consumed.
- Encourage self-feeding (if able) or feed the patient slowly (delegate to UAP, if desired).
- Eliminate or minimize interruptions during mealtime for nonurgent procedures or rounds.

- Ensure best practices with enteral feeding
    1. Total enteral nutrition (TEN) or tube feedings can be administered through one of the available gastrointestinal (GI) tubes.
        - A nasoenteric tube (NET) is any feeding tube inserted nasally and advanced into the GI tract. These tubes are used for short-term enteral feedings (less than 4 weeks).
        - Enterostomal feeding tubes are used for long-term enteral feeding, directly accessing the GI tract using various surgical, endoscopic, and laparoscopic techniques.
        - Tube feedings are administered by bolus feeding, continuous feeding, and cyclic feeding.

2. Complications of TEN include:
- Obstructed tube
- Tube misplacement or dislodgment
- Abdominal distention
- Nausea or vomiting
- Diarrhea
- Refeeding syndrome

 BEST PRACTICE FOR PATIENT SAFETY AND QUALITY CARE

Tube-Feeding Care and Maintenance

- If nasogastric or nasoduodenal feeding is prescribed, use a soft, flexible, small-bore feeding tube (smaller than 12 Fr).
- Recognize that tubes with ports minimize contamination by eliminating the need to open the feeding system to administer drugs.
- *The initial placement of the tube should be confirmed by x-ray study* even if another method of confirmation is available, such as an electromagnetic tube-placement device (ETPD). Evidence shows that chest x-ray is still preferable to an ETPD.
- If correct tube placement is ever in question, chest x-ray should again be performed.
- Secure the tube with tape or a commercial attachment device after applying a skin protectant; change the tape regularly.
- If a gastrostomy or jejunostomy tube is used, assess the insertion site for signs of infection or excoriation (e.g., excessive redness/hyperpigmentation, drainage). Rotate the tube 360 degrees each day and check for in-and-out play of about ¼ inch (0.6 cm).
- Check and document residual volume every 6 hours or per agency policy by aspirating stomach contents into a syringe. If residual feeding is obtained, check with the health care provider for the appropriate intervention (usually to slow or stop the feeding for a time) or consult the American Society of Parenteral and Enteral Nutrition (ASPEN) (2023) best practice recommendations.
- Check the feeding pump to ensure proper mechanical operation.
- Ensure that the enteral product is infused at the prescribed rate (mL/hr).
- Change the feeding bag and tubing every 24 to 48 hours; label the bag with the date and time of the change with your initials. Use an irrigation set for no more than 24 hours.
- For continuous or cyclic feeding, add only 4 hours of product to the bag at a time to prevent bacterial growth. *A closed system is preferred, and each set should be used no longer than 24 hours.*
- Wear clean gloves when changing or opening the feeding system or adding product; wipe the lid of the formula can with clean gauze; wear sterile gloves for critically ill or immunocompromised patients.

Continued

BEST PRACTICE FOR PATIENT SAFETY AND QUALITY CARE—cont'd

Tube-Feeding Care and Maintenance

- Label open cans with date and time opened; cover and keep refrigerated. Discard any unused open cans after 24 hours.
- Do not use blue (or any color) food dye in formula because it can cause serious complications.
- To prevent aspiration, keep the head of the bed elevated at least 30 degrees during the feeding and for at least 1 hour after the feeding for bolus feeding; continuously maintain semi-Fowler's position for patients receiving cyclic or continuous feeding.
- Monitor laboratory values, especially blood urea nitrogen (BUN), serum electrolytes, hematocrit, prealbumin, and glucose.
- Monitor for complications of tube feeding, especially diarrhea.
- Monitor and document the patient's weight, and intake and output, per the health care provider's order or agency policy.

! NURSING SAFETY PRIORITY

Action Alert

If enteral tubes are misplaced or become dislodged, the patient is likely to aspirate. *Aspiration pneumonia is a life-threatening complication associated with TEN, especially for older adults.* Observe for fever and signs of dehydration, such as dry mucous membranes and decreased urinary output. Auscultate lungs every 4 to 8 hours to check for diminishing breath sounds, especially in lower lobes. Patients may become short of breath and report chest discomfort. If a chest x-ray confirms this diagnosis, treatment with antibiotics is started.

Parenteral Nutrition

- When a patient cannot effectively use the GI tract for *nutrition*, either partial or total parenteral nutrition therapy may be needed. This form of nutrition is introduced into the veins, and differs from standard IV therapy in that any or all nutrients (carbohydrates, proteins, fats, vitamins, minerals, electrolytes, and trace elements) can be given.
- *Peripheral parenteral nutrition* (PPN) is administered through a cannula or catheter in a large distal vein of the arm on a short-term basis. PPN is fat-based and does not contain all of the carbohydrates a patient needs, so it is not used on a long-term basis (Baiu & Spain, 2019).
- When the patient requires intensive *nutrition* support for an extended time, the health care provider prescribes centrally administered *total parenteral nutrition* (TPN). TPN is delivered through

a temporary central line inserted in the neck or chest, a long-term tunneled catheter or implanted part inserted in the chest, or via a PICC line (Baiu & Spain, 2019).

BEST PRACTICE FOR PATIENT SAFETY AND QUALITY CARE

Care and Maintenance of Total Parenteral Nutrition

- Check each bag of total parenteral nutrition (TPN) solution for accuracy by comparing it with the original prescription.
- Administer insulin as prescribed.
- Monitor the IV pump for accuracy in delivering the prescribed hourly rate.
- If the TPN solution is temporarily unavailable, collaborate with the health care provider so that 10% dextrose/water ($D_{10}W$) or 20% dextrose/water ($D_{20}W$) can be administered until the TPN solution can be obtained.
- If the TPN administration is not on time ("behind"), do not attempt to "catch up" by increasing the rate.
- Monitor and document the patient's weight daily or according to facility protocol.
- Monitor serum electrolytes and glucose daily or per facility protocol.
- Monitor for, report, and document complications, including problems with ***fluid and electrolyte balance.***
- Monitor and carefully record the patient's intake and output.
- Assess the patient's IV site for signs of infection or infiltration.
- Change the IV tubing every 24 hours or per facility protocol.
- Change the dressing around the IV site every 48 to 72 hours or per facility protocol.
- Before administering TPN, have a second nurse check the prescription and solution to prevent patient harm.

U

Care Coordination and Transition Management

- The patient with undernutrition, once stabilized, can be cared for in a variety of settings, including the acute care hospital, transitional care unit, nursing home, or the patient's own home.
- The patient with undernutrition will need resources at home to continue consistent nutritional support.
- It is important to educate the patient and family about the following:
  1. Reinforce the importance of adhering to the prescribed diet.
  2. Review any drugs the patient may be taking.
  3. If taking an iron preparation, teach the importance of taking the drug immediately before or during meals.
  4. Caution the patient that iron can cause constipation.

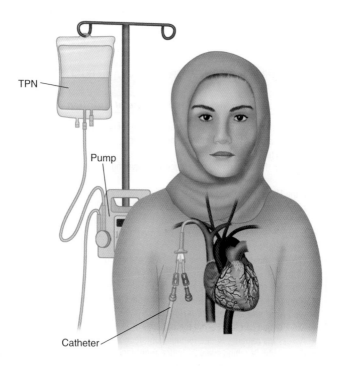

Total parenteral nutrition (TPN).

5. For the patient already susceptible to constipation, emphasize ways to prevent constipation, including adequate fiber intake, adequate fluids, and exercise.

Evaluate Outcomes: Evaluation

- Evaluate the care of the patient with undernutrition based on the identified priority patient problems. The primary expected outcomes are that the patient:
  1. Will consume available nutrients to meet the metabolic demands for maintaining weight and total protein
  2. Has adequate hydration

See Chapter 52 in the main text for more information on undernutrition.

URINARY INCONTINENCE: ELIMINATION CONCEPT ✳ EXEMPLAR

Overview

- Urinary incontinence (UI) is an involuntary loss of urine severe enough to cause social or hygienic problems. It is *not* a normal consequence of aging or childbirth, and often is a stigmatizing and underreported health problem.
- Common forms of UI are:
  1. *Stress incontinence,* the loss of small amounts of urine during coughing, sneezing, jogging, or lifting. Patients are unable to tighten the urethra sufficiently to overcome the increased detrusor pressure, and leakage of urine results.
  2. *Urge incontinence,* the involuntary loss of urine associated with a sudden, strong desire to urinate. Patients are unable to suppress the signal for bladder contractions. It is also known as *overactive bladder.*
  3. *Overflow incontinence,* when the bladder becomes overdistended. Urine leaks once the maximum capacity of the bladder is reached. It is also known as *reflex incontinence* or *underactive bladder* and can be caused by obstruction (e.g., kidney stone) or loss of detrusor muscle/reflex activity (e.g., a neurologic condition such as spinal cord injury).
  4. *Functional incontinence,* or leakage of urine caused by factors other than abnormal function of the bladder and urethra, such as cognitive dysfunction, impaired vision, or inability to reach a toilet

U

👤 PATIENT-CENTERED CARE: OLDER ADULT HEALTH

Urinary Incontinence

Many factors contribute to urinary incontinence in older adults. An older adult may have decreased mobility from many causes. In inpatient settings, mobility is limited when the older patient is placed on bed rest. Vision and hearing impairments may also prevent the patient from locating a call light to notify the nurse or unlicensed assistive personnel of the need to void. Assess for these factors and minimize them to prevent urinary incontinence. Getting out of bed to urinate is a common cause of falls among older adults in the home and other settings (Touhy & Jett, 2023).

👤 PATIENT-CENTERED CARE: HEALTH EQUITY

Urinary Incontinence

Evidence indicates that over 50% of females do not seek treatment for urinary incontinence (AHRQ, 2022). Understanding barriers to treatment for urinary incontinence is a key step in promoting health equity. The existing evidence indicates that barriers to care vary across racial groups, with Latina women experiencing more barriers. A few studies also indicate that access to pelvic floor physical therapy is inconsistent and that patients with Medicaid or no insurance were less likely to receive this treatment, which is proven to be beneficial in the treatment of urinary incontinence (Brown & Simon, 2021). It is important for the nurse to assess all patients for urinary health and for signs of incontinence. In addition, teaching patients that most urinary incontinence is very treatable may encourage those who are reluctant to discuss this condition to talk to the provider about treatment options.

Interprofessional Collaborative Care

Recognize Cues: Assessment

- Obtain patient information.
  1. Determine the presence and severity of incontinence with effective screening questions. Ask the patient to respond with *always*, *sometimes*, or *never* to the following questions:
     - Do you ever leak urine when you do not want to?
     - Do you ever leak urine or water when you cough, laugh, or exercise?
     - Do you ever leak urine on the way to the bathroom?
     - Do you ever use pads, tissue, or cloth in your underwear to catch urine?
  2. Risk factors for UI
     - Age, menopausal status
     - History of vaginal delivery; vaginal prolapse
     - Urologic procedures
     - Stress or anxiety level
     - Central or peripheral neurologic disease with associated impairment in cognition or mobility
     - Chronic conditions or use of medications that affect nerve conduction or elimination, such as diabetes, diuretic use, obesity, or spinal cord or nerve damage
- Assess for and document the findings of the following:
  1. Palpate the abdominal area for evidence of bladder fullness and to rule out constipation.
  2. Evaluate the force and character of the urine stream during voiding.

3. Ask the patient to cough while wearing a perineal pad; a wet pad may indicate stress incontinence.
4. Inspect the external genitalia of women to determine whether uterine prolapse, cystocele, or rectocele is present.
5. Describe any secretions or discharge from the genitourinary openings.
6. Query the patient regarding the effects of incontinence on socialization, family relationships, and emotional status.
7. Monitor the urine for color, odor, and presence of sediment or cloudiness, and report abnormal results of a urinalysis in a timely manner to the provider.
8. Review the results of the voiding cystourethrogram or urodynamic testing that detect the anatomic structure and function of the bladder.

Analyze Cues and Prioritize Hypotheses: Analysis
- The priority collaborative problems for patients with urinary incontinence include:
  1. Altered urinary elimination due to incontinence
  2. Potential for altered tissue integrity due to incontinence

Generate Solutions and Take Actions: Planning and Implementation
Promoting Urinary Elimination
Nonsurgical Management
- Nutrition therapy
  1. Weight reduction is helpful for patients who are obese because stress incontinence is made worse by increased abdominal pressure from obesity.
  2. Avoid bladder irritants, such as caffeine and alcohol.
  3. Maintain adequate fluid intake, especially water.
- Drug therapy

U

Common Examples of Drug Therapy
Urinary Incontinence

Drug Category	Nursing Implications
Hormones—Thought to enhance nerve conduction to the urinary tract, improve blood flow, and reduce tissue deterioration of the urinary tract	
Estrogen vaginal cream "daily or an estrogen-containing ring inserted monthly	Teach patients to use only a thin application of the cream. Teach patients that it takes 4 to 6 weeks to achieve continence benefits and that benefits disappear about 4 weeks after discontinuing regular use.

Continued

Common Examples of Drug Therapy—cont'd

Urinary Incontinence

Drug Category	Nursing Implications

Anticholinergics—Suppress involuntary bladder contraction and increase bladder capacity

Darifenacin Fesoterodine Oxybutynin Solifenacin Tolterodine Trospium	Ask whether the patient has glaucoma before starting any drugs from this class. Suggest that patients increase fluid intake and use hard candy to moisten the mouth. Teach patients to increase fluid intake and the amount of dietary fiber *to prevent constipation.* Teach patients to monitor urine output and to report an output significantly lower than intake to the primary health care provider *because all of these drugs can cause urinary retention.*

Alpha-Adrenergic Agonists—Increase contractile force of the urethral sphincter, increasing resistance to urine outflow

Midodrine[a]	Teach the patient to monitor their blood pressure periodically when starting the drug *because this drug can cause severe supine hypertension and should not be used in patients with severe cardiac disease.*

Beta₃ Agonists—Relax the detrusor smooth muscle to increase bladder capacity and urine storage

Mirabegron	Teach the patient to periodically obtain a blood pressure and to inform the health care provider if the systolic or diastolic values increase more than 10 mm Hg or measure above 180/110 If the patient is taking warfarin, avoid this drug or schedule additional blood testing for a potential increase in the risk for bleeding *because this drug uses the same metabolic pathway as warfarin and can potentiate warfarin's effects, leading to a prolonged international normalized ratio (INR) and increase in the risk for bleeding.*

Antidepressants: Tricyclics and Serotonin-Norepinephrine Reuptake Inhibitors (SNRIs)—Increase norepinephrine and serotonin levels, which are thought to strengthen the urinary sphincters; also have anticholinergic actions

Tricyclics Imipramine Amitriptyline SNRI Duloxetine[a]	Warn patients not to combine these drugs with other antidepressant drugs *to avoid a drug-drug interaction that can lead to a hypertensive crisis.* Instruct patients to inform their primary health care provider if they take drugs to manage hypertension. Teach patients to change positions slowly, especially in the morning, *to avoid dizziness from orthostatic hypotension, which increases the risk for falls.* Teach patients the same interventions as for anticholinergic agents *because these drugs have anticholinergic activity and can produce the same side effects.*

[a]This drug is used off label and do not have U.S. Food and Drug Administration (FDA) approval for use to treat incontinence. However, they are commonly used to manage incontinence syndromes.

NURSING SAFETY PRIORITY

Drug Alert

> Teach patients taking the extended-release forms of anticholinergic drugs to swallow the tablet or capsule whole without chewing or crushing. Chewing or crushing the tablet/capsule destroys the extended-release feature, allowing the entire dose to be absorbed quickly, which increases adverse drug side effects.

- **Devices:** Devices can be used to assist with continence.
  1. A **pessary** (a plastic device, often ring-shaped, that helps hold internal organs in place) inserted into the vagina may help with a prolapsed uterus or bladder when this condition is contributing to urinary incontinence.
  2. Urethral occlusion devices (urethral plugs) can be helpful for activity-induced incontinence.
  3. A penile clamp can be applied around the outside of the penis to compress the urethra and prevent urine leakage.
- **Electrical stimulation:** Electrical stimulation with either an intravaginal or intrarectal electrical stimulation device is available to treat urge, stress, and mixed incontinence. Treatment consists of stimulating sensory nerves to decrease the sensation of urgency.
- **Pelvic muscle therapy:** Pelvic muscle (Kegel) exercise therapy for women with stress incontinence strengthens the muscles of the pelvic floor (circumvaginal muscles).
  1. The most important step in teaching pelvic muscle exercises is to help the patient learn which muscles to exercise.
- **Vaginal cone therapy:** *Vaginal cone weight therapy* involves using a set of five small, cone-shaped weights (Touhy & Jett, 2020). They are of equal size but of varying weights and are used together with pelvic muscle exercise.
  1. Starting with the lightest weight, the patient inserts the cone into the vagina; if the patient can hold the cone in place while walking around, the patient proceeds to the second cone with a higher weight and repeats the procedure.
  2. Treatment periods are 15 minutes twice a day.
  3. Weighted vaginal cones can strengthen pelvic muscles and decrease stress incontinence.
- Behavioral interventions
  1. Habit training (scheduled toileting) is a type of bladder training that is successful in reducing incontinence in cognitively impaired patients. To use habit training, caregivers help the patient void at specific times (e.g., every 2 hours on the even hours).
  2. *Intermittent self-catheterization* is often used to help patients with long-term problems of incomplete bladder emptying.

U

PATIENT AND FAMILY EDUCATION

Pelvic Muscle Exercises

- Like any other muscles in your body, you can make your pelvic muscles stronger by alternately contracting (tightening) and relaxing them in regular exercise periods. By strengthening these muscles, you will be able to stop your urine flow more effectively.
- To identify your pelvic muscles, sit on the toilet with your feet flat on the floor about 12 inches apart. Begin to urinate, and then try to stop the urine flow. Do not strain down, lift your bottom off the seat, or squeeze your legs together. When you start and stop your urine stream, you are using your pelvic muscles.
- To perform pelvic muscle exercises, tighten your pelvic muscles for a slow count of 10 and then relax for a slow count of 10. Do this exercise 15 times while you are lying down, sitting up, and standing (a total of 45 exercises). Repeat the exercise, this time rapidly contracting and relaxing the pelvic muscles 10 times. This should take no more than 10 to 12 minutes for all three positions, or 3 to 4 minutes for each set of 15 exercises.
- Begin with 45 exercises a day in three sets of 15 exercises each. You will notice faster improvement if you can do this twice a day, or a total of 20 minutes each day. After you have been doing the exercises for several weeks, you will notice improvement in your control of urine. However, many people report that improvement may take as long as 3 months.

! **NURSING SAFETY PRIORITY**

Action Alert

Habit training is undermined when absorbent briefs are used in place of timed toileting. Do not tell patients to "just wet the bed." A common cause of falls in health care facilities is related to patients' efforts to get out of bed unassisted to use the toilet. Collaborate with all staff members, including unlicensed assistive personnel (UAP), to consistently implement the toileting schedule for habit training.

- Surgical interventions
  1. Surgical sling or bladder suspension: used to treat stress incontinence
  2. Injection of bulking agents into the urethral wall to provide resistance to urine outflow
  3. For patients with overflow (reflex) incontinence caused by obstruction of the bladder outlet, interventions may include surgery to relieve the obstruction. The most common procedures are prostate removal and repair of uterine prolapse.

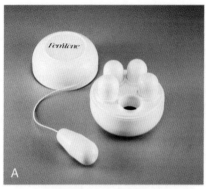

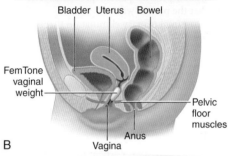

(A) FemTone vaginal weights, or cones. The number on the top of each cone represents increasing weight up to the heaviest cone, number 5. (B) Diagram showing the correct positioning of a vaginal weight, or cone, in place. (A courtesy ConvaTec, A Bristol-Meyers Squibb Company, a Division of E. R. Squibb & Sons, Inc., Princeton, NJ.)

Maintaining Tissue Integrity
- A major concern with the use of wearable protective pads is the risk for skin breakdown (loss of *tissue integrity*).
- Containment is achieved with absorbent pads and briefs designed to collect urine and keep the patient's skin and clothing dry. Many types and sizes of pads are available:
  1. Shields or liners inserted inside the undergarment
  2. Undergarments that are full-size pads with waist straps
  3. Plastic-lined protective underpants
  4. Combination pad and pant systems
  5. Absorbent bed pads

Care Coordination and Transition Management
- Community-based care for the patient with urinary incontinence considers personal, physical, emotional, and social resources.

- Teach the patient and family about the specific type of incontinence, and discuss available treatment options.
- Instruct the patient and family about the importance of weight reduction and dietary modification to help control incontinence of urine *elimination*.
- Remind the patient who smokes that nicotine can contribute to bladder irritation and that coughing can cause urine leakage.
- Referral of patients to home care agencies for help with personal care and to continence clinics that specialize in evaluation and treatment may be helpful.

Evaluate Outcomes: Evaluation

- Evaluate the care of the patient with urinary incontinence based on the identified priority patient problems. The expected outcomes are that the patient will:
  1. Maintain optimal urinary elimination through a reduction in the number of urinary incontinence episodes
  2. Maintain tissue integrity of the skin and mucous membranes in the perineal area

See Chapter 58 in the main text for more information on urinary incontinence.

UROLITHIASIS

- Urolithiasis is the presence of calculi (stones) in the urinary tract. Stones often do not cause symptoms until they pass into the lower urinary tract, where they can cause excruciating pain. *Nephrolithiasis* is the formation of stones in the kidney. *Ureterolithiasis* is the formation of stones in the ureter.
- The most common condition associated with stone formation is dehydration.
- Formation of stones involves two conditions:
  1. Supersaturation of the urine with the particular element (e.g., calcium, uric acid) that first becomes crystallized and later becomes the stone
  2. Formation of a *nidus* (deposit of crystals that can be the point of infection) along the lining of the kidney and urinary tract
- Calculi may be formed from calcium, phosphate, oxalate, uric acid, struvite, and cystine crystals, but most stones contain calcium as one component.

PATIENT-CENTERED CARE: GENETICS/GENOMICS

Kidney Stone Formation

Family history has a strong association with stone formation and recurrence because of inherited metabolic variations. More than 30 genetic variations are associated with the formation of kidney stones, although single gene disorders are rare. More commonly, nephrolithiasis is a complex disease, with genetic variation in intestinal calcium absorption, kidney calcium transport, or kidney phosphate transport all associated with stone formation (Online Mendelian Inheritance in Man [OMIM], 2022). Always ask a patient with a renal stone whether other family members also have this problem.

Interprofessional Collaborative Care

Recognize Cues: Assessment
- Obtain patient information about:
  1. Personal and family history of kidney stones
  2. Metabolic disorders and diet history, including fluid intake
- Assess for and document:
  1. The location and duration of pain, which is often described as severe, unbearable, spasmodic (colic), and in the region of the trunk, back, and thighs ("flank" pain)
  2. Nausea and vomiting
  3. Hematuria, oliguria, or anuria
  4. Increased turbidity and odor of urine
  5. Bladder distention

Take Actions: Interventions
Managing Pain
Nonsurgical Management
- Administer drugs to manage severe pain and assess patient response, including:
  1. Opioid analgesics for severe pain
  2. NSAIDs, such as ketorolac
  3. Spasmolytic agents, such as oxybutynin chloride
  4. Drugs to aid in stone expulsion
- When infection occurs, a stone has not passed in 1 to 2 months, or when kidney function is at risk, antibiotics or lithotripsy may be used.
- Lithotripsy, or extracorporeal *shock wave lithotripsy* (SWL), is the application of ultrasound or dry shock wave energies to break the stone. The patient receives conscious sedation as the lithotripter and fluoroscope locate and break up the calculus. After lithotripsy, implement routine postoperative care with additional monitoring for urine output (quantity, quality, and presence of sediment or stones).

U

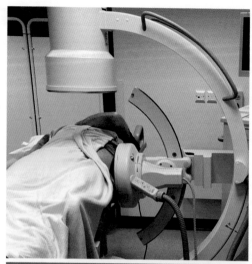

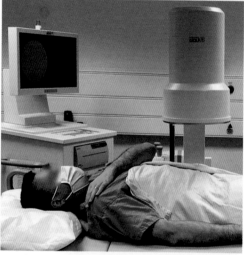

A patient undergoing extracorporeal shock wave lithotripsy (ESWL). (From Hobson, R.P., et. al. [2023]. *Davidson's Principles and practice of medicine* [24th ed.]. St. Louis: Elsevier.)

Surgical Management

- Minimally invasive surgical and open surgical procedures are used if urinary obstruction occurs or if the stone is too large to be passed and include stenting, ureteroscopy, percutaneous ureterolithotomy, and percutaneous nephrolithotomy.
- When other stone removal attempts have failed or when risk for a lasting injury to the ureter or kidney is possible, an *open ureterolithotomy* (into the ureter), *pyelolithotomy* (into the kidney pelvis), or *nephrolithotomy* (into the kidney) procedure may be performed. These procedures are used for a large or impacted stone.
- Preoperative care includes routine care and the delivery of individualized instructions, depending on the procedure to be performed.
- Postoperative care includes routine care and:
  1. Monitoring the urine amount and character (color, presence of sediment or clots, volume) every 1 to 2 hours for 24 hours and preventing urinary obstruction from stone fragments or clots
  2. Monitoring intake to provide adequate hydration
  3. Preventing infection or detecting signs of infection early to avoid complications of surgical site or urinary tract infection
  4. Evaluating effects of intervention with a 24-hour urine collection and chemical analysis

Care Coordination and Transition Management

- Inform the patient that:
  1. Extensive bruising may occur after lithotripsy and may take several weeks to resolve
  2. Urine may be bloody for several days after surgical intervention
- Instruct the patient about:
  1. The importance of following the prescribed drug regimen
  2. The rationale for preventing dehydration, stressing the importance of dilute urine from adequate fluid intake and any dietary restrictions to reduce recurrent stone formation
  3. The importance of reporting symptoms of infection or formation of another stone, such as pain, fever, chills, and difficulty with urination

 See Chapter 58 in the main text for more information on urolithiasis.

UTERINE FIBROIDS (LEIOMYOMAS)

- See *Leiomyomas (Uterine Fibroids).*

VASCULAR DISEASE, PERIPHERAL

- Peripheral vascular disease (PVD) includes disorders that change the natural flow of blood through the arteries and veins of the peripheral circulation.
- It affects the legs much more commonly than the arms.
- A diagnosis of PVD usually implies arterial disease (peripheral arterial disease [PAD]) rather than venous involvement. Some patients have both arterial and venous disease.

See *Peripheral Arterial Disease.*

See Chapter 30 in the main text for more information on vascular disease.

VEINS, VARICOSE

- Varicose veins are distended, protruding veins that appear darkened or tortuous.
- The vein walls weaken and dilate. Venous pressure increases, and the valves become incompetent. Incompetent valves contribute to venous insufficiency. Both superficial and deep veins can become dilated.
- Varicose veins are also frequently seen in patients with systemic problems (e.g., heart disease), obesity, high estrogen states, and a family history of varicose veins.

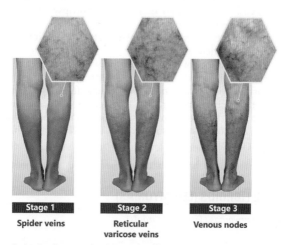

Stage 1	Stage 2	Stage 3
Spider veins	**Reticular varicose veins**	**Venous nodes**

Stages in the development of varicose veins. (Used with permission from istockphoto. com, 2021, Marina113.)

Interprofessional Collaborative Care

- The overall purpose of management for patients with varicose veins is to improve and maintain optimal venous return to the heart and prevent disease progression.
- Conservative treatment measures include (the three *E*s):
  1. Elastic compression hose
  2. Exercise
  3. Elevating the legs as often as possible
- Surgical management includes endovenous ablation to occlude the varicose vein.
  1. This is generally completed as a same-day surgery with routine perioperative care and restrictions to weight bearing for several days.
- Collateral veins take over supplying blood to tissues after laser, radiofrequency, or surgical interventions.

See Chapter 30 in the main text for more information on varicose veins.

VENOUS THROMBOEMBOLISM: CLOTTING CONCEPT ✳ EXEMPLAR

Overview

- Venous thromboembolism (VTE) is one of health care's greatest challenges and includes both thrombus and embolus complications.
- A thrombus (also called a thrombosis) is a blood clot believed to result from an endothelial injury, venous stasis, or hypercoagulability.
- When a thrombus develops, immunity is altered, causing **inflammation** to occur around the clot, thickening of the vein wall, and possible embolization (the formation of an embolus).
  1. Pulmonary embolus (PE) is the most common type of embolus.
- Deep vein thrombophlebitis, commonly referred to as deep vein thrombosis (DVT), is the most common type of thrombophlebitis (a thrombus associated with inflammation). It is more serious than superficial thrombophlebitis because it presents a greater risk for PE.
- With PE, a dislodged blood clot travels to the pulmonary artery—a medical emergency!

V

Interprofessional Collaborative Care
Recognize Cues: Assessment

- Obtain patient information about:
  1. History of VTE

2. Risks associated with the development of VTE
   - Prolonged periods of sitting or bed rest
   - Recent surgery
   - Factors affecting coagulation
- Assess for signs and symptoms:
  1. Patients may be asymptomatic.
  2. The classic signs and symptoms of DVT are calf or groin tenderness and pain and sudden onset of unilateral leg swelling.
  3. Gently palpate the site; observe for induration (hardening) along the blood vessel.
  4. Redness/hyperpigmentation may be present.
- The preferred diagnostic test for DVT is venous duplex ultrasonography.
- A D-dimer test is the global marker of coagulation activation and measures fibrin degradation products produced from fibrinolysis (clot breakdown). Used as an adjunct to noninvasive testing.

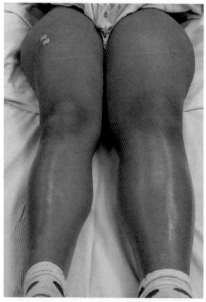

Deep vein thrombosis (DVT) of lower left leg. (Found in Olshansky, E. F. [2023]. *Maternal-child nursing* [7th ed.]. St. Louis: Elsevier. From Murphy, E. H., Davis, C. M., Journeycake, J. M., et al. [2009]. Symptomatic ileofemoral DVT after onset of oral contraceptive use in women with previously undiagnosed May-Thurner syndrome. *Journal of Vascular Surgery, 49*[3], 697–703.)

Analyze Cues and Prioritize Hypotheses: Analysis
- The priority collaborative problem for most patients with VTE is:
  1. Potential for injury due to complications of VTE and anticoagulation therapy.

Generate Solutions and Take Actions: Planning and Implementation
Preventing Injury
- The focus of managing thrombophlebitis is to prevent complications such as pulmonary emboli, further thrombus formation, or an increase in the size of the thrombus.

Nonsurgical Management
- Prevention of DVT and other types of VTE is crucial for patients at risk. Initiate the following interventions to prevent VTE:
  1. Patient education
  2. Leg exercises
  3. Early ambulation
  4. Adequate hydration
  5. Graduated compression stockings
  6. Intermittent pneumatic compression, such as sequential compression devices (SCDs)
  7. Venous plexus foot pump
  8. Anticoagulant therapy

Drug Therapy
- Anticoagulants are the drug of choice for actual DVT and for patients at risk for DVT.
- The conventional treatment has been IV unfractionated heparin followed by oral anticoagulation with warfarin (Coumadin).
- Unfractionated heparin can be problematic because each patient's response to the drug is unpredictable; hospital admission is usually required for laboratory monitoring and dose adjustments.
- The use of low-molecular-weight heparin (LMWH) and the development of direct oral anticoagulants (DOACs) has changed the management of both DVT and PE.

V

✚ NURSING SAFETY PRIORITY

Critical Rescue

Notify the health care provider if the activated partial thromboplastin time (aPTT) value is greater than 70 seconds, or follow hospital protocol for reporting critical laboratory values. Assess patients for signs and symptoms of bleeding, which include hematuria, frank or occult blood in the stool, ecchymosis (bruising), petechiae, an altered level of consciousness, or pain. If bleeding occurs, stop the anticoagulant immediately and call the primary health care provider or Rapid Response Team!

BEST PRACTICE FOR PATIENT SAFETY AND QUALITY CARE

Anticoagulant Therapy

- Carefully check the dosage of anticoagulant to be administered, even if the pharmacy prepared the drug.
- Monitor the patient for signs and symptoms of bleeding, including hematuria, frank or occult blood in the stool, ecchymosis, petechiae, altered mental status (indicating possible cranial bleeding), or pain (especially abdominal pain, which could indicate abdominal bleeding).
- Monitor vital signs frequently for decreased blood pressure and increased pulse (indicating possible internal bleeding).
- Have antidotes available as needed (e.g., protamine sulfate for heparin; vitamin K for warfarin).
- Monitor aPTT for patients receiving unfractionated heparin. Monitor prothrombin time (PT)/ international normalized ratio (INR) for patients receiving warfarin or LMWH. Anti-factor Xa can also be used to monitor LMWH or DOACs.
- Apply prolonged pressure over venipuncture sites and injection sites.
- When administering subcutaneous heparin, apply pressure over the site and do not massage.
- Teach the patient going home while taking an anticoagulant to:
  1. Use only an electric razor
  2. Take precautions to avoid injury; for example, do not use tools such as hammers or saws, where accidents commonly occur
  3. Report signs and symptoms of bleeding, such as blood in the urine or stool, nosebleeds, ecchymosis, or altered mental status
  4. Take the prescribed dosage of drug at the precise time that it was prescribed to be taken
  5. Avoid an abrupt stop in taking the drug; the health care provider usually tapers the anticoagulant gradually

 NURSING SAFETY PRIORITY

Drug Alert

For patients taking warfarin, assess for any bleeding, such as hematuria or blood in the stool. Ensure that vitamin K, the antidote for warfarin, is available in case of excessive bleeding. Report any bleeding to the primary health care provider and document in the patient's health record. Teach patients to avoid foods with high concentrations of vitamin K, especially dark green leafy vegetables. These foods interfere with the action of warfarin, which is a vitamin K synthesis inhibitor.

Surgical Management

- Surgical removal of a DVT is rare unless there is a massive occlusion that does not respond to medical treatment.
- A thrombectomy is the surgical procedure used for clot removal.
- For patients with recurrent DVT or pulmonary emboli that do not respond to medical treatment or that cannot tolerate anticoagulation, inferior vena cava filtration may be indicated.
    1. The surgeon or interventional radiologist inserts a filter device into the femoral vein or jugular vein. The device is meant to trap emboli in the inferior vena cava before they progress to the lungs. Holes in the device allow blood to pass through, without interfering with the return of blood to the heart.
    2. Provide standard preoperative care and collaborate with the primary health care provider if the patient has been taking anticoagulants to avoid hemorrhage.
    3. After surgery, inspect the groin insertion site for bleeding and signs or symptoms of infection. Provide standard postoperative care.

Care Coordination and Transition Management

- Patients recovering from thrombophlebitis or DVT are ambulatory when they are discharged from the hospital.
- The primary focus of planning for discharge is to educate the patient and family about anticoagulation therapy.
- Teach patients recovering from DVT:
    1. Stop smoking.
    2. Avoid the use of oral contraceptives.
    3. Discuss alternative methods of birth control.
    4. Most patients are discharged on warfarin or LMWH.

Evaluation: Evaluate Outcomes

- Evaluate the care of the patient with VTE on the basis of the identified priority problem. The expected outcome is that the patient:
    1. Remains free of injury associated with VTE complications such as pulmonary embolism and bleeding associated with anticoagulation therapy.

See Chapter 30 in the main text for more information on venous thromboembolism.

Electrocardiographic Complexes, Segments, and Intervals

The electrocardiogram (ECG) is a graphic record of electrical activity of the heart. The spread of electrical current in the heart is detected by surface electrodes, and the amplified electrical signals are recorded on calibrated paper.

Cardiac dysrhythmias are abnormal rhythms of the heart's electrical system that can affect its ability to effectively pump oxygenated blood throughout the body. Some dysrhythmias are life-threatening, whereas others are not. They are the result of disturbances of cardiac electrical impulse formation, conduction, or both. When the heart does not work effectively as a pump, perfusion to vital organs and peripheral tissues can be impaired, resulting in organ dysfunction or failure.

Complexes that make up a normal ECG consist of a P wave, a QRS complex, a T wave, and possibly a U wave. Segments include the PR segment, the ST segment, and the TP segment. Intervals include the PR interval, the QRS duration, and the QT interval (see Figure). *Assess the patient to differentiate artifact from actual lethal rhythms! Do not rely only on the ECG monitor!*

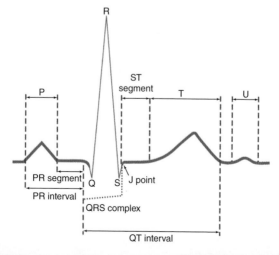

1. **P wave** represents atrial depolarization.
2. **PR segment** represents the time required for the impulse to travel through the atrioventricular (AV) node (where the impulse is delayed).
3. **PR interval** represents the time required for atrial depolarization and impulse travel through the AV node, inclusive of the P wave and PR segment. It is measured from the beginning of the P wave to the end of the PR segment, and a normal time in adults is 0.12 to 0.20 of a second. It is measured from the beginning of the P wave to the beginning of the QRS complex.
4. **QRS complex** represents depolarization of both ventricles and is measured from the point at which the complex first leaves the baseline to the end of the last appearing wave (from the end of the PR interval to the J point). This is normally less than 0.11 second (2½ small blocks). A wide QRS complex indicates a delay in the conduction time in the ventricles. Delay in ventricular depolarization (i.e., a wide QRS) can be the result of myocardial ischemia, injury, or infarct; it may also result from ventricular hypertrophy or electrolyte imbalances. It is measured from the beginning of the Q or R wave to the end of the R or S wave (not all leads have a Q, R, and S.)
5. **J point** represents the junction where the QRS complex ends and the ST segment begins.
6. **ST segment** represents early ventricular repolarization. It is measured from the J point to the beginning of the T wave.
7. **T wave** represents ventricular repolarization.
8. **U wave** represents late ventricular repolarization. It is not normally seen in all leads.
9. **QT interval** represents the total time required for ventricular depolarization and repolarization. It is measured from the beginning of the QRS complex to the end of the T wave. It varies with age, sex, and heart rate. It may be prolonged by certain medications, electrolyte disturbances, or subarachnoid hemorrhage. A prolonged QT interval may lead to a unique type of ventricular tachycardia called *torsades de pointes*.

Analysis of an ECG rhythm strip requires a systematic approach using an eight-step method:

1. ***Determine the heart rate.*** The most common method is to count the number of QRS complexes in 6 seconds and multiply that number by 10 to calculate the rate for a full minute. Normal heart rates fall between 60 and 100 beats/min. A rate of less than 60 beats/min is called **bradycardia**. A rate of greater than 100 beats/min is called **tachycardia**.
2. ***Determine the heart rhythm.*** Assess for atrial and/or ventricular regularity. Heart rhythms can be either regular or irregular. Irregular

rhythms can be regularly irregular, occasionally irregular, or irregularly irregular. A slight irregularity of no more than three small blocks between intervals is considered essentially regular if the QRS complexes are all of the same shape.

3. *Analyze the P waves.* Ask these questions; a response of yes indicates normality:
   - Are P waves present?
   - Are the P waves occurring regularly?
   - Is there one P wave for each QRS complex?
   - Are the P waves smooth, rounded, and upright in appearance?
   - Do all P waves look similar?

4. *Measure the PR interval.* The normal PR interval is between 0.12 and 0.20 second and should be a constant value in the strip. The PR interval cannot be determined if there are no P waves or if P waves occur after the QRS complex.

5. *Measure the QRS duration.* The QRS duration normally measures between 0.06 and 0.11 second and should be a constant value and consistently shaped throughout the strip. When the QRS complex is narrow, this indicates that the impulse was not formed in the ventricles and is referred to as *supraventricular* or *above the ventricles.* When the QRS complex is wide (greater than 0.11 second), this indicates that the impulse is either of ventricular origin or of supraventricular origin with aberrant conduction. More than one QRS complex pattern or occasionally missing QRS complexes indicates a dysrhythmia.

6. *Examine the ST segment.* The normal ST segment begins at the isoelectric line. ST elevation or depression is significant if displacement is 1 mm (one small box) or more above or below the line and is seen in two or more leads. ST *elevation* may indicate a problem, such as myocardial infarction, pericarditis, or hyperkalemia. ST *depression* is associated with hypokalemia, myocardial infarction, or ventricular hypertrophy.

7. *Assess the T wave.* Note the shape and height of the T wave for peaking or inversion. Abnormal T waves may indicate problems such as myocardial infarction and ventricular hypertrophy.

8. *Measure the QT interval.* A normal QT interval should be equal to or less than one-half the distance of the R-to-R interval.

Sinus Rhythm

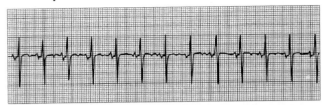

A

(A) Sinus tachycardia is defined as a heart rate (HR) faster than 100 beats/min with normal waves and intervals (HR = 100 beats/min, PR = 0.12 second, QRS = 0.08 second).

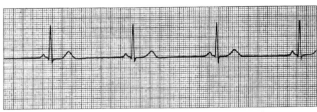

B

(B) Sinus bradycardia is defined as a heart rate of less than 60 beats/min with all other waves and segments within normal values (HR = 35 beats/min, PR = 0.16 second, QRS = 0.10 second).

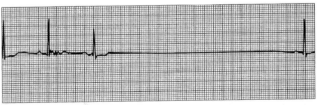

C

(C) Sinus pause (underlying HR = 60 beats/min, PR = 0.20 second, QRS = 0.08 second, with just under a 5-second pause.)

Normal Sinus Rhythm With a Premature Contraction

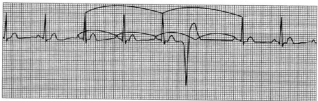

A

(A) Normal sinus rhythm with a premature ventricular contraction (PVC). A complete compensatory pause follows the PVC, indicated by the fact that the sinus P wave after the pause comes exactly when it was due to occur.

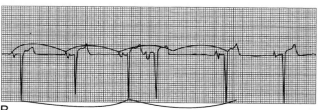

B

(B) Normal sinus rhythm with a premature atrial contraction (PAC). An incomplete or noncompensatory pause follows the PAC, indicated by the sinus P wave after the pause coming before it was originally due to occur. The QRS complex also comes before it was due.

Atrial Dysrhythmias

An atrial dysrhythmia implies that the source of the irregular rate or rhythm originates in the atria.

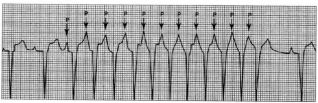

A

(A) Normal sinus rhythm with an 11-beat run of paroxysmal atrial tachycardia (PAT) with 1:1 conduction.

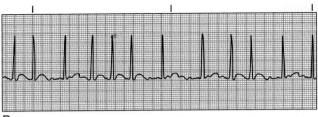

B

(B) Atrial fibrillation (AF). Multiple pacemaker sites in the atria cause atrial depolarization at 350 to 600 times per minute. The result is an irregular, wavy baseline between each QRS rather than organized P waves. Atrial fibrillation is often but not universally characterized by an irregular ventricular response, as seen in this figure.

Ventricular Dysrhythmias

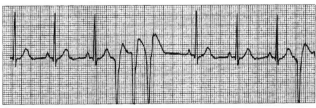

A

(A) Normal sinus rhythm with a three-beat run of ventricular tachycardia and one unifocal premature ventricular complex.

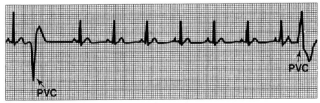

B

(B) Normal sinus rhythm with multifocal PVCs (one negative and the other positive).

Ventricular Dysrhythmias

The dysrhythmia originates in the ventricle. Sustained ventricular tachycardia, ventricular fibrillation, and asystole are all associated with sudden cardiac death; they do not support a blood pressure or perfusion.

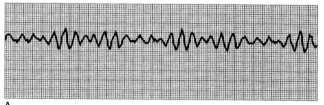

A

(A) Coarse ventricular fibrillation.

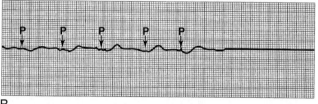

B

(B) Ventricular asystole, initially with five P waves and then with no P waves (arterial and ventricular standstill).

Atrioventricular Block

A heart block implies a disruption in the normal conduction of a pacemaker signal that originates in the sinoatrial (SA) node.

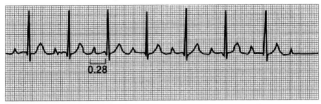

A

(A) Normal sinus rhythm with a first-degree AV block (PR interval = 0.28 second). First- and second-degree heart block imply a delay at the AV node.

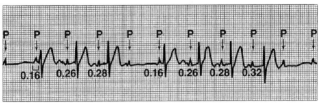

B

(B) Second-degree AV block type 1 (Wenckebach) with an irregular rhythm, grouped beating, and progressive prolongation of the PR interval until a P wave is completely blocked and not followed by a QRS complex.

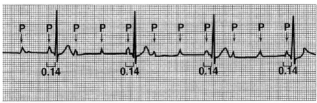

C

(C) Second-degree AV block type 2 (Mobitz III) with 3:1 conduction and a constant PR interval. A type 2 second-degree block is more serious and indicates the need for more urgent intervention, such as placing a transcutaneous pacemaker and anticipating the placement of a permanent pacemaker.

Atrioventricular Block

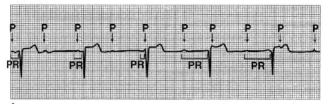

A

(A) Third-degree AV block (complete heart block) with regular atrial and ventricular rhythms. This dysrhythmia indicates no communication between the atria and ventricles at the AV node and is typically treated with a pacemaker. Note the inconsistent PR intervals (AV dissociation) and a junctional escape focus (normal QRS complexes) pacing the ventricles at a rate of 38 beats/min.

B

(B) Third-degree AV block with regular atrial and ventricular rhythms, inconsistent PR intervals (AV dissociation), and ventricular escape focus pacing the ventricles at a rate of 35 beats/min, with wide QRS complexes. Third-degree heart block implies a more serious condition and a delay low in the AV node or along the bundle of His. New onset of this rhythm should be communicated to the health care provider immediately, and a transcutaneous pacemaker should be placed until the patient can be fully evaluated for possible permanent pacemaker placement.

---

b indicates boxed material, *f* indicates illustrations, and *t* indicates tables.

CONTENTS—cont'd